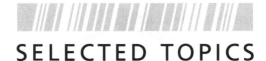

SELECTED TOPICS

Toward a Better Understanding of
Physical Fitness and Activity

The papers included in this book
were previously published in
THE PRESIDENT'S COUNCIL FOR PHYSICAL FITNESS
AND SPORTS *RESEARCH DIGEST*

EDITED BY

CHARLES B. CORBIN
ARIZONA STATE UNIVERSITY

ROBERT P. PANGRAZI
ARIZONA STATE UNIVERSITY

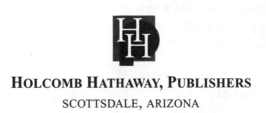

HOLCOMB HATHAWAY, PUBLISHERS
SCOTTSDALE, ARIZONA

Library of Congress Cataloging-in-Publication Data

Toward a better understanding of physical fitness and activity :
  selected topics / edited by Charles B. Corbin, Robert P. Pangrazi.
        p.   cm.
      "The papers included in this book were previously published in The
  President's Council for Physical Fitness and Sport research digest."
      Includes bibliographical references and index.
      ISBN 1-890871-08-7
      1. Exercise. 2. Physical fitness. 3. Health. I. Corbin,
  Charles B. II. Pangrazi, Robert B.
  √RA781.T69   1999
    613.7—dc21   98-38693
                                                           CIP

Publisher: Gay L. Pauley
Editor: Colette Kelly
Marketing: Renee Rosen
Production: Laurie Orr
Composition: Aerocraft Charter Art Service
Cover Design: Didona Design

Holcomb Hathaway, Publishers
6207 North Cattle Track Road
Scottsdale, Arizona 85250

10 9 8 7 6 5 4 3 2 1

ISBN 1-890871-08-7

Printed in the United States of America.

Contents

SECTION IV
FITNESS, ECONOMIC, AND MENTAL HEALTH BENEFITS OF PHYSICAL ACTIVITY   117

SECTION V
PHYSICAL ACTIVITY AND CHILDREN   151

SECTION VI
PHYSICAL ACTIVITY AND ERGOGENIC AIDS   193

Foreword

This edited volume contains 22 papers by some of the world's leading authorities on physical activity. These papers, covering a wide variety of topics, were originally prepared for The President's Council on Physical Fitness and Sports (PCPFS) *Physical Activity and Fitness Research Digest* (later renamed the PCPFS *Research Digest*) and were published in quarterly issues of the *Digest*. Many readers have collected an entire set of the papers. These collectors and other readers who were not subscribers to early issues suggested that a compendium of the papers would be useful as a reference source and as a reader for students. Thus, this text will be important for those who would like the entire set in their library. In addition, it will serve as a valuable educational tool for instructors who wish to adopt the text for classroom use.

For these reasons we, as the PCPFS *Research Digest*'s editors, have pulled together the full set of manuscripts into this edited collection. To make the book more readable and useful, the papers have been grouped into six sections. Since papers have been gathered according to similarity of topic, they do not appear in the same order in which they were published.

When the papers were originally published, we as editors frequently included "Editors' Notes." In many cases, we have retained these notes in this volume to help readers interpret the papers. Notes have also been added to improve the readability of the complete collection.

It is our hope that this complete volume of papers covering physical activity will greatly expand the audience that is able to read works by leaders in the field.

ACKNOWLEDGMENTS

As co-editors of this collection of The President's Council on Physical Fitness and Sports *Research Digest,* we have had the opportunity to work with some of the most well-known and prolific scholars in our field. We are indebted to all of the authors for making the PCPFS *Research Digests* a success and appreciate the efforts of Holcomb Hathaway, Publishers, for making this volume a reality.

Of course, no project can be a success without the efforts of people behind the scenes. Christine Spain, Director of Research, Planning and Special Projects of the President's Council on Physical Fitness and Sports, was instrumental in obtaining support for the PCPFS *Research Digests*. Her tireless efforts have resulted in continued public service sponsorship from 1993 through 1998. Together, Sandra Perlmutter, Executive Director of the Council, and Ms. Spain have given this project the leadership it deserves.

Specific thanks should be extended to Chiquita Brands International, Inc. for their supporting Series 1 and to the Advil Forum on Health Education for sponsoring Series 2 of the PCPFS *Research Digest*. The generous public service support of these two companies allowed for the dissemination of the *Digest* to thousands of fitness leaders, educators, physicians, and laypeople.

Finally, we would like to thank the U.S. Department of Health and Human Services and, specifically, the Office of Public Health and Science, for their continued support of physical activity/fitness as a means to improve and maintain the health of our nation.

Chuck Corbin and Bob Pangrazi

A TRIBUTE TO H. HARRISON CLARKE

For eight and one-half years, Dr. H. Harrison Clarke edited the PCPFS *Physical Fitness Research Digest.* Many people benefited from this effort during the 1970s. Dr. Clarke is also known for his other significant contributions to the field of physical fitness. It is appropriate, in this compendium of the new PCPFS *Research Digest,* that we pay tribute to Dr. Clarke for his many contributions.

A graduate of Springfield College in 1925, Dr. Clarke started his career as a physical education teacher and coach in New York. Later, he received masters (1931) and doctoral (1940) degrees from Syracuse University. During World War II, he served as an officer in the Army Air Force working in a physical conditioning assignment. Subsequently, he served as a professor at Springfield College and in 1953 became a Research Professor of Physical Education at the University of Oregon. He is identified with the Medford Growth Study, which followed the fitness and growth of boys in Medford, Oregon, throughout their schooling. It is the most comprehensive growth and development study that has been done in our country. It resulted in many different publications, including a monograph. Dr. Clarke has published more than 160 articles and several books, most of which are related to physical fitness. He is a past president of the American Academy of Physical Education and has received numerous awards, including the Luther Halsey Gulick Medal of the American Alliance for Health, Physical Education, Recreation and Dance and the Hetherington Award, the highest honor bestowed by the American Academy of Physical Education. In 1983, he was named a Healthy American Fitness Leader. Dr. Clarke is one of the best known scholars in physical education/physical fitness in the United States. We thank Dr. Clarke for starting the original *Physical Fitness Research Digest* and are pleased to dedicate this volume to him.

About the Contributors

ODED BAR-OR. Oded Bar-Or is professor of pediatrics and director of the Children's Exercise and Nutrition Centre, McMaster University, Canada. He was the founder and director of the Department of Research and Sports Medicine at the Wingate Institute in Israel.

Dr. Bar-Or has published extensively on responses of children to exercise in health and disease, and has written and edited several books. He has been an invited speaker to numerous national and international conferences.

Dr. Bar-Or has held leadership roles in several organizations. He has served as president of the Canadian Society of Sports Sciences, president of the International Council for Physical Fitness Research, vice president of the American College of Sports Medicine, and board member of the Sports Medicine Council of Canada. He also chaired a task force of the American Medical Association on the participation of children in sports. He recently received a Citation Award from the American College of Sports Medicine.

CLAUDE BOUCHARD. Claude Bouchard, Ph.D. is professor of kinesiology in the Department of Social and Preventive Medicine and director of the Biology of Physical Activity Research Group at Universite Laval, Quebec, Canada. He has an M.Sc. in Exercise Physiology and a Ph.D. in anthropological genetics. His research work focuses primarily on the genetic and molecular basis of obesity and the metabolic complications associated with obesity, as well as the genetic and molecular basis of the responsiveness to regular physical activity in terms of the risk factors for heart disease and diabetes mellitus.

Dr. Bouchard is a fellow of the American College of Sports Medicine and a member of the American Society of Human Genetics and of the North American Association for the Study of Obesity. He has been elected as a foreign member of the Royal Academy of Medicine of Belgium. He has also received a number of awards, including the Citation Award from the American College of Sports Medicine, the Award of Excellence from the Canadian Society for Exercise Physiology, the Prix Benjamin Delessert de Nutrition (France), the Willendorf Award from the International Association for the Study of Obesity, and an Honoris Causa Doctorate from the University of Leuven, Belgium.

Dr. Bouchard has published over 600 scientific papers and book chapters. He has also written and edited several books regarding obesity and the biological aspects of physical activity.

LINDA BUNKER. Linda Bunker is a Professor of Human Services (Physical Education) at the University of Virginia, where she directs the Motor Learning program. She earned her Ph.D. from the University of Illinois and has published over 100 scholarly articles and co-authored 15 books, including *The Courtside Coach, Parenting Your Superstar, Motivating Kids through Play,* and *Golf: Steps to Success.* Her research interests include a blend of topics related to sport psychology and motor learning, with particular interest in girls and women in sport. Dr. Bunker serves on the Advisory Committee of the Women's Sports Foundation, the Melpomene Institute, and *SHAPE* magazine. She has received the NASPE Hall of Fame Award, the NAGWS Honor Award, the R. Tait McKenzie Award, and the President's Award from the Women's Sports Foundation. At the University of Virginia, she has been recognized with the Algernon Sydney Sullivan Award for outstanding service, the Raven Distinguished Professor Award, and in 1995 received the University's highest faculty distinction, the Thomas Jefferson Award.

CHARLES B. CORBIN. Charles (Chuck) Corbin is a professor in the Department of Exercise Science and Physical Education at Arizona State University. He has more than 200 published papers and books, including *Concepts of Physical Fitness,* 10th ed., and *Fitness for Life,* 4th ed., co-authored with Dr. Ruth Lindsey. *Fitness for Life,* 4th ed., received the Texty Award from the Textbook Authors Association in 1997.

Dr. Corbin is a fellow in the American College of Sports and has made presentations worldwide, including the Prince Phillip Lecture (London), The Delphine Hanna Lecture (NAPEHE), T. K. Cureton Lecture (ACSM), the Raymond Weiss Lecture (AAHPERD), as well as keynote lectures to the ICHPER World Congress in Limerick, Ireland. He has served as president of the American Academy of Kinesiology Physical Education and editor of *Quest,* and is current co-editor of the PCPFS *Research Digest.* Among the honors bestowed on Dr. Corbin are the AAHPERD Honor Award, the Physical Fitness Council Honor Award

(AAHPERD), Better Health and Living National Award, Centennial Distinguished Alumnus Award (University of New Mexico), and Healthy American Fitness Leader (President's Council on Physical Fitness and Sports, Allstate Co., and the National Jaycees). In1995, he received the Distinguished Scholar Award from the National Association for Physical Education in Higher Education and in 1998 was named Alliance Scholar by the AAHPERD.

MARTHA E. EWING.   Martha Ewing earned her bachelor's degree in physical education from Kansas State University and both a master's in athletic administration and a Ph.D. in sport psychology from the University of Illinois. Dr. Ewing taught and coached basketball, volleyball, and tennis at Iowa State University, Western Washington University, and Purdue University. She is currently an Associate Professor at Michigan State University, where she conducts research on youth in sport. Dr. Ewing's research interests include achievement motivation, parental pressure, and improving sport opportunities in urban areas. She has also been active in developing a program for coaches' education and has served as a sport psychology consultant with numerous youth and sport teams. Dr. Ewing maintains active memberships in the North American Society for Psychology of Sport and Physical Activity, the Association for the Advancement of Applied Sport Psychology, and the American Alliance for Health, Physical Education, Recreation and Dance.

B. DON FRANKS.   Don Franks, Ph.D. University of Illinois; M.Ed. and B.S.E., University of Arkansas, is professor and chair of the Department of Kinesiology, University of Maryland. His past professional experience includes positions at Louisiana State University, University of Tennessee, Temple University, University of Illinois, and Paine College.

Dr. Franks has served as fellow and past president of American Academy of Kinesiology and Physical Education and of the Research Consortium (AAHPERD). The major focus of Dr. Franks' research has been on interactions of physical activity, fitness, stress, and health. He has been an advocate for health-related physical fitness.

LARRY R. GETTMAN.   Larry Gettman is director of Clinical Analytical Services for the HBOC National Health Call Center in Phoenix, Arizona. His Ph.D. includes the specialties of health science, statistics, and research methods.

Dr. Gettman has developed a series of health assessments during his 30 years of experience and is an expert in outcomes research and the economics of health promotion, wellness, and health/fitness in the corporate, clinical, community, and commercial settings. He has authored 10 books and more than 50 major peer-reviewed publications, and has made more than 70 major professional presentations.

Dr. Gettman was the co-developer of *Heart At Work,* the American Heart Association's worksite health promotion program, and has been recognized for his achievements in impacting the health of hundreds of thousands of Americans by receiving the prestigious Healthy American Fitness Leader Award in 1994.

WILLIAM L. HASKELL.   William L. Haskell, Ph.D., is professor of medicine and Deputy Director of the Stanford Center for Research in Disease Prevention, Stanford University. He has been an investigator on numerous studies on the prevention or management of various chronic degenerative diseases. A major focus of his research has been the role of physical activity in the etiology of heart disease. The results of these studies have made a substantial contribution to the understanding of the role of physical activity in heart disease prevention and rehabilitation. Dr. Haskell has served as a consultant to help develop exercise guidelines for health promotion for various medical/fitness organizations including the American Heart Association, American College of Cardiology, President's Council on Physical Fitness and Sports, and Heart Foundation of Australia. He is past president of the American College of Sports Medicine and a founder and past president of the American College of Sports Medicine Foundation.

Dr. Haskell is the author or co-author of more than 240 scientific articles, reviews, chapters, and books in the areas of preventive cardiology, cardiac rehabilitation, health promotion, and physical activity/performance.

ANDREA KRISKA.   Dr. Andrea Kriska is involved both locally and internationally in examining the role of physical inactivity in the development of chronic diseases, mainly involving minority populations. She has participated in many of the national physical activity efforts over the past decade including the Surgeon General's Report on Physical Activity and Health, the NIH Consensus Development Conference on Physical Activity and Cardiovascular Health, the American College of Sports Medicine Position Stand on Physical Activity and Type 2 Diabetes Mellitus, the Women's Health National Leadership Conference on Physical Activity and Women's Health, and the expert panel organized by the CDC and the American College of Sports Medicine to develop the national physical activity recommendations.

Dr. Kriska is currently the principal investigator of an NIH grant whose purpose is to investigate the role of physical inactivity in NIDDM development in the Pima Indians of Arizona. She also serves as co-investigator or consultant for various other NIH funded studies such as the NIDDK Diabetes Prevention Trial currently underway in the US; NIDDM in the South Pacific, Environmental/Genetic Determinants; the Strong Heart Study (Cardiovascular Disease in American Indians); and the Epidemiological Transition and NIDDM in the Virgin Islands. The activity questionnaire that she has developed is being used in all of the above populations as well as others around the world.

On faculty in the Department of Epidemiology at the University of Pittsburgh, Dr. Kriska also trains graduate students in the area of physical activity epidemiology, providing them with hands-on experience in an area that is in great demand.

DANIEL M. LANDERS.   Daniel M. Landers is a regents' professor of exercise science and physical education at Arizona State University. After receiving graduate degrees from the University of Illinois, he was on the faculty at the University of Illinois, Champaign-Urbana, the University of Washington, and the Pennsylvania State University. Dr. Landers' chief research interest deals with psychophysiological theory and methodology applied to sport and exercise, with a focus on understanding how athletes control arousal and focus concentration so as to maximize performance. Dr. Landers is a fellow of the American Psychological Association, the American College of Sports Medicine, the Research Consortium of AAHPERD, and the American Academy of Physical Education. Dr. Landers is former president of the North American Society for Psychology of Sport and Physical Activity and the Division of Exercise Sport Psychology of APA. His advisory work has included membership on education and training committees for national sports governing bodies, the Sport Psychology and Sport Vision and Enhancement committees for the U.S. Olympic committee, the *Research Quarterly* for Exercise and Sport editorial board, and the National Academy of Sciences' Committee on Techniques for the Enhancement of Human Performance. Dr. Landers was the cofounder and editor of the *Journal for Sports and Exercise Psychology.* He has edited or authored seven books, contributed chapters to 27 books, and authored more than 100 journal articles.

I-MIN LEE.   I-Min Lee, M.D., Sc.D., is assistant professor of medicine at Harvard Medical School and assistant professor of epidemiology at the Harvard School of Public Health. She grew up in Malaysia and received her medical training in Singapore. She received her training in epidemiology at the Harvard School of Public Health.

Dr. Lee's main research interest is in the role of physical activity in promoting health and enhancing longevity. She is also concerned with issues related to women's health. She contributed to the writing of the Surgeon General's report on physical activity and health, served on the expert panel of the NIH Consensus Development Conference on Physical Activity and Cardiovascular Health, and presented at numerous other national and international conferences highlighting physical activity as a means towards health and longevity. Dr. Lee is author or co-author of over 60 publications.

ROBERT P. PANGRAZI.   Robert Pangrazi is a professor in the Department of Exercise Science and Physical Education at Arizona State University. Professionally, he has served as an elementary teacher, university teacher, and researcher and as a university administrator. Dr. Pangrazi is an Honor Fellow of the AAHPERD and a Fellow in the American Academy of Kinesiology and Physical Education. He was honored by NASPE with the Margie Hanson Distinguished Service Award.

One of Dr. Pangrazi's books, *Dynamic Physical Education for Elementary School Children,* 12th ed., is used for teacher preparation courses in many colleges and universities. He has authored 32 other textbooks, more than 55 research/journal articles, and has served as editor of three professional journals. In addition, Dr. Pangrazi has produced five professional 16mm films, a series of educational videotapes, and two fitness-related videos for national television. Dr. Pangrazi has been the keynote speaker for many state and district conventions, delivered three international presentations, and presented approximately 150 speeches at the local, state, and national level. Dr. Pangrazi has worked with teachers throughout the U.S. He regularly conducts training sessions in schools and universities and is regarded as a motivational speaker. His approach to elementary school physical education has been adopted worldwide by the Department of Defense Dependents Schools, nationally by the Edison Project, and is used in hundreds of public, private, and charter schools. He currently is working with the President's Council on Physical Fitness and Sports to develop an activity promotion program for America's youth.

SHARON ANN PLOWMAN.   Sharon Ann Plowman is a professor in the Department of Physical Education at Northern Illinois University and Director of the Human Performance Laboratory. During her 29 year tenure she has taught physical fitness activity classes, exercise physiology, training and conditioning, stress testing, fitness programming, and exercise bioenergetics. She received the University Excellence in Teaching Award in 1975.

Dr. Plowman has published approximately 50 research-based articles, numerous articles on physical fitness, and is co-author of two books: Anshel, M.H., et al. (1991) *Dictionary of the Sport and Exercise Sciences,* and Plowman, S.A. and Smith, D.L. *Exercise Physiology for Health, Fitness and Performance.*

Dr. Plowman is a fellow of the American College of Sports Medicine and the American Academy of Kinesiology and Physical Education. She served as a member on the 1975-77 Task Force to Study the Feasibility for a Revision of the AAHPER Youth Fitness Test, which resulted in the AAHPERD Health-Related Fitness Test, and is currently a member of the FITNESSGRAM Advisory Council. She is the recipient of AAHPERD's Mable Lee Award and the Physical Fitness Council Award.

MICHAEL L. POLLOCK. Michael Pollock, Ph.D., has been professor in the Department of Medicine (Cardiology), University of Florida, College of Medicine, and professor in the Department of Exercise Sport Sciences, University of Florida, Gainesville, Florida from 1986 to present. He is the Director of the Center for Exercise Science. He earned his B.S. from the University of Arizona and both his M.S. and Ph.D. from the University of Illinois, Champaign-Urbana.

Dr. Pollock served as assistant professor and director of the Adult Fitness Program, Wake Forest University from 1967 to 1973, director of research for the Institute for Aerobics Research, Dallas, Texas from 1973 to 1977, director of the Cardiac Rehabilitation Program and Human Performance Laboratory, Mount Sinai Medical Center, Milwaukee, Wisconsin from 1977 to 1984, professor of medicine, University of Wisconsin Medical School from 1980 to 1984, director of the Cardiac Rehabilitation Program, Sports Medicine and Human Performance Laboratory, Travis Medical Center, Houston, Texas from 1984 to 1985.

He is a fellow and past-president of the American College of Sports Medicine and a fellow of American Association of Cardiovascular and Pulmonary Rehabilitation, American Heart Association, American College of cardiology, American Physiological Society, and AAHPERD. He has authored more than 300 articles, three books, and two monographs in the areas of exercise physiology, physical fitness, cardiac rehabilitation, and sports medicine.

JAMES F. SALLIS. James Sallis received his doctorate in clinical psychology from Memphis State University, with an internship at Brown University. He was a post-doctoral fellow in cardiovascular disease prevention and epidemiology at the Stanford Center for Research in Disease Prevention, where he began work on physical activity issues and pursued his interest in public health programs. He is currently Professor of Psychology at San Diego State University and Adjunct Professor of Pediatrics at University of California, San Diego.

Dr. Sallis's primary research interest is promoting physical activity throughout the lifespan, with an emphasis on youth. Over the past six years Dr. Sallis has been awarded over $5 million by the National Institutes of Health and Centers for Disease Control and Prevention to study the effects of physical activity interventions and other health promotion programs. These programs are being carried out in the real world settings of elementary schools, physician offices, middle schools, and university campuses.

Dr. Sallis is the author of over 190 scientific publications and is on the editorial boards of several journals. He served on the editorial committee for the 1996 U.S. Surgeon General's Report, *Physical Activity and Health.* Dr. Sallis is co-author of a health psychology textbook titled *Health and Human Behavior* (McGraw-Hill, 1993) and a forthcoming book *Physical Activity and Behavioral Medicine* (Sage, 1999). He is a frequent consultant to government agencies, research programs, health organizations, and corporations throughout the United States and internationally.

VERN D. SEEFELDT. Vern Seefeldt began his career as an educator by teaching biological science and physical education in the public schools of Wisconsin. He also coached high school interscholastic football, basketball, and baseball in Wisconsin and the U.S. Army in Karlsruhe, Germany. Vern received his B.S. degree with joint majors in biological science and physical education from the University of Wisconsin-LaCrosse and his Ph.D. degree from the University of Wisconsin-Madison in 1966. Dr. Seefeldt's professional interests include the interrelationship of physical growth, biological maturity, and motor skill acquisition of children and youth. As founder and Director of the Institute for the Study of Youth Sports at Michigan State University, Vern devoted his professional time to the study of beneficial/detrimental effects of athletic competition on children and youth. Vern is a past president of the National Association for Sport and Physical Education and retains a keen interest in the status and content of physical education programs in the United States.

JANET M. SHAW. Janet Shaw received her undergraduate degree at Indiana University. Upon completing her master's degree at the University of North Carolina in exercise science, she pursued her doctoral degree at Oregon State University under the direction of Dr. Christine M. Snow. Dr. Shaw's doctoral work focused on the effects of long-term resistance training on multiple indices of fracture risk and psychological variables in postmenopausal women.

Dr. Shaw is currently an Assistant Professor in the Department of Exercise and Sport Science at the University of Utah, where she teaches exercise physiology, fitness evaluation and exercise prescription, and exercise programming in the community. She continues to conduct research on exercise programming for improving physical function and reducing fall and fracture risk in older women as well as on determining the types of exercise that are best for bone health.

R. J. SHEPHARD. Dr. R. J. Shephard is presently professor emeritus of applied physiology in the School of Physical and Health Education and the Department of Preventive Medicine and Biostatistics, Faculty of Medicine, University of Toronto. He is also a visiting scientist at the Defence and Civil Institute of Environmental Medicine and a consultant to the Toronto Rehabilitation Centre, the Gage Research Institute, the Directorate of Active Living, Health and Welfare Canada, the Institute for Aerobics, Dallas, and the State University of New York at Brockport. Dr. Shephard was director of the School of Physical and Health Education at the University of Toronto from 1979 to 1991 and Canadian Tire Acceptance Limited Resident Scholar in Health Studies at Brock University from 1994 to 1998.

Dr. Shephard holds four scientific and medical degrees from London University (B.Sc., M.B.B.S., Ph.D. and M.D.) and honorary doctorates from Gent University (Belgium) and the Universite de Montreal, together with the Honour Award of the Canadian Society of Exercise Physiology and a Citation from the American College of Sports Medicine. He is a former president of the Canadian Association of Sports Sciences, a former president of the American College of Sports Medicine, editor-in-chief of the *Year Book of Sports Medicine* and of *Exercise Immunology Review,* a former editor-in-chief of the *Canadian Journal of Sport Sciences,* and a member of the editorial board of many other journals. He is the author of some 70 books on exercise physiology, fitness, and ergonomics, and has published over 1200 scientific papers on related topics.

CHRISTINE SNOW. Christine Snow, Ph.D., is an associate professor in the Department of Exercise and Sport Science, director of the Bone Research Laboratory at Oregon State University, and is part-time visiting associate professor at the Orthopedic biomechanics Laboratory, Beth Israel Deaconess Medical Center, Harvard Medical School. She received her Ph.D. in exercise science from University of Oregon in 1985 and was a post-doctoral fellow in the Department of Medicine at Stanford University from 1987 to 1990.

At Oregon State University, Dr. Snow developed and now directs the Bone Research Laboratory where she has supervised numerous cross-sectional and longitudinal research projects. She also teaches in the area of exercise physiology, mentors an average of 5 graduate students per year, and directs a clinical program for community patient referrals.

As a part of the ACSM-NASA Countermeasures Roundtable in November, 1995, Dr. Snow served a major role in the development of the bone-specific recommendations and assisted in finalizing the report. She has authored chapters, peer-reviewed publications, and given presentations nationally and internationally. She has received research funding from the National Institutes of Health, the AARP Andrus Foundation, the Medical Research Foundation, NASA, the Erkkila Foundation, and the American College of Sports Medicine.

KEVIN R. VINCENT. Kevin Vincent, M.S., is a doctoral candidate in the College of Health and Human Performance at the University of Florida. He earned his B.S. in Sports Medicine/Athletic Training from the University of Connecticut, and his M.S. in Exercise Science from the University of Massachusetts. He is currently the Coordinator of Strength and Conditioning for the Recreation and Fitness Centers at the University of Florida.

Vincent has served as instructor of cardiopulmonary pharmacology, for Santa Fe Community College 1997 to present, coordinator of Low Back Testing and Rehabilitation, University of Florida from 1996 to 1997, assistant editor for *International Journal of Sport Nutrition,* 1995, editorial assistant for *International Journal of Sport Nutrition,* from 1993 to 1994. He is a member of the American College of Sports Medicine, National Strength and Conditioning Association, and the American Heart Association. He has published in the areas of sport nutrition, resistance training, physical fitness, muscle soreness/damage, neurological adaptations to exercise, and exercise prescription.

GREG WELK. Greg Welk received his M.S. in exercise physiology from the University of Iowa and his Ph.D. in exercise and wellness from Arizona State University. He currently works at the Cooper Institute for Aerobics Research in Dallas, a research and education center devoted to the study and promotion of physical activity. In this position, he serves as the director of Childhood and Adolescent Health Division and the scientific director of the FITNESSGRAM

Youth Fitness Program. He also serves as the director of the Clinical Applications Laboratory, coordinating various research projects.

Dr. Welk's research interests focus on the assessment and promotion of physical activity in children. He has authored (or co-authored) 15 papers and has made 22 presentations at regional and national meetings.

CHRISTINE L. WELLS. Christine Wells, Ph.D., is professor emerita of exercise science and physical education at Arizona State University. She earned degrees from the University of Michigan, Smith College, and The Pennsylvania State University, and she completed two years of post-doctoral studies at the Institute of Environmental Stress of The University of California, Santa Barbara. She has held several elected offices including president of the Research Consortium of the American Alliance for Health, Physical Education, Recreation, and Dance; board of trustees and vice president for Education of the American College of Sports Medicine, and president of the Southwest Chapter of the American College of Sports Medicine.

She is listed in *Who's Who of American Women, Foremost Women of the Twentieth Century,* and *Who's Who in the West.* She is an Active Fellow of the American Academy of Kinesiology and Physical Education.The second edition of her book *Women, Sport and Performance: A Physiological Perspective* was published by Human Kinetics Publishers in 1991. The book has been translated into Japanese, Spanish, and Korean. Dr.Wells was also recognized as a Master's Triathlete.

JAMES R. WHITEHEAD. James Whitehead taught physical education in England for 13 years before returning to school at Arizona State University, where he completed his M.S. and Ed.D. degrees. Since 1988 he has been at the University of North Dakota, where he is currently an associate professor of health and physical education. His teaching specialties are exercise psychology and fitness education. In his research, he is particularly interested in motivation and physical self-perceptions, and in the application of theory in those areas to fitness promotion and education. Dr. Whitehead is a fellow of the AAHPERD Research Consortium, and of the American College of Sports Medicine.

MELVIN H. WILLIAMS. Eminent Scholar Emeritus Melvin Williams received his Ph.D. in physical education from the University of Maryland. He joined the faculty at Old Dominion University in Norfolk, Virginia, establishing both the Human Performance Laboratory and the Wellness Institute and Research Center within the Department of Exercise Science, Physical Education and Recreation.

His major research focus has been the effect of nutritional, pharmacological, and physiological ergogenic aids on exercise and sports performance, culminating in over fifty research-related publications. He is also an author and editor of several books on ergogenic aids, nutrition, and health and fitness, the most recent being *The Ergogenics Edge: Pushing the Limits of Sports Performance* (1998) and *Nutrition for Health, Fitness, and Sport* (1999). He is the founding editor of the *International Journal of Sport Nutrition,* and has presented research findings internationally in over a dozen countries.

JACK H. WILMORE. Jack Wilmore received his B.S. and M.S. degrees in physical education from the University of California, Santa Barbara, and his Ph.D. in physical education from the University of Oregon. Dr. Wilmore is presently the department head and professor in the Department of Health and Kinesiology at Texas A&M University. From 1985 to 1997, he was the Margie Gurley Seay Centennial Professor and former chair of the Department of Kinesiology and Health Education at the University of Texas at Austin. From 1976 to 1985, he was the director of the Exercise and Sports Sciences Laboratory, and professor and head of the Department of Exercise and Sport Sciences at the University of Arizona. He also held a joint appointment in the Department of Surgery, College of Medicine. His present research interests include exercise in the prevention and control of obesity, exercise in the prevention and control of coronary heart disease, alterations in physiological function with training and detraining, and factors limiting the performance of elite athletes.

A former president of the American College of Sports Medicine, Dr. Wilmore has chaired many ACSM organizational committees. He is a former member of the United States Olympic Committee's Sports Medicine Council, having chaired their Research Committee; and is currently a member of the American Physiological Society and a Fellow and President-Elect of the American Academy of Kinesiology and Physical Education.

Dr. Wilmore has published 52 chapters, over 190 peer-reviewed research papers, and 14 books. He is also a member of the Editorial Board for several journals. Dr. Wilmore has served as a consultant for several professional sports teams, including the L. A. Lakers and the San Francisco 49ers, and for the California Highway Patrol, the PCPFS, NASA, and the U. S. Air Force.

Physical Activity Antecedents

The papers included in this section cover a variety of topics. Each discusses factors worthy of consideration prior to a person's entry into physical activity. It is fitting that the paper by Roy Shephard is first because medical readiness is essential to safe participation in physical activity. Claude Bouchard's paper is included because heredity has been shown to be a powerful factor influencing fitness and physical activity. The third paper, by B. Don Franks, discusses physical activity guidelines that should be considered before participation in activity. Finally, James Sallis discusses intrinsic motivation and other determinants or antecedents of physical activity.

Readiness for Physical Activity

Roy J. Shephard
UNIVERSITY OF TORONTO

Current practice in physical education and sports medicine emphasizes the twin goals of reducing the risk of illness and increasing quality-adjusted life expectancy through the development of health-related fitness (Bouchard et al., 1990; Bouchard et al., 1994; US Surgeon General, 1996). The average city-dweller currently takes insufficient habitual physical activity to realize these goals, but involvement in a regular, well-designed program of aerobic training, supplemented by moderate resisted muscle exercises, could satisfy both objectives (American College of Sports Medicine (ACSM), 1991; ACSM, 1993). What are the risks of engaging in such activity, and how can a person determine if he or she is ready to undertake such a program?

RISKS OF EXERCISE

Excessive physical activity can provoke a variety of musculoskeletal injuries, but the big fear, highlighted by such events as the sudden death of Jim Fixx and other high-profile exercisers, is that the program will provoke a fatal heart attack. Studies from our own laboratory and elsewhere (Cobb & Weaver, 1986; Northcote & Ballantyne, 1984; Sadaniantz & Thompson, 1990; Shephard, 1974, 1981, 1995; Siscovick, 1990; Thompson & Fahrenbach, 1994; Vuori, 1995) show that (at least in symptom-free men) the risk of fatal and nonfatal heart attacks during physical activity is from 4 to 56 times higher than it is while sitting at home reading a book. The issue of hypertrophic cardiomyopathy and sudden death is controversial (Maron, Isner, & McKenna, 1994; Rost & Hollman, 1992; Shephard, 1996a, b). Maron et al. (1986) suggested that the main causes of sudden death in exercisers under 35 years of age were hypertrophic cardiomyopathy (48%: particularly a thickening of the septum between left and right ventricles) and unexplained enlargement of the left ventricle (18%). However, the norms of wall thickness are still not agreed upon, and the prevalence of the disorder is so low that routine electrocardiographic and/or echocardiographic screening of young adults is not warranted; indeed, such an approach yields many false positive diagnoses, with resulting anxiety and iatrogenic invalidism (Shephard, 1996a, b). In those over the age of 35 years, 80% of exercise-related deaths were attributed to disease of the coronary arteries. The overall risk that

ORIGINALLY PUBLISHED AS SERIES 1, NUMBER 5, OF THE PCPFS RESEARCH DIGEST.

HIGHLIGHT ||▊| ||▊▊▊ ▊▊ |▊▊▊| || ▊||| ▊█| | |▊|||▊|| ▊▊||||||▊| | | ||▊| ||▊ || |▊▊|||▊|▊ ▊▊▊||| |▊

"The risk that exercise will induce a cardiac catastrophe is low and many screening tests are costly and time consuming. The revised PAR-Q has shown remarkable success as an exercise screening procedure and is recommended for symptom-free adults with no more than one major cardiac risk factor."

---

vigorous physical activity will provoke a cardiac emergency is quite low, about one death per 400,000 hours of jogging (Thompson et al., 1982), and furthermore the risk seems even lower in regular than in occasional exercisers (Siscovick et al., 1984).

IMPLICATIONS FOR PRE-EXERCISE SCREENING

Ideally, regular physical activity should be conceived as a simple, safe, and natural part of healthy living, a lifestyle to which the human body has adapted over many centuries of evolutionary struggle as a hunter and primitive agriculturalist (Shephard, 1993), rather than as a dangerous medical intervention that requires extensive, high-technology pre-exercise evaluation.

For a long period, physicians in the United States adopted a somewhat restrictive approach to exercise prescription, suggesting that a stress electrocardiogram was needed in all men over the age of 35 years who wanted to increase their habitual physical activity (Cooper, 1970). Their starting point was the now largely discredited assumption (Shephard, 1984; Siscovick et al., 1991) that echocardiography and/or a medically supervised exercise stress ECG could predict and thus avert the occasional exercise-induced cardiac arrest. Northcote and Ballantyne (1984) have pointed out that it would cost $13 billion to screen even current athletes over the age of 35 years; moreover, it would be necessary to screen 10,000 potential exercisers to find one who might die, and four other individuals who had been cleared by exercise stress testing would die unexpectedly while exercising (Epstein & Maron, 1986). Finally, the stress test itself has a significant morbidity and mortality (Van Camp, 1988), and a heavy emotional, financial, and medical burden is generated by the high proportion of false positive test results.

The need for extensive preliminary screening is particularly questionable, given that moderate exercise decreases rather than increases a person's overall risk of cardiac death (Siscovick et al., 1984). The Swedish physiologist P. O. Astrand has often suggested in his lectures that it would be more logical to focus detailed medical attention on sedentary people than on those who are about to enter a conditioning program. Nevertheless, potential exercisers can be offered some practical advice that will reduce the likelihood of an exercise catastrophe. A review of such incidents (Johnson, 1992; Shephard, 1974, 1981, 1995) suggests that risks are increased if:

1. There is a history of fainting or chest pain during exercise.

2. There is a family history of sudden death at a young age.

3. The intensity and duration of activity are much greater than the subject has recently experienced.

4. Competition, publicity, or pride encourages persistence with exercise in the face of warning symptoms.

5. The individual exercises while under pressure of time, or when oppressed by business or social problems.

6. The activity involves heavy lifting or prolonged isometric effort.

7. The weather is unduly hot or cold.

8. The participant has a viral infection, senses chest discomfort or cardiac irregularity, or feels "unwell."

9. Exercise soon after rising from bed (Willich, 1995).

The corresponding precautions are all matters of common sense, readily understood by the general public, but rarely discussed in the course of the usual clinical examination. There has thus been increasing acceptance of the Canadian viewpoint (Shephard, 1976, 1988, 1994), that (in symptom-free people from adolescence through to early old age) simple advice and self-administered question-naires provide the most appropriate method of determining readiness for a modest increase of physical activity.

Current U.S. Screening Recommendations

The current U.S. recommendation for pre-exercise screening has moved much closer to the Canadian position (Table 1.1). It looks at the age of the subject (males >40 and females >50 years, American College of Sports Medicine, 1991, p. 37), the proposed intensity of effort, and associated symptoms or major cardiac risk factors.

If the subject is planning no more than a moderate increase of habitual activity (an intensity of less than 60% of peak aerobic effort, which the person can sustain comfortably for an hour or longer), is symptom-free and has no more than one major coronary risk factor, then a preliminary medical examination is no longer recommended. Indications for medical advice are (1) the presence of disease,

TABLE 1.1

Indications for preliminary medical screening among those who wish to increase their habitual physical activity (based on the recommendations of the American College of Sports Medicine, 1991; see original article for details).

Variable	Indication for Medical Screening
Known disease	Yes, if cardiac, pulmonary, or metabolic
Symptoms or signs suggesting disease[a]	Yes, if cardiac, pulmonary, or metabolic
Major cardiac risk factors[b]	Yes, if two or more
Vigorous exercise[c]	Yes, if man >40 yr or woman >50 yr

[a]Pain or discomfort in chest, shortness of breath with mild exertion, dizziness or sudden loss of consciousness, shortness of breath while sleeping, swelling of the ankles, palpitations or racing heart beat, pain in the calves on walking, or known heart murmur.

[b]Blood pressure higher than 160 mm Hg systolic or 90 mm Hg diastolic on two occasions, or use of medication to reduce blood pressure; serum cholesterol higher than 6.2 mmol/L (240 mg/dL); cigarette smoking; diabetes mellitus; family history of coronary or atherosclerotic disease in parents or siblings before the age of 55 years.

[c]Exercise that represents a substantial challenge; usually higher than 60% of maximal oxygen intake, and causing fatigue within 20 minutes or less.

(2) the intent to undertake vigorous exercise above the specified age limit, and (3) two or more major risk factors, or symptoms suggestive of cardiopulmonary or metabolic disease.

Simple Approaches to Screening

Although the expense and anxiety associated with a formal medical examination are unwarranted for the great majority of people who plan to begin a simple exercise program, there remains merit in simple screening procedures, either self-administered or carried out by the staff of a fitness center.

Bailey et al. (1976) first suggested such an approach when screening candidates for the Canadian Home Fitness Test. In the following year, Chisholm and associates (1975, 1978) surveyed 1,253 apparently healthy adults who were attending an exhibition. They evaluated a potential list of some 19 self-administered screening questions against a medical examination that included a physical examination, the measurement of resting blood pressure, and recordings of resting and exercise electrocardiograms. As a result of this research, a brief self-administered questionnaire (the Physical Activity Readiness Questionnaire, or PAR-Q) was developed. This incorporated the seven questions they judged had been the most effective in identifying individuals who needed a medical examination prior to exercise testing or conditioning.

The original version of the PAR-Q was quickly endorsed by the Canadian federal government fitness agency (Fitness Canada), and it has since been widely used, both in Canada and abroad (Shephard, 1986). Indeed, the American College of Sports Medicine recently recommended adoption of the PAR-Q procedure for healthy adults (men >40, women >50 years) who wish to increase their habitual physical activity (American College of Sports Medicine, 1991). Nearly two decades of experience has shown that the original PAR-Q procedure is remarkably safe (Shephard 1988, 1991). Given the low inherent risk of exercise for the healthy adult, and the fact that even clinical examination and an exercise stress ECG provide a rather dubious "gold standard" of exercise readiness, it is difficult to assess the sensitivity (the percentage of subjects unready for exercise who are detected) and the specificity (the percentage of individuals who are screened needlessly) of the PAR-Q procedure. Sensitivity seems adequate, since the PAR-Q has been used to screen as many as half a million people, without any reported adverse events in subsequent exercise testing or programs. On the other hand, about 20% of would-be exercisers "fail the test" by responding positively to one or more questions (Shephard et al., 1981), and in those aged 60–69 years, as many as 55% are "screened out" (Fitness Canada, 1983; Shephard, 1986). Moreover, subsequent examination of the medical records, blood pressure readings, and electrocardiograms on positive responders suggests that at all ages from adolescence onward, many of the PAR-Q exclusions are unnecessary (Shephard et al., 1981).

Accordingly, the detailed wording of individual PAR-Q questions has recently been reviewed and revised by an expert committee of Fitness Canada (Figure 1.1). Given the absence of any clear gold standard of exercise readiness, the rewording was agreed through the Delphic process of circulating repeated drafts of the questionnaire for critical comment. The principal objective was to increase specificity without an undue sacrifice of sensitivity. The revised wording of the questionnaire reduced the overall number of individuals who were "screened out" from 17% to 12%. In all, 7.3% who had originally made positive responses were cleared by the rPAR-Q, but 2.3% of new candidates were cautioned about exercising (Shephard, Thomas, & Weller, 1991).

The trend was for the revised format to allow exercise in a higher proportion of elderly subjects. The largest change of response patterns occurred on the question relating to blood pressure, which had been a major cause of erroneous exercise exclusions when using the original PAR-Q (Shephard et al., 1981).

Current Evaluation of Screening Questionnaires

The specificity of any screening test can only be improved at the price of some loss of sensitivity. A further decade of usage will be needed to decide whether the shift in this balance has been gauged correctly in the rPAR-Q, although preliminary data are encouraging in this regard. Unfortunately, there are major obstacles to an objective comparison of the two questionnaire wordings. Cost is a significant barrier, given the required sample size, but the

FIGURE 1.1

Revised physical activity readiness questionnaire (rPAR-Q).

Yes   No

☐ ☐ 1. Has a doctor said that you have a heart condition and recommended only medically supervised activity?

☐ ☐ 2. Do you have chest pain brought on by physical activity?

☐ ☐ 3. Have you developed chest pain in the past month?

☐ ☐ 4. Do you tend to lose consciousness or fall over as a result of dizziness?

☐ ☐ 5. Do you have a bone or joint that could be aggravated by the proposed physical activity?

☐ ☐ 6. Has a doctor ever recommended medication for your blood pressure or a heart condition?

☐ ☐ 7. Are you aware through your own experience, or a doctor's advice, of any other physical reason against your exercising without medical supervision?

NOTE: If you have a temporary illness, such as a common cold, or are not feeling well at this time—POSTPONE.

From Shephard, R.J., Thomas, S., & Weller, I. (1991). "The Canadian Home Fitness Test: 1991 Update," *Sports Medicine.* 1: page 359, used by permission.

cost/effectiveness of a validation against clinical examination is also questionable, given the lack of agreement between doctors on appropriate criteria for exclusion from conditioning programs, and the high proportion of false positive stress ECGs in symptom-free adults (Shephard, 1981). Physician-exclusion rates can range from 1% to 15% in comparable samples of the general adult population (Shephard, 1988). Moreover, high physician exclusion rates apparently lack validity, since they do not reduce the number of electrocardiographic abnormalities and other minor complications that are encountered during exercise testing.

When developing the original PAR-Q, Chisholm et al. (1975, 1978) did attempt to validate their list of 19 potential questions against physician records, blood pressures and electrocardiographic tracings. The final, reduced list of seven questions did not receive any formal clinical validation. Nevertheless, less direct validation has been possible, coupling the International Classification of Diseases (ICD) codings reported in a national health survey (Health & Welfare, Canada, 1982) with PAR-Q responses. Trial of this approach has shown remarkable success (Arraiz et al., 1992). Over a seven-year follow-up, 1,644 of 31,668 subjects died. PAR-Q responses were divided into three categories: pass (no positive responses), conditional pass (positive response about hypertension, not under treatment or supervision for elevated blood pressure), and failure (other positive response). In those failing the test (Table 1.2), the crude overall mortality risk ratio was 2.2 (or 2.1, after adjustment for age, sex, body mass index, and smoking behavior). Moreover, the relative risk of cardiovascular death was 9.1 (or 7.8 after adjusting for age, sex, body mass index, and smoking behavior). Interestingly, the relative risk was moderately greater than that associated with a poor performance on the Canadian Home Fitness Test, and was much greater than would have been obtained by use of an exercise stress ECG. Siscovick et al. (1991) found a relative risk of only 2.6 when asymptomatic hypercholesterolemic men with exercise-induced ST segmental depression were followed for a seven-year period. The PAR-Q responses remained of prognostic value when cases with known heart disease, stroke, and high blood pressure were deleted (Table 1.2).

When the Canadian governmental committee revised the PAR-Q, changes from the original format were deliberately held to minor clarifications of wording, and the number of questions was unchanged. It already seems a very useful screening tool. However, the questionnaire may pass through several further revisions and refinements of wording before all of its potential has been realized. Issues that remain to be addressed include the need for age-specific questionnaires for children and for the very old, the level of certification needed by paramedical professionals who are now urged to discuss client responses to questions 5 and 6, the need to caution those cleared by the rPAR-Q against large and sudden increases in habitual activity, the value of additional questions, and the potential to add information about lifestyle and conditioning techniques to the back of the questionnaire.

SUMMARY

The risk that exercise will induce a cardiac catastrophe is low, and a medically supervised exercise ECG is not a cost-effective approach to the preexercise screening of symptom-free adults. However, a questionnaire (whether self-administered, or completed by fitness center staff) is a useful safety precaution. The Canadian Physical Activity Readiness Questionnaire (PAR-Q) has proven a very safe screening tool, and comparison of responses with findings from the Canada Health Survey has shown remarkable success in detecting potential contraindications to exercise. Nevertheless, the PAR-Q also "screens out" an excessive proportion of apparently healthy older adults. To reduce unnecessary exclusions, the questionnaire wording has now been revised (rPAR-Q). The balance of sensitivity to specificity is apparently improved in the revised questionnaire, particularly in regard to the question about an elevation of blood pressure. The rPAR-Q is thus the currently recommended method of determining exercise readiness in symptom-free adults with no more than one major cardiac risk factor.

TABLE 1.2

Validation of the original PAR-Q test against a 7-year prospective study of data from the Canada Health Survey (data abstracted from the paper of Arraiz et al., 1992).

Source of Risk	Relative Risk if Failed PAR-Q	
	Crude	*Adjusted*
All causes	2.2	2.1
Cardiovascular disease	9.1	7.8
CVD (omitting if history of CVD)	5.4	
CVD (omitting if history of CVD, stroke, HBP)	2.9	
Cancer	2.1	1.6
Other causes	2.4	2.1

REFERENCES

Adams, R. (1991). *Report of Expert Committee on Revision of the Physical Activity Readiness Questionnaire*. Ottawa: Fitness and Amateur Sport.

American College of Sports Medicine. (1991). *Guidelines for Graded Exercise Testing and Prescription*. 4th ed. Philadelphia: Lea & Febiger.

American College of Sports Medicine. (1993). Summary Statement: Workshop on Physical Activity and Public Health. *Sports Medicine Bulletin*, October–November, p. 7.

Arraiz, G.A., Wigle, D.T., & Mao, Y. (1992). Risk assessment of physical activity and physical fitness in the Canada Health Survey mortality follow up. *Journal of Clinical Epidemiology, 45*, 419–428.

Bailey, D.A., Shephard, R.J., & Mirwald, R.L. (1976). Validation of a self-administered home test for cardio-respiratory fitness. *Canadian Journal of Applied Sport Sciences, 1*, 67–78.

Bailey, D.A., Shephard, R.J., Mirwald, R.L., & McBride, G.A. (1974). A current view of Canadian cardio-respiratory fitness. *Canadian Medical Association Journal 111*, 25–30.

Bouchard, C., Shephard, R.J., & Stephens, T. (1994). *Physical Activity, Fitness, and Health*. Champaign, IL: Human Kinetics Publishers.

Bouchard, C., Shephard, R.J., Stephens, T., Sutton, J., & McPherson, B. (1990). *Exercise, Fitness and Health*. Champaign, IL: Human Kinetics Publishers.

Chisholm, D.M., Collis, M.L., Kulak, L.L., Davenport, W., & Gruber, N. (1975). Physical activity readiness. *British Columbia Medical Journal, 17*, 375–378.

Chisholm, D.M., Collis, M.L., Kulak, L.L., Davenport, W., Gruber, N., & Stewart, G. (1978). *PAR-Q Validation Report: The evaluation of a self-administered pre-exercise screening questionnaire for adults*. Vancouver, BC: Ministry of Health.

Cobb, L.A., & Weaver, W.D. (1986). Exercise a risk for sudden death in patients with coronary heart disease. *Journal of the American College of Cardiology, 7*, 215–219.

Cooper, K.H. (1970). Guidelines in the management of the exercising patient. *Journal of the American Medical Association, 211*, 1163–1167.

Epstein, S.E., & Maron, B.J. (1986). Sudden death and the competitive athlete: Perspectives on preparticipation screening studies. *Journal of the American College of Cardiology, 7*, 220–230.

Fitness Canada. (1983). *Fitness and Lifestyle in Canada*. Ottawa: Fitness and Lifestyle Research Institute.

Health & Welfare Canada (1982). *Canada Health Survey*. Ottawa: Health & Welfare Canada.

Maron, B.J., Epstein, S.E., & Roberts, W.C. (1986). Causes of sudden death in competitive athletes. *Journal of the American College of Cardiology, 7*, 204–214.

Maron, B.J., Isner, J.M., & McKenna, W.J. (1994). Hypertrophic cardiomyopathy, myocarditis and other myopericardial diseases and mitral valve prolapse. *Medicine and Science in Sports and Exercise, 26*, S261–S267.

Northcote, R.J., & Ballantyne, D. (1984). Sudden death and sport. *Sports Medicine, 1*, 181–186.

Rost, R., & Hollman, W. (1992). Cardiac problems in endurance sport. In R.J. Shephard & P.O. Astrand (Eds.). *Endurance in Sport*. Oxford: Blackwell Scientific, pp. 438–452.

Sadaniantz, A., & Thompson, P.D. (1990). The problem of sudden death in athletes as illustrated by case studies. *Sports Medicine, 9*, 199–204.

Shephard, D.A.E. (1976). Home fitness testing of Canadians. *Canadian Medical Association Journal, 114*, 662–663.

Shephard, R.J. (1974). Sudden death—A significant hazard of exercise? *British Journal of Sports Medicine, 8*, 101–110.

Shephard, R.J. (1981). *Ischemic Heart Disease and Exercise*. London: Croom Helm.

Shephard, R.J. (1984). Can we identify those for whom exercise is hazardous? *Sports Medicine, 1*, 75–86.

Shephard, R.J. (1986). *Fitness of a Nation: Lessons from the Canada Fitness Survey*. Basel: Karger Publications.

Shephard, R.J. (1988). PAR-Q, Canadian Home Fitness Test and exercise screening alternatives. *Sports Medicine, 5*, 185–195.

Shephard, R.J. (1991). Safety of exercise testing—The role of the paramedical specialist. *Clinical Journal of Sports Medicine, 1*, 8–11.

Shephard, R.J. (1993). *Physical Activity and Health-Related Fitness*. Champaign, IL: Human Kinetics Publishers.

Shephard, R.J. (1994). *Aerobic Fitness and Health*. Champaign, IL: Human Kinetics Publishers.

Shephard, R.J. (1995). Exercise and sudden death: An overview. *Sport Science Review, 4(2)*, 1–13.

Shephard, R.J. (1996a). The athlete's heart: Is big beautiful? *British Journal of Sports Medicine, 30*, 5–10.

Shephard, R.J. (1996b). Sudden cardiac death in young athletes: A critical reevaluation. *Perspectives in Cardiology, 12(6)*, 35–43.

Shephard, R.J., Cox, M., & Simper, K. (1981). An analysis of PAR-Q responses in an office population. *Canadian Journal of Public Health, 72*, 37–40.

Shephard, R.J., Thomas, S., & Weller, I. (1991). The Canadian Home Fitness Test: 1991 Update. *Sports Medicine, 11*, 358–366.

Siscovick, D. (1990). Risks of exercising: Sudden cardiac death and injuries. In C. Bouchard, R.J. Shephard, T. Stephens, J. Sutton, & B. McPherson (Eds.): *Exercise, Fitness, and Health*. Champaign, IL: Human Kinetics Publishers.

Siscovick, D.S., Ekelund, L.G., Johnson, J.L., Truong, Y., & Adler, A. (1991). Sensitivity of exercise electrocardiography for acute cardiac events during moderate and strenuous physical activity. *Archives of Internal Medicine, 151,* 325–330.

Siscovick, D.S., Weiss, N.S., Fletcher, R.H., & Lasky, T. (1984). The incidence of primary cardiac arrest during vigorous exercise. *New England Journal of Medicine, 311,* 874–877.

Thompson, P.D., & Fahrenbach, M.C. (1994). Risks of exercising: Cardiovascular, including sudden cardiac death. In C. Bouchard, R.J. Shephard, & T. Stephens (Eds.). *Physical Activity, Fitness, and Health.* Champaign, IL: Human Kinetics Publishers.

Thompson, P.D., Funk, E.J., Carleton, R.A., et al. (1982). Incidence of death during jogging in Rhode Island from 1975 through 1980. *Journal of the American Medical Association, 247,* 2535–2538.

US Surgeon General. (1996). *Physical Activity and Health.* Washington, DC: Dept. of Health and Human Services.

Van Camp, S.P. (1988). Exercise-related sudden death: Risks and causes. *Physician and Sportsmedicine, 16(5),* 97–112.

Vuori, I. (1995). Sudden death and exercise: Effects of age and type of activity. *Sport Science Review, 4(2),* 46–84.

Vuori, I., Suurnakki, L., & Suurnakki, T. (1982). Risk of sudden cardiovascular death (SCVD) in exercise. *Medicine and Science in Sports and Exercise, 14,* 114–115.

Willich, S.N. (1995). Circadian influences and possible triggers of sudden cardiac death. *Sport Science Review, 4(2),* 31–45.

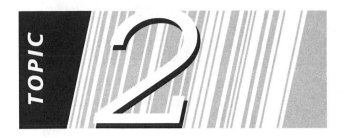

Heredity and Health-Related Fitness

Claude Bouchard
UNIVERSITÉ LAVAL

A NOTE FROM THE EDITORS

This paper, "Heredity and Health-Related Fitness," is written by the most prominent scholar in the area. While we have known for some time that heredity was a factor affecting fitness performances, it was not until Dr. Bouchard and his colleagues began their in-depth studies in the area that we really began to know the extent of hereditary influences.

Dr. Bouchard has studied families, especially families with twins, to learn how heredity affects fitness. Heredity (genotypes) affects different fitness components (phenotypes) in different ways. For example, two people of the same age and sex with similar lifestyles could vary in health-related fitness just because of the genes they inherited. As noted later in this paper, the heritability for body fatness is 25%+, muscle fitness 20-40%, and CV fitness 10 to 25%.

But heritability only accounts for differences that heredity might make when comparing two people who have not trained. Bouchard and colleagues have been the pioneers who have demonstrated that not only do people differ in fitness based on heredi-

ty, but people of different genetic backgrounds respond differently to training. In other words, two people of different genetic background could do the exact same exercise program and get quite different benefits (see Figure 2.1). Some people get as much as 10 times as much benefit from activity as others who do the same program.

Though quite technical in some places, the following paper has many practical implications for teachers and professionals in physical activity and fitness. Some of these are listed below:

- Recognizing individual differences is critical in helping students, clients, and patients with fitness achievement. People do not enter our programs with similar backgrounds, nor do they respond similarly to training.

- Assumptions about a person's fitness cannot always be indicative of their current activity levels. The conclusion that the lower fitness of one person compared to another is a result of inactivity is a dangerous one. Those who do not adapt quickly to physical activity need encouragement to keep them involved, not discourage-

ORIGINALLY PUBLISHED AS SERIES 1, NUMBER 4, OF THE PCPFS *RESEARCH DIGEST*.

"Not only is it important to recognize that there are individual differences in the response to regular physical activity, but research indicates that there are nonresponders in the population. Heredity may account for fitness differences as large as three- to tenfold when comparing low and high responders who have performed the same physical activity program."

ment associated with conclusions about their level of activity and effort.

- Different people (genotypes) respond differently to each part of fitness (phenotype). A person who has less hereditary predisposition to one type of fitness may respond well to another. For this reason we should be careful not to expect people to perform well on all health-related fitness tests just because they score well on one test.

Even those with little technical background can benefit from the paper that follows. Read on!

INTRODUCTION

Health is the culmination of many interacting factors, including the genetic constitution. Humans are genetically quite diverse. Current estimates are that each human being has about one variable DNA base for every 300 bases out of a total of about 3 billion base pairs. Variations in DNA sequence constitute the molecular basis of genetic individuality. Given genetic individuality, an equal state of health and of physical and mental well-being is unlikely to be achieved for all individuals even under similar environmental and lifestyle conditions. Some will thrive better than others and will remain free from disabilities for a longer period of time. Allowing for such individuality, it should thus come as no surprise that there is a minority of adults who remain relatively fit in spite of a sedentary lifestyle.

Genetic differences do not operate in a vacuum. They constantly interact with existing cellular and tissue conditions to provide a biological response commensurate with environmental demands. Genes are constantly interacting with everything in the physical environment as well as with lifestyle characteristics of the individual that translate into signals capable of affecting the cells of the body. For instance, overfeeding, a high fat diet, smoking, and regular endurance exercise are all powerful stimuli that may elicit strong biological responses. However, because of inherited differences at specific genes, the amplitude of adaptive responses varies from one individual to another. Inheritance is one of the important reasons why we are not equally prone to become diabetic or hypertensive or to die from a heart attack. It is also one major explanation for individual differences in the response to dietary intervention or regular physical activity.

HEALTH-RELATED FITNESS

There is no universally agreed-upon definition of fitness and of its components. In the present context, we are particularly interested in what is now referred to as health-related fitness, i.e., in the physical and physiological components of fitness that impact more directly on health status. Health-related fitness refers to the state of physical and physiological characteristics that define the risk levels for the premature development of diseases or morbid conditions presenting a relationship with a sedentary mode of life (Bouchard & Shephard, 1993). Important determinants of health-related fitness include such factors as body mass for height, body composition, subcutaneous fat distribution, abdominal visceral fat, bone density, strength and endurance of the abdominal and dorso-lumbar musculature, heart and lung functions, blood pressure, maximal aerobic power and tolerance to submaximal exercise, glucose and insulin metabolism, blood lipid and lipoprotein profile, and the ratio of lipid to carbohydrate oxidized in a variety of situations. A favorable profile for these various factors presents a clear advantage in terms of health outcomes as assessed by morbidity and mortality statistics. The components of health-related fitness are numerous and are determined by several variables, including the individual's pattern and level of habitual activity, diet, and heredity.

THE GENETIC PERSPECTIVE

In general, genetic issues can be considered from two different perspectives. The first is from the genetic epidemiology perspective. Here the evidence is derived from samples of human subjects, particularly families, large pedigrees, relatives by adoption or twins. The data can be epidemiological in nature or be enriched by molecular studies. The second perspective is frankly molecular and pertains to transcription, translation, and regulatory mechanisms and how the genes adapt or come into play in response to various forms of acute exercise and of training. In this case, the tissue (generally heart muscle or skeletal muscle) is perturbed by an acute or a chronic stress and the changes are monitored. The emphasis is therefore on the molecular mechanisms involved in the adaptation.

Both approaches are very useful in delineating how important genes are for a given phenotype. However, they differ considerably in the type of information they can provide. The first approach is asking whether individual differences for a given phenotype are caused by DNA sequence variation, gene-environment interactions and gene-gene interactions seen among human beings and, ultimately, what are the genes involved and the specific DNA variants accounting for human heterogeneity. The second approach relies heavily on animal models with a focus on the role of various DNA sequences on regulatory mechanisms with no particular interest for the differences that may exist among members of the species.

The genetic epidemiology approach is of particular interest to us here because it deals with individual differences caused by inherited DNA sequence differences. Results available from the genetic epidemiology perspective will therefore constitute the essence of this review.

HEREDITY AND HEALTH-RELATED FITNESS

Although the literature presents evidence for a role of genetic factors in most of the health-related fitness phenotypes, the quality of the evidence varies according to the phenotype considered. Four major components of health-related fitness will be considered here.

TABLE 2.1

An overview of trends in heritability data for selected factors of morphological fitness.

Phenotype	Heritability[a]	Familial environment[b]
Body fat content	~ 25%	Weak
Distribution of subcutaneous fat	30–50%	Weak
Visceral fat	30–60%	Unknown
Bone density	30–60%	Weak

[a] Approximate proportion of the variation in the phenotype compatible with a genetic transmission after removing the effects of age and sex.

[b] Conditions shared by individuals living together.

Morphological Component

Obesity (body fat content) and regional fat distribution are the phenotypes of morphological fitness that have been studied most by geneticists. Table 2.1 summarizes the trends emerging from several reviews regarding the contribution of genetic factors to obesity, regional subcutaneous fat distribution, abdominal visceral fat, and bone density. The body mass index (BMI), subcutaneous fat (sum of skinfold thicknesses), and percent body fat derived from underwater weighing are among the most commonly used phenotypes in genetic studies of obesity. They are characterized by heritability levels reaching about 25% and at times higher. Results from a few studies suggest that BMI and percent body fat may be influenced by variation at a single or a few genes, although there are conflicting results. The phenotypes associated with regional fat distribution are generally characterized by slightly higher heritability levels with values reaching about 30% to 50% of the phenotypic variance. The trunk to extremity skinfolds ratio as a marker of regional subcutaneous fat distribution has been found to be influenced by major effects, possibly associated with variation at a single gene, suggesting that the pattern of fat deposition between the trunk and the limbs is significantly conditioned by genetic factors.

Muscular Component

This fitness component is probably the one for which the evidence for a contribution of genetic factors is the least abundant. Two studies used family data to study familial transmission of muscular fitness. In one study (Pérusse et al., 1988), muscular endurance and muscular strength measurements were obtained in 13,804 subjects who participated in the 1981 Canada Fitness Survey. The results showed that about 40% of the phenotypic variance in muscular endurance and muscular strength could be accounted for by factors transmitted from parents to offspring. In the Quebec Family Study (Pérusse et al., 1987), we found a genetic effect of 21% for muscular endurance and 30% for muscular strength. These results suggest that the heritability of muscular fitness is significant and ranges from low to moderate.

Cardiorespiratory Component

Cardiorespiratory fitness is a major component of health-related fitness and depends on a large number of phenotypes associated primarily with cardiac, vascular, and respiratory functions. Measurements of submaximal exercise capacity and maximal aerobic power are generally performed to assess cardiorespiratory fitness. The contribution of genetic factors to these two phenotypes has been recently reviewed (Bouchard et al., 1992) and estimates of heritability were found to be lower for submaximal exercise capacity (about 10%) than for maximal aerobic power (about 25%). These inherited differences in cardiorespiratory fitness may be partly explained by interindividual differences in heart structures and functions, but relatively little is known about the role of heredity on these determinants despite evidence for significant familial aggregation.

Because of the high prevalence of hypertension in most developed countries and its association with an increased risk of death from myocardial infarction or stroke, the genetic and non-genetic determinants of blood pressure have been extensively studied in various populations. Overall, it is clearly established that blood pressure aggregates in families and heritability estimates reported from various populations are remarkably similar, accounting for about 30% of the interindividual differences. More recently, several specific genes have been implicated in the determination of the susceptibility to hypertension.

Metabolic Component

There is increasing evidence that the metabolic component of health-related fitness should be con-

sidered as an important element of the relationship between physical activity and health. The metabolic component refers to normal blood and tissue carbohydrate and lipid metabolisms and adequate hormonal actions, particularly insulin. A large number of studies have been reported on the genetics of blood lipids and lipoproteins, because of their predominant role in the etiology of cardiovascular disease. Briefly, genetic factors contribute to interindividual differences in blood lipids and lipoproteins with heritability estimates generally accounting for about 25% to as much as 98% of the phenotypic variance, depending on the trait considered with an average value of 50%. Major gene effects have been reported for most of the phenotypes including total cholesterol, LDL-cholesterol, HDL-cholesterol, various apolipoprotein concentrations, and Lpa. Highly significant genetic effects have also been reported for fasting glucose and insulin values as well as for plasma fibrinogen, a protein involved in blood clotting. The glucose and insulin responses to a carbohydrate meal appear to be characterized by lower heritability estimates (<25%) than for fasting values.

The contribution of heredity to the various health-related fitness components thus ranges from low to moderate and, except for some phenotypes pertaining to muscular fitness and metabolic fitness, it rarely exceeds 50% of the phenotypic variance and is often below 25%. These low to moderate heritabilities should not be interpreted as an indication that genes are not important in the determination of these phenotypes. These highly complex phenotypes are undoubtedly influenced by a variety of interactions. There is increasing evidence to the effect that interactions between genes and environmental factors or between various genes are common and contribute to interindividual differences in health-related fitness phenotypes and, consequently, cannot any longer be ignored in the field of physical activity, fitness, and health.

HEREDITY AND RESPONSE TO EXERCISE

Research has amply demonstrated that aerobic performance, stroke volume, skeletal muscle oxidative capacity, and lipid oxidation rates are phenotypes that can adapt to training. For instance, the VO_2max of sedentary persons increases, on the average, by about 20 to 25 percent after a few months of train-

FIGURE 2.1

Individual differences in the response of 47 young men to training programs lasting from 15 to 20 weeks. Results are expressed as gains of VO₂max in liters of O₂ per min.

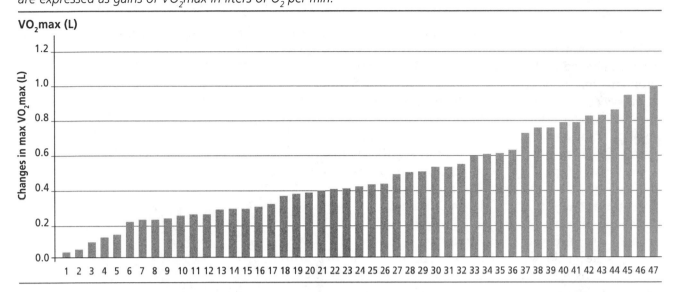

VO₂max (L)

ing. The skeletal muscle oxidative potential can easily increase by 50 percent with training and, at times, it may even double. However, if one is to consider a role for the genotype in such responses to training, there must be evidence of individual differences in trainability. There is now considerable support for this concept (Bouchard, 1986; Lortie et al., 1984). Some indications about the extent of individual differences in the response of maximal oxygen uptake to training are shown in Figure 2.1. Following exposure to training programs lasting from 15 to 20 weeks in 47 young men, some exhibited almost no change in VO₂max, while others gained as much as one liter of O₂ uptake. Such differences in trainability could not be accounted for by age (all subjects were young adults, 17 to 29 years of age) or gender (all young men). The initial (pre-training) level accounted for about 25% of the variance in the response of VO₂max; the lower the initial level the greater the increase with training. Thus about 75% of the heterogeneity in response to regular exercise was not explained.

Similar individual differences were observed for other relevant phenotypes such as indicators of endurance, markers of skeletal muscle oxidative metabolism, markers of adipose tissue metabolism, relative ratio of lipid and carbohydrate oxidized, fasting glucose and insulin levels as well as in their response to a glucose challenge, and fasting plasma lipids and lipoproteins (Bouchard et al., 1992). All

these phenotypes respond to regular exercise in the young adults of both sexes. However, there are considerable individual differences in the response of these biological markers to exercise-training, some exhibiting a high responder pattern, while others are almost non-responders and with a whole range of response phenotypes between these two extremes.

What is the main cause of the individuality in the response to training? We believe that it has to do with as yet unidentified genetic characteristics (Bouchard, 1986). To test this hypothesis, we have now performed several different training studies with pairs of identical (MZ) twins, the rationale being that the response pattern can be observed for individuals having the same genotype (within pairs) and for subjects with differing genetic characteristics (between pairs). We have concluded from these studies that the individuality in trainability of cardiovascular fitness phenotypes and in response to exercise-training of cardiovascular risk factors is highly familial and most likely genetically determined. The data are expressed in terms of the ratio of the variance between genotypes to that within genotypes in the response to standardized training conditions. The similarity of the training response among members of the same MZ pair is illustrated in Figure 2.2 for the VO₂max phenotype based on the results of our first study on this issue (Prud'homme et al., 1984). In this case, 10 pairs of MZ twins were subjected to a fully standardized and laboratory-controlled training program for 20 weeks and gains of absolute VO₂max showed almost 8 times more variance between pairs than within pairs.

Over a period of several years, 26 pairs of MZ twins were trained in our laboratory with standardized endurance and high-intensity cycle exercise programs for periods of 15 or 20 weeks (Bouchard et al., 1992). After 10 weeks of training, the twins were exercising 5 times per week, 45 minutes per session at the same relative intensity in each program. These training programs caused significant increases in VO₂max and other indicators of aerobic performance. They were also associated with a decrease in the intensity of the cardiovascular and metabolic responses at a given submaximal power output. For instance, when exercising in relative steady state at 50 watts, there were decreases in heart rate, oxygen uptake, pulmonary ventilation, ventilatory equivalent of oxygen, and with an increase in the oxygen pulse. These various metabolic improvements were, however, all characterized by a significant within-pair resemblance (Bouchard et al., 1992). We have made the same observation for the alterations seen in skeletal muscle metabolism following training studies performed on skeletal muscle biopsies obtained before and after the training program in a good number of MZ twin pairs (Simoneau et al., 1986).

Nonpharmacological interventions designed to improve the cardiovascular risk profile center around the cessation of smoking, weight loss by means of dietary restriction and at times regular physical activity, dietary modifications aimed at fat, sodium and fiber intake, and regular exercise in order to improve health-related fitness. Among the expected changes associated with a regular exercise regimen, one finds in a group of sedentary and unfit adults a decrease in resting heart rate and blood pressure, a reduction in fasting plasma insulin level and in its response to a glucose load, a decrease in plasma triglycerides and, occasionally, in LDL-cholesterol and total cholesterol, and an increase in plasma HDL-cholesterol. Little is known about the individual differences in the response of these important clinical markers to regular exercise and about the role of genetic variation. We have used the MZ twin design to explore these issues in two studies. In one experiment, 6 pairs of young adult male MZ twins exercised on the cycle er-

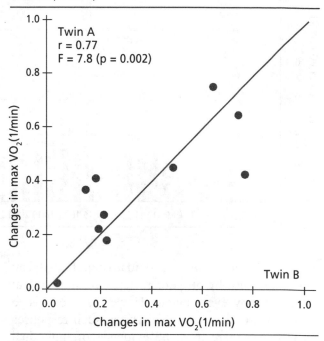

FIGURE 2.2

Intrapair resemblance in 10 pairs of monozygotic twins for training changes in VO₂max (liters of O₂ per min) after 20 weeks of endurance training. (Adapted from Prud'homme et al., Medicine and Science in Sports and Exercise, *1984.)*

gometer 2 hours per day for 22 consecutive days (Poehlman et al., 1986). The mean intensity of training reached 58% of VO₂max and the program was designed to induce an energy deficit of about 1,000 kcal per day. Baseline energy intake was assessed and prescribed for the 22 days of the training program. The diet prescription was fully enforced for each subject in the metabolic ward where they lived for the duration of the experiment. The second study was performed on 7 pairs of MZ twins who followed the same regimen for 100 days. The results of both studies are quite concordant. The program induced a significant increase in VO₂max and a significant decrease in body fat content. Significant changes were observed in fasting plasma insulin and in the insulin response to an oral glucose tolerance test. Plasma triglycerides, total cholesterol, LDL-cholesterol, and apo B as well as the HDL-cholesterol to total cholesterol ratio were also modified. However, again, significant within MZ pair resemblance was observed for the response of fasting plasma insulin, and LDL-cholesterol, HDL-cholesterol, the HDL-cholesterol to total cholesterol ratio and for the improvement in body fat content and in fat topography. Thus being genetically different translates into heterogeneity in the adaptation to exercise programs.

CONCLUSIONS

Genetic individuality is important because it has an impact on the physical activity, fitness, and health paradigm. The results summarized here reveal that there is highly suggestive evidence that genetic variation accounts for most of the individual differences in the response to regular exercise of health-related fitness components and of various risk factors for cardiovascular disease and diabetes. Not only is it important to recognize that there are individual differences in the response to regular physical activity but research also indicates that there are nonresponders in the population. Typically, there is a three- to tenfold difference between low responders and high responders, depending upon the phenotype considered, as a result of exposure to the same standardized physical activity regimen for a period of 15 to 20 weeks.

An appreciation of the critical role of DNA sequence variation in human responses to a variety of challenges and environmental conditions has become essential to those interested in the physical activity, fitness and health paradigm. It can only augment our understanding of human individuality and make us more cautious when defining fitness and health benefits that may be anticipated from a physically active lifestyle. Incorporating biological individuality into our thinking will increase the relevance of our observations to the true human situation.

REFERENCES

Bouchard, C. (1986). Genetics of aerobic power and capacity. In R.M. Malina & C. Bouchard (Eds.), *Sport and human genetics* (pp. 59–88). Champaign, IL: Human Kinetics Publishers.

Bouchard, C., Dionne, F.T., Simoneau, J.A., & Boulay, M.R. (1992). Genetics of aerobic and anaerobic performances. *Exercise and Sport Sciences Reviews, 20,* 27–58.

Bouchard, C., & Shephard, R.J. (1993). Physical activity, fitness and health: The model and key concepts. In C. Bouchard, R.J. Shephard, & T. Stephens (Eds.), *Physical activity, fitness, and health: Consensus statement* (pp. 11–20). Champaign, IL: Human Kinetics Publishers.

Lortie, G., Simoneau, J.A., Hamel, P., Boulay, M.R., Landry, F., & Bouchard, C. (1984). Responses of maximal aerobic power and capacity to aerobic training. *International Journal of Sports Medicine, 5,* 232–236.

Pérusse, L., Leblanc, C., & Bouchard, C. (1988). Inter-generation transmission of physical fitness in the Canadian population. *Canadian Journal of Sport Sciences, 13,* 8–14.

Pérusse, L., Lortie, G., Leblanc, C., Tremblay, A., Thériault, G., & Bouchard, C. (1987). Genetic and environmental sources of variation in physical fitness. *Annals of Human Biology, 14,* 425–434.

Poehlman, E.T., Tremblay, A., Nadeau, A., Dussault, J., Thériault, G., & Bouchard, C. (1986). Heredity and changes in hormones and metabolic rates with short-term training. *American Journal of Physiology: Endocrinology and Metabolism, 250,* E711–E717.

Prud'homme, D., Bouchard, C., Leblanc, C., Landry, F., & Fontaine, E. (1984). Sensitivity of maximal aerobic power to training is genotype-dependent. *Medicine and Science in Sports and Exercise, 16,* 489–493.

Simoneau, J.A., Lorlie, G., Boulay, M.R., Marcotte, M., Thibault, M.C., & Bouchard, C. (1986). Inheritance of human skeletal muscle and anaerobic capacity adaptation to high-intensity intermittent training. *International Journal of Sports Medicine, 7,* 167–171.

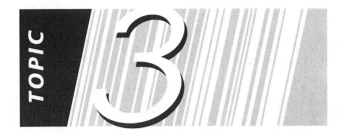

Personalizing Physical Activity Prescription

B. Don Franks
UNIVERSITY OF ILLINOIS

INTRODUCTION

An explosion of recent scientific research findings has provided the basis for numerous reports that document the health benefits of regular physical activity. These reports have been issued by varied public and private organizations, including the Office of the Surgeon General, the National Institutes of Health, the Centers for Disease Control and Prevention, the President's Council on Physical Fitness and Sports, the American Medical Association, the National Coalition for Promoting Physical Activity (including the American College of Sports Medicine, the American Alliance for Health, Physical Education, Recreation and Dance, and the American Heart Association), as well as many other organizations in both the public and the private domain (see box at the end of this article for a description of some of these reports). However, there remain several unresolved issues regarding physical activity prescription that require further study. These include intensity, duration, frequency, type of activity, and whether or not activity must be done in one session or can be divided into several shorter sessions throughout the day.

The purpose of this paper is to describe how coherent recommendations for physical activity can be provided to individuals based on, and consistent with, the current research and the expert judgment of professionals in the field. Although "how much activity to recommend?" seems like a simple question, there is confusion about its answer both in the research and the popular literature. *The confusion is the result of the failure to consider two factors: the physical activity status of the individual and the health, fitness, and performance goals that are desired by the individual.*

A MODEL FOR MAKING PHYSICAL ACTIVITY RECOMMENDATIONS

It is possible to harmonize all the various research studies and position statements by using the model described earlier. There are certain activities that can be universally recommended. Other activities depend on the current activity level of the individual. After a modest level of physical activity is included in a person's lifestyle, then the

ORIGINALLY PUBLISHED AS SERIES 2, NUMBER 9, OF THE PCPFS *RESEARCH DIGEST.*

Coherent individualized recommendations for physical activity can be consistent with the research data and expert judgment by using the individual's current activity status and the health/fitness/performance goals in the following sequence:

Activity Status	Recommended Activities
Everyone	*Include activity in everyday life*
Sedentary	*Accumulate at least 30 min. of daily moderate-intensity activities*
Moderately active	*Include activities based on Health and Fitness Goals*
Vigorously active	*Perform activities based on Performance Goals*

recommendations for additional activity depend largely on the specific health, fitness, and/or performance goals of the individual. Figure 3.1 summarizes this model for recommending physical activity.

1. Activities for Everyone

Recommendation: Activities for everyone should be of the type that can be done as part of an individual's routines at home, work, and during leisure time. In order to promote general health and well-being and the ability to handle routine tasks, there are common activities recommended

FIGURE 3.1

Model for physical activity recommendations.

1. Activities recommended for everyone
2. Activities for sedentary individuals
3. Activities for moderately active individuals interested in health
   - Cardiovascular
   - Bone
   - Low Back
   - Psychological
4. Activities for moderately active individuals interested in physical fitness
   - Aerobic fitness
   - Relative leanness
   - Muscular strength and endurance
   - Flexibility
5. Activities for vigorously active individuals interested in performance
   - Sport
   - Physical task(s)

for everyone. Each person can increase activity as part of her or his lifestyle.

To increase physical activity as part of daily life, individuals should walk rather than ride when possible; climb stairs rather than taking the elevator or escalator; park farther away from the store or office for a short walk to and from the car; get off the bus or train one stop earlier for a short walk to the office, store, or home. Emphasize weight-bearing activities to use more energy and to enhance bone health. Include a daily routine of stretching aimed at preventing low back problems.

2. Activities for Sedentary Individuals

Recommendation: Inactive individuals should continue to find ways to include activity in their daily routine and should accumulate at least 30 minutes of moderate-intensity activity daily. Most experts agree that in addition to those daily activities included in Recommendation 1, additional activities are desirable to improve one's health. This second recommendation is designed for sedentary individuals—those who currently **do no regular physical activity,** or who cannot walk for 30 minutes continuously without discomfort or pain. (Individuals who are unable to walk can substitute moving in a wheelchair, swimming, etc. See American Association for Active Lifestyles, 1995, for recommendations for activity modifications for individuals with disabilities.)

These activities for sedentary individuals include walking, yardwork, cycling, slow dancing, and low-impact exercise to music. The activity can be broken into 2–4 segments, for example, taking two 10-minute exercise breaks during the workday, and another exercise break in the morning or at night during the week, with a 30-minute walk on weekend days. Weight-bearing activities should be included with the emphasis on either being active or accumulating activity and not the intensity level.

3. Activities for Moderately Active People with Health Goals

Recommendation: Those individuals who have specific health goals should perform the activities in Figure 3.2 based on the health goal desired. Moderately active individuals are those who currently accumulate 30 minutes of activity daily, or who can walk 30 minutes continuously without pain or discomfort, but could not jog three miles (or walk six miles at a brisk pace, cycle 12 miles, or swim 3/4 mile) continuously without discomfort and undue fatigue. These individuals should continue to include activity in their normal routine, and accumulate 30 minutes of moderate-intensity activity every day. At this point, the individual's desired goals are essential in making additional recommendations. Different activities need to be recommended depending on an individual's health and fitness goals.

The consensus statement by Bouchard, Shephard, and Stephens (1994) and the Surgeon General's report both deal with the relationship between physical activity and cardiovascular and other health issues. In addition, recent issues of the *PCPFS Physical Activity and Fitness Research Digest* deal

FIGURE 3.2
Physical activity for health goals.

These activities should be considered **after** an individual is already doing those activities recommended for sedentary individuals. The activities should be done *in addition* to these activities.

Health Goal	Recommended Activity
Cardiovascular	Accumulate at least 30 min. of daily moderate-intensity activities
	Include longer duration and/or higher intensity
Bone	Weight-bearing activities
	Resistance exercises
Low Back	Static stretching in mid-trunk and thigh regions
	Abdominal curl-ups
Psychological	Enjoyable activities and fun atmosphere

with activity recommendations for specific health goals, including cardiovascular (Haskell, 1995), bone (Shaw and Snow-Harter, 1995), cancer (Lee, 1995), healthy low back (Plowman, 1993), and obesity (Wilmore, 1994).

For those individuals who want to prevent cardiovascular and other diseases and to **promote general health,** the emphasis should be on including activity as part of the daily routine and accumulating 30 minutes of moderate-intensity activity daily. There is good evidence that this type of activity will reduce risk of cardiovascular disease. There is additional gain with longer duration of activity and/or the addition of vigorous-intensity activity. For **healthy bones,** weight-bearing activities and those activities designed to improve muscular strength and endurance are emphasized. For a **healthy low back,** static stretching in the mid-trunk area and abdominal curl-ups (slow, without feet held) are recommended. A major part of one's overall health is **psychological well-being.** Feeling good, a positive outlook on life, healthy levels of depression or anxiety, and the ability to capture the positive aspects of stress while minimizing its negative side are all components of psychological health. There is increasing evidence that an active lifestyle is associated with improved psychological well-being, although the specific activity recommendations for psychological health cannot be precisely defined at this time. Moreover, it seems logical that the emphasis for psychological health is selecting enjoyable activities and environment. The desired activities and atmosphere will, of course, vary with individuals. For example, many individuals enjoy the social interaction of being part of a group jogging, playing games, or exercising to music, while others look forward to time alone with one's own thoughts. Relaxation techniques can also be helpful for psychological well-being.

Physical activity may help prevent or minimize many other health problems that are not listed above. More research is needed before definitive exercise prescriptions can be made for each specific potential health problem. In general, the activities recommended for cardiovascular health are appropriate for a variety of health concerns.

Although the emphases for health goals are on including more activity as part of one's routine and accumulating 30 minutes of daily activity, there is additional benefit in more activity. It appears that either doing more activity (longer duration) and/or activities that are more intense can result in additional health benefits. The nature of the additional activities can often be determined by looking at specific physical fitness goals.

4. Activities for Moderately Active People with Fitness Goals

Recommendation: Those individuals who have specific fitness goals should perform the activities in Figure 3.3 based on the fitness goal desired. Health-related physical fitness includes aerobic fitness, relative leanness, muscular strength and endurance, and flexibility. Individuals interested in one or more of these fitness goals should continue to do activities as part of the daily lifestyle and accumulate 30 minutes of daily activity. In addition, improvement in these fitness elements requires different types of activity.

A. Aerobic fitness: The aerobic fitness goal is related to the health goal for cardiovascular health and performance goals involving endurance activities. These individuals should schedule at least 20 minutes of vigorous-intensity activity (preceded and followed by 5–10 minutes of moderate-intensity activity) 3–4 days per week. These activities can include fast walking, jogging, cycling, fast

FIGURE 3.3

Physical fitness goals and recommended activities.

These activities should be considered only **after** an individual is doing the activities for sedentary individuals. The activities should be done *in addition* to these activities.

Physical Fitness Goals	Recommended Activities
Aerobic fitness	20–40 min vigorous-intensity activity, 3–5 days/week
Relative leanness	
Too little fat	Eat more calories, especially carbohydrates
	Include resistance exercise
Too much fat	Reduce calories, especially fat
	Increase duration of aerobic activities
	Include resistance exercise
Muscular strength/ endurance	Include resistance exercise 1–2 sets, 10–15 reps, each muscle group 2–3 days/week
Flexibility	Daily static stretching, 10–30 sec, 2–3 times, each joint

dancing, low- to moderate-impact exercise to music, and swimming. The heart rate (HR) during these activities should be 70–85% of maximal heart rate (HR) (calculated by: (220 b/min − age) × .7; (220 b/min − age) × .85. For example, a 40-year-old individual would have an estimated maximum heart rate of 180 b/min (220 b/min − 40). The target heart rate would range from 126 b/min (180 b/min × .7) to 153 b/min (180b/min × .85). The individual can learn how hard to work out by stopping and counting the heart rate for 10 seconds (beats/min divided by 6). Thus in the 40-year-old example, the 10 sec HR should be from 21 b/10 sec (126/6) to 25–26 b/10 sec (153/6). As always, it is important for these individuals to warm up and cool down for 5–10 minutes before and after the vigorous-intensity workout. The low back routine can be included as part of the warm-up or cool-down. These activities will increase maximal oxygen uptake, make current submaximal tasks less stressful, and reduce resting and submaximal heart rate. These activities are related to additional reductions in the risk of cardiovascular disease, and provide the basis for a number of endurance-type sports and activities.

B. Relative leanness: The amount of fat related to the total body weight is a key health ingredient. Too little fat can have serious health consequences. Too much fat is related to the development and aggravation of numerous health problems. The healthy range for children prior to puberty and for men is 5–18%, and for women, 15–28%. Children before puberty and men have a necessary amount of fat of about 3%. Women after puberty have approximately 12% of fat that is necessary for normal body function.

Recommendations for relative leanness obviously include both nutrition and activity. For those with too little fat, increased caloric intake, especially carbohydrates, and resistance exercises for increasing body mass are recommended. In addition, the possibility of eating disorders should be checked in these individuals. Individuals with too much fat need to reduce the total calories and the percent of fat in their diet. These individuals should be encouraged to include activity as part of their routines, accumulate at least 30 minutes of moderate-intensity activity daily, and either continue the moderate-intensity activity for longer duration or include vigorous-intensity activities such as those recommended for aerobic fitness. The main emphasis is on activities that use energy (calories). Resistance exercise also should be included to increase the lean tissue mass, thereby increasing the number of calories burned throughout the day.

C. Muscular strength and endurance: Although elite performers need to distinguish between strength (one contraction) and endurance (repeated contractions), from health and fitness perspectives, strength and endurance can be considered together for health and fitness goals. Individuals need modest levels of strength and endurance to be able to function in normal routines that include lifting, moving, carrying, etc. Abdominal endurance is an important factor in the prevention of low back problems. Resistance activities to maintain muscle mass are particularly important for individuals who are restricting their caloric intake (Pollock, *PCPFS Digest,* 1996).

Improvement in strength and endurance includes resistance exercise, where individuals lift greater weights than normal for the major muscle groups. A routine of 10–15 repetitions of the lift for each muscle group, with 1–2 sets, done 2–3 alternate days per week is recommended. It can be done in conjunction with the vigorous-intensity aerobic activities, or on separate days.

D. Flexibility: The ability to move all joints through their complete range of motion without pain is important for daily tasks. In addition, flexibility in the mid-trunk and thigh region is important for low back health. A routine of daily static stretches (moving the joint to its extreme position and holding for 10–30 sec) for all the joints, repeated 2–3 times is recommended. Individuals often include these flexibility activities as part of their warm-up and cool-down.

5. Activities for Vigorously Active Individuals with Performance Goals

Recommendation: Those individuals who are vigorously active and who have specific performance goals should consider the information in Figure 3.4 and the discussion below. Individuals who can run 3 miles continuously (or walk fast 6

FIGURE 3.4

Recommended activity for performance goals.

These activities should be considered only **after** an individual is doing activities recommended in Figure 3.3. These activities should be done *in addition* to activities in Figure 3.3.

Performance Goals	Recommended Activities
Sport or physical task(s)	Develop and/or maintain fitness levels
	Interval training
	Motor tasks related to performance
	Specific skills related to performance
	Strategy and mental readiness

miles, cycle 12 miles, or swim $^3/_4$ mile) within their target HR, 3–4 times per week without discomfort or pain can, if interested, engage in a variety of sport and performance activities. Some individuals have specific performance goals, such as being a better tennis player, or running a 10K race in a certain time.

These individuals should continue to include activity as part of their lives, accumulate 30 minutes daily of moderate-intensity activity, and include vigorous-intensity activity at target HR those days when not engaging in sport/performance activities. Performance activities include a wide range such as soccer, basketball, racquetball, badminton, high-intensity exercise to music, road races, etc. It is not possible to make general recommendations for performance. Different sports or tasks need additional fitness levels as well as elements and skills of the game. For example, running, cycling, or swimming races demand high levels of aerobic fitness in that mode of activity, specific form to increase efficiency of movement, and strategy and mental readiness for the event. Racquetball requires aerobic and anaerobic energy, court agility and coordination, different types of strokes (serve, kill, lob, hitting after the ball rebounds from the wall), plus strategy and mental readiness for the match. Being a fire fighter requires the ability to respond quickly to emergencies, repeated anaerobic energy production in smoke-filled air, muscular endurance for carrying heavy loads up and down ladders or stairs, etc. All activities require energy sources, but the aerobic/anaerobic mix is quite different. Interval training that mimics the energy demands of the performance is one important aspect of training. The point is that each performance has its own needs for underlying fitness levels and specific skills.

ACHIEVING QUALITY OF LIFE

Perhaps everyone's overall goal is to be able to participate in and enjoy life fully. For most individuals, that will include several health, fitness, and performance goals. Thus, it seems logical to **start with the health goals, then progress to the fitness goals, adding performance goals for those interested.** In this way, the overall quality of one's life can be enhanced.

SUMMARY

Two factors for physical activity prescription have been considered—current activity status and health/fitness/performance goals. Initial recommendations for activity should be based on the individual's activity status—getting each person involved in routine activities and daily moderate-intensity activities. Then after an individual is engaging in the daily activities on a regular basis, without any problems of discomfort or fatigue, activities for health and fitness goals should be included. After daily physical activity and fitness activities have been included as part of a person's lifestyle, then a variety of performance goals, based on personal interests, can be considered.

Selected Reports on Physical Activity: A Brief History

The American College of Sports Medicine has been the major public voice regarding exercise recommendations for the last 20 years. Its 1978 recommendations (ACSM, 1978) have been the most quoted source in this regard. These recommendations (3-5 times per week, at least 20 minutes of vigorous-intensity aerobic activity—60-80% of maximal functional capacity) represented a good summary of the experimental literature on the effects of physical activity on cardiovascular fitness (maximal oxygen uptake). The more recent recommendations from ACSM (ACSM, 1995) and others expand the earlier statement to include evidence from epidemiological studies (e.g., Blair et al., 1989; Paffenbarger, Hyde, & Wing, 1986) on risk reduction of cardiovascular disease, encouraging everyone to accumulate at least 30 minutes of daily moderate-intensity activity. The July 1996 issue of the *PCPFS Physical Activity and Fitness Research Digest* (Now *PCPFS Research Digest*) (Corbin & Pangrazi, 1996) includes an excellent summary of the recent report on *Physical Activity and Health* by the Office of the Surgeon General. The Surgeon General's report (USDHHS, 1996) and the *PCPFS Physical Activity and Fitness Research Digest* synthesize the research findings related to physical activity and health. Its conclusions are similar to the more focused report from the NIH Consensus Conference on Physical Activity and Cardiovascular Health (NIH, 1996). Other resources for those interested in the scientific basis for this *PCPFS Research Digest* can be found in papers from the conference reported by Bouchard et al. (1994), and the statement from the ACSM, CDC, and PCPFS, published by ACSM and CDC by Pate et al. (1995). Similar recommendations for adolescents are reported by Sallis and Patrick (1994).

In recent years, professionals have modified the original ACSM recommendation in order to engage a greater proportion of the general public in regular physical activity. This was done because evidence continues to mount showing that sedentary individuals can reduce their risk of cardiovascular disease with moderate activity and a rather small percentage of people in the United States are active at the level suggested in the original ACSM position statement. The current activity status is well documented in the recent update of the **Midcourse Review of Healthy People 2000** (USDHHS, 1995) and the **Surgeon General's Report on Physical Activity and Health.** In the U.S. adult population, about 15% engage in activities recommended by the original ACSM position statement, 22% accumulate moderate-intensity activity, and 24% are completely sedentary, leaving 39% who do some activity but less than the minimum recommended (USDHHS, 1996).   *(continued)*

However, despite these official statements and reports that have received wide recognition in the media, there is still confusion about how to answer the question, What and how much activity should be recommended? The general answer given in many reports and in the mass media seems to be "something is better than nothing," and "although some is good, more is better." Although this accurately reflects the research and professional opinion, it is inadequate to provide helpful guidance for physical activity patterns for individuals.

REFERENCES

American Association for Active Lifestyles. (1995). *Physical Best and Individuals with Disabilities.* Reston, VA: Author.

American College of Sports Medicine. (1978). The recommended quality and quantity of exercise for developing and maintaining fitness in healthy adults. *Medicine and Science in Sports and Exercise, 10,* vii.

American College of Sports Medicine. (1995). *ACSM's Guidelines for exercise testing and prescription* (5th edition). Baltimore: Williams and Wilkins.

American Heart Association. (1992). Statement on exercise. *Circulation, 86,* 340–344.

Blair, S.N., et al. (1989). Physical fitness and all-cause mortality. *Journal of the American Medical Association, 262,* 2395–2401.

Bouchard, C., Shephard, R.J., & Stephens, T. (Eds.) (1994). *Physical activity, fitness, and health.* Champaign, IL: Human Kinetics Publishers.

Corbin, C.B., & Pangrazi, R.P. (1994). Toward an understanding of appropriate physical activity levels for youth. *PCPFS Physical Activity and Fitness Research Digest, 1(8).*

Corbin, C.B., & Pangrazi, R.P. (1996). What you need to know about the Surgeon General's Report on Physical Activity and Health. *PCPFS Physical Activity and Fitness Research Digest, 2(6).*

Haskell, W.L. (1995). Physical activity in the prevention and management of coronary heart disease. *PCPFS Physical Activity and Fitness Research Digest, 2(1).*

Lee, I.M. (1995). Physical activity and cancer. *PCPFS Physical Activity and Fitness Research Digest, 2(2).*

National Institutes of Health. (1996). Physical activity and cardiovascular health: Consensus Development Conference Statement. Washington, DC: Author.

Paffenbarger, R.S., Hyde, R.T., & Wing, A.L. (1986). Physical activity, all-cause mortality, and longevity of college alumni. *New England Journal of Medicine, 314,* 605–613.

Pate, R.R., et al. (1995). Physical activity and public health: A recommendation from the Centers for Disease Control and Prevention and the American College of Sports Medicine. *Journal of the American Medical Association, 273,* 402–407.

Plowman, S.A. (1993). Physical fitness and healthy low back function. *PCPFS Physical Activity and Fitness Research Digest, 1(3).*

Pollock, M.L., & Vincent, K.R. (1996). Resistance training for health. *PCPFS Research Digest, 2(8).*

Sallis, J.F., & Patrick, K. (1994). Physical activity guidelines for adolescents: Consensus statement. *Pediatric Exercise Science, 6,* 302–314.

Shaw, J.M., & Snow-Harter, C. (1995). Osteoporosis and physical activity. *PCPFS Physical Activity and Fitness Research Digest, 2(3).*

U.S. Department of Health and Human Services. (1994). *Healthy people 2000: National health promotion and disease prevention objectives, 1994 update.* Washington, DC: Author.

U.S. Department of Health and Human Services. (1996). *Surgeon General's Report: Physical activity and health.* Washington, DC: Author.

U.S. Department of Agriculture. (1995). *Dietary guidelines for American adults.* Washington, DC: Author.

Wilmore, J.H. (1994). Exercise, obesity, and weight control. *PCPFS Physical Activity and Fitness Research Digest, 1(6).*

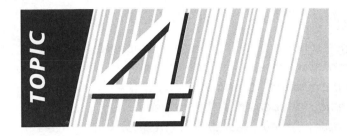

Influences on Physical Activity of Children, Adolescents, and Adults

James F. Sallis

SAN DIEGO STATE UNIVERSITY

The U.S. Department of Health and Human Services has adopted a policy of increasing regular physical activity of children, adolescents and adults, because of the numerous health benefits that have been documented through research (Bouchard et al., 1994). The physical activity guidelines are published in *Healthy People 2000* (USDHHS, 1990). The Surgeon General's Report, *Physical Activity and Health* (USDHHS, 1996) concludes that most Americans are not physically active enough to optimize their health, and a sizable percent of adults are extremely sedentary.

Before launching large-scale programs to stimulate more physical activity, it is widely accepted that a better understanding of the various influences on physical activity habits is needed. If the most important influences can be identified, then they could be targeted for change in educational or other intervention programs. In this paper, some of the theory and research on "determinants" of physical activity are summarized, and both the commonalities and differences between youth and adults are described. An attempt is made to apply these findings to the improvement of physical activity intervention programs.

EXPLAINING HUMAN BEHAVIOR

Human behavior is complex enough to frustrate all attempts to explain it, but the attempts continue because of the importance of the task. Efforts to explain individual differences in physical activity are further complicated by variations in frequency, intensity, duration, and type. The objectives in *Healthy People 2000* (USDHHS, 1990) call for decreases in sedentary behaviors and increases in light-to-moderate, vigorous, strength-building, and flexibility-promoting activities. The influences may differ for each of these categories of physical activity. Most of the research work to date has focused on vigorous exercise in leisure time, but some studies are beginning to examine the influences on moderate-intensity activities, like walking (Hovell et al., 1992), that are now emphasized in public health recommendations because of their health benefits (Pate et al., 1995). There are many studies of special populations, such as cardiac patients, but the present paper focuses on physical activity in the general population.

Theoretical models are the starting point for research on human behavior, because theories simplify

ORIGINALLY PUBLISHED AS SERIES 1, NUMBER 7, OF THE PCPFS *RESEARCH DIGEST*.

HIGHLIGHT

"Understanding the many factors that influence physical activity may help improve the effectiveness of physical activity intervention programs. Research suggests that the effectiveness of programs should be maximized when participants' confidence about their ability to continue physical activities is nurtured, they enjoy the activities they have chosen, receive encouragement and assistance from other people in their lives, and reside in a supportive environment that provides convenient, attractive, and safe places for physical activity."

the complex phenomena under study by suggesting which factors should be studied. Psychological models that emphasize the role of knowledge, beliefs, attitudes, motivations, and emotions have been dominant and have inspired studies that have shown many psychological factors influence physical activity patterns of adults and youth. These models include the theory of planned behavior (Godin & Shephard, 1990) and the intrinsic motivation model (Whitehead, 1993).

Other models take into consideration that beliefs and perceptions are not the only influences on physical activity. The behavior of others and factors in the external environment can also play a role in influencing physical activity. Social cognitive theory (Bandura, 1986) emphasizes multiple influences from within the person, the social environment, and the physical environment.

Over 300 studies of the influences on physical activity have produced a scientific literature rich with information, but the picture is not yet entirely clear. The following sections summarize some of the major findings, and readers desiring more detailed information can consult recent reviews (Dishman & Sallis, 1994; Sallis & Owen, 1998; USDHHS, 1996).

BIOLOGICAL AND PSYCHOLOGICAL INFLUENCES

Biologic factors are strongly associated with level of physical activity, even though it is not clear these factors actually "cause" physical activity to vary. Age is a potent predictor, and the level of physical activity is known to decrease throughout the entire age span, beginning at least with entry into school. During the school years, the activity level declines about 50% (Sallis, 1993), and the decline continues until the typical elderly person is almost entirely sedentary (USDHHS, 1996). Females are less physically active

than males at virtually all ages (Pate et al., 1994; USDHHS, 1996), but many people feel this difference is due to socialization rather than biology.

A biological reason why adults drop out of vigorous exercise programs is musculoskeletal injuries. In one study, injuries were the most common reason for dropping out (Sallis et al., 1990), and the history of injuries is a good predictor of future injuries. Though most people believe the obese are less active than the normal weight, it is difficult to find evidence to support this notion in either adults or youth. However, recent studies indicate that a substantial portion of physical activity may be explained by genetic factors (Pérusse et al., 1989).

The personal characteristics of being well educated and affluent are consistently associated with higher levels of leisure time physical activity. African Americans and Latinos are usually found to be less active than Anglos, even in childhood (McKenzie et al., 1992). However, these ethnic differences are largely due to socioeconomic factors (Shea et al., 1991). It is surprising that health behaviors such as cigarette smoking, dietary habits, and alcohol consumption are not consistently related to physical activity habits, but it appears that people selectively choose their health behaviors. Recent physical activity predicts future activity in leisure time, but activity levels in childhood are not reliable predictors of exercise habits in adulthood. One explanation is that children may be taught activities, like team sports, that are difficult to carry over to adulthood.

A wide variety of psychological factors appear to influence participation in physical activity among adults. Much of our current understanding can be summarized by stating that beliefs and perceptions that are not personal in nature, such as knowledge about exercise, personality traits, and general attitudes, are weakly related to behavior. Personal beliefs about one's own physical activity are usually found to be significant influences on physical activity. One of the strongest predictors of future activity is perceptions of personal efficacy, or confidence regarding one's ability to be active on a regular basis. Simple ratings are useful in predicting activity levels among adolescents (Reynolds et al., 1990) and adults of all ages (Garcia & King, 1991; McAuley, 1992; Sallis, Hovell, Hofstetter, et al., 1992). Program leaders could use such ratings to estimate which participants are likely to continue activity and which are at risk of dropping out.

There is a growing literature that supports the common belief that people must enjoy physical activity if they are to continue. Enjoyment appears to influence the activity levels of both children (Stucky-Ropp & DiLorenzo, 1993) and adults (Garcia & King, 1991). One of the main influences on enjoyment is the amount of exertion required by the activity. Children (Epstein et al., 1991) and adults (Garcia & King, 1991) prefer activities with lower levels of exertion, and dropout rates are higher from vigorous activity than from moderate-intensity activity (Dishman & Sallis, 1994). One of the reasons behind the recent emphasis on encouraging people to engage in moderate activities (USDHHS, 1990) is that more people are expected to adhere.

Every sedentary person seems to have a reason for not being active, and knowing what those reasons are can provide clues about how to design an intervention. It is well known that the most common reason is "lack of time." In addition, the number and strength of perceived barriers to activity are consistently related to physical activity in both adults (Sallis, Hovell, Hofstetter, et al., 1992) and adolescents (Tappe et at., 1989).

Psychological influences on children's physical activity have not been widely researched, in part because of the difficulties of assessing psychological states in children, and in part because parents and teachers select and control many of children's physical activities. Most children enjoy "playing," but our research group has encountered many children in elementary schools who complain, in the same way adults do, they do not have the time for physical activity.

SOCIAL AND PHYSICAL ENVIRONMENT INFLUENCES

Significant others can make it more or less likely that a person is active on a regular basis. Social influences on physical activity are strong for people of all ages, but the nature of the support varies with developmental level. Social support for adults can come from friends, coworkers, or family members, and the main types of support are encouragement, participating m physical activities, and providing assistance, such as child care (Dishman & Sallis, 1994). For adolescents, the influence of peers is paramount. If a given adolescent identifies with a peer group that values and participates in physical activity, the group creates a supportive environment for its members. If the main peer group devalues physical activity, this is an effective deterrent.

The younger the child, the more influential parents are. Studies of children aged 9 to 13 years have shown there are several ways that parents can support children's physical activity. Serving as active role models and providing encouragement may have limited influence, but two studies show that parents can have the most impact by directly helping children be active. Parents who participate in activities with their children (Stucky-Ropp & DiLorenzo, 1993), organize activities (Anderssen & Wold, 1992), or transport children to places where they can be active are the most effective supporters (Sallis, Alcaraz, et al., 1992). For preschool children, prompts and encouragement to be active can be helpful (Sallis et al., 1993).

It seems self-evident that physical environmental factors such as climate and weather can have a major effect on physical activities, but few of many possible environmental factors have been documented in research. It is probable that changes in the environment have made it necessary to focus attention on increasing physical activity. Automobiles, television, computers, labor-saving devices, and sedentary jobs have created an environment that makes possible a profoundly sedentary lifestyle for large numbers of people, maybe for the first time in history. Thus, it is critical to be aware of the effect of our artificial environments on physical activity levels (Sallis & Owen, 1998).

A supportive environment for adults might consist of a safe and attractive space for outdoor activities, exercise equipment or supplies in or near the home, and convenient access to exercise facilities and programs. One study showed that adults were more likely to be active if they had a number of exercise facilities within a short distance from their homes (Sallis et al., 1990). For adolescents, it may be especially important to have organized activities in convenient locations, such as afterschool intramural teams.

A supportive environment is essential for younger children. Because it is difficult for children to be active indoors, time spent outdoors is highly correlated with physical activity levels (Klesges et al., 1990; Sallis et al., 1993). Many parents are concerned about the safety of the their neighborhoods and prohibit children from going outside to play. Unfortunately, the more parental rules that limit children's play, the less physically active young children are (Sallis et al., 1993). The more places the child can play that are within walking distance from home, the more active the child is (Sallis et al., 1993). Balancing safety concerns with the need to let children play outdoors is a serious challenge.

Television is a ubiquitous part of the environment of children, adolescents, and adults that encourages sedentary behavior. However, there is little indication that children or adults who watch the most television are the least active. There is reason to limit the hours per week children watch television, because of associations between amount of television viewing and obesity (Robinson et al., 1993).

APPLYING THE RESEARCH TO THE IMPROVEMENT OF PROGRAMS

The research on influences on physical activity provides information that may be useful in more effectively promoting physical activity in individuals or groups of adults and youth. Figure 4.1 is a checklist that can be used to assess some of the key influences. Steps can then be taken to modify these influences so that physical activity is facilitated.

The biological and demographic influences are not easily changeable, but they provide some index of risk. A person or group with a low score on this section may need additional assistance in developing regular physical activity habits.

The higher the scores on the Psychological, Social, and Physical Environment sections, the more likely the person or group is to be physically active. Ideally, there are some checks in all of the sections. If there are few checks in a section, consider how to make changes in some of the influences listed. This checklist provides a rough assessment of existing resources and strengths as well as an indication of areas that need improve-

FIGURE 4.1

Assessing influences on physical activity.

Check those that apply. Each check represents an influence that supports physical activity.

Biological and Demographic Influences

_____ Age. One check if less than 50; two checks if less than 18 years.

_____ Male sex.

_____ No (or minor) history of activity-related injuries.

_____ Genetics. Both parents led active lifestyles.

_____ Graduated college (for children, one parent graduated college).

_____ White-collar occupation (for children, parents have white-collar occupation).

Psychological Influences

_____ Self-efficacy. High level of confidence in ability to do regular physical activity.

_____ Enjoy physical activity.

_____ Belief that time for physical activity can be found.

_____ Perceive few barriers to doing regular physical activity.

_____ Strong intentions to be physically active.

_____ Belief that personal benefits of physical activity outweigh the costs.

Social Influences

_____ Friends or family are active role models.

_____ Friends or family encourage physical activity.

_____ Friends or family participate in physical activity with you.

_____ Friends or family directly help you be physically active.

Physical Environment

_____ Weather or climate is favorable for preferred activities.

_____ Feel safe being active outdoors near home.

_____ Attractive outdoor space is convenient.

_____ Exercise facilities or programs are convenient and affordable.

_____ Exercise equipment or supplies in home.

ment. The reader is challenged to use this assessment to guide appropriate changes in personal or other physical activity programs.

SUMMARY

Many health benefits of physical activity are documented, but large numbers of Americans are not engaging in the recommended levels of physical activity. Understanding the many factors that influence physical activity may help improve the effectiveness of physical activity intervention programs. Research suggests that the effectiveness of programs should be maximized when participants' confidence about their ability to continue physical activities is nurtured, they enjoy the activities they have chosen, receive encouragement and assistance from other people in their lives, and reside in a supportive environment that provides convenient, attractive and safe places for physical activity.

REFERENCES

Anderssen, N., & Wold, B. (1992). Parental and peer influences on leisure-time physical activity in young adolescents. *Research Quarterly for Exercise and Sport, 63,* 341–348.

Bandura, A. (1986). *Social foundations of thought and action.* Englewood Cliffs, NJ: Prentice-Hall.

Bouchard, C., Shephard, R.J., & Stephens, T. (Eds.) (1994). *Physical Activity, Fitness, and Health: International Proceedings and Consensus Statement.* Champaign, IL: Human Kinetics Publishers.

Dishman, R.K., & Sallis, J.F. (1994). Determinants and interventions for physical activity and exercise. In C. Bouchard, R.J. Shephard, & T. Stephens (Eds.), *Physical Activity, Fitness, and Health: International Proceedings and Consensus Statement* (pp. 214–238). Champaign, IL: Human Kinetics Publishers.

Epstein, L.H., Smith, J.A., Vara, L.S., & Rodefer, J.S. (1991). Behavioral economic analysis of activity choice in obese children. *Health Psychology, 10,* 311–316.

Garcia, A.W., & King, A.C. (1991). Predicting long-term adherence to aerobic exercise: A comparison of two models. *Journal of Sport and Exercise Psychology, 13,* 394–410.

Godin, G., & Shephard, R.J. (1990). Use of attitude-behaviour models in exercise promotion. *Sports Medicine, 10,* 103–121.

Hovell, M.F., Hofstetter, C.R., Sallis, J.F., Rauh, M.J.D., & Barrington, E. (1992). Correlates of change in walking for exercise: An exploratory analysis. *Research Quarterly for Exercise and Sport, 63,* 425–434.

Kiesges, R.C., Eck, L.H., Hanson, C.L., Haddock, C.K., & Klesges, L.M. (1990). Effects of obesity, social interactions, and physical environment on physical activity in preschoolers. *Health Psychology, 9,* 435–449.

McAuley, E. (1992). The role of efficacy cognitions in the prediction of exercise behavior in middle-aged adults. *Journal of Behavioral Medicine, 15,* 65–88.

McKenzie, T.L., Sallis, J.F., Nader, P.R., Broyles, S.L., & Nelson, J.A. (1992). Anglo- and Mexican-American preschoolers at home and at recess: Activity patterns and environmental influences. *Journal of Developmental and Behavioral Pediatrics, 13,* 173–180.

Oldridge, N.B., Paffenbarger, R.S., Powell, K.E., & Yeager, K.K. (1992). Determinants of physical activity and interventions in adults. *Medicine and Science in Sports and Exercise, 24,* S221–S236.

Pate, R.R., Long, B.J., & Heath, G. (1994). Descriptive epidemiology of physical activity in adolescents. *Pediatric Exercise Science, 6,* 434–447.

Pate, R.R., Pratt, M., Blair, S.N., Haskell, W.L., Macera, C.A., Bouchard, C., Buchner, D., Ettinger, W., Heath, G.W., King, A.G., Kriska, A., Lion, A.S., Marcus, B.H., Morris, J., Paffenbarger, R.S., Patrick, K., Pollock, M.L., Rippe, J.M., Sallis, J., & Wilmore, J.H. (1995). Physical activity and public health: A recommendation from CDC and ACSM. *Journal of the American Medical Association, 273,* 402–407.

Pérusse, L., Tremblay, A., Leblanc, C., & Bouchard, C. (1989). Genetic and environmental influences on level of habitual physical activity and exercise participation. *American Journal of Epidemiology, 129,* 1012–1022.

Reynolds, K.D., Killen, J.D., Bryson, S.W., Maron, D.J., Taylor, C.B., Maccoby, N., & Farquhar, J.W. (1990). *Preventive Medicine, 19,* 541–551.

Robinson, T.N., Hammer, L.D., Killen, J.D., Kraemer, H.C., Wilson, D.M., Hayward, C., & Taylor, C.B. (1993). Does television viewing increase obesity and reduce physical activity? Cross-sectional and longitudinal analyses among adolescent girls. *Pediatrics, 91,* 273–280.

Sallis, J. F. (1993). Epidemiology of physical activity and fitness in children and adolescents. *Critical Reviews in Food Science and Nutrition, 33,* 403–408.

Sallis, J.F., Alcaraz, J.E., McKenzie, T.L., Hovell, M.F., Kolody, B., & Nader, P.R. (1992). Parent behavior in relation to physical activity and fitness in 9-year-olds. *American Journal of Diseases of Children, 146,* 1383–1388.

Sallis, J.F., Hovell, M.F., Hofstetter, C.R., Elder, J.P., Caspersen, C.J., Hackley, M., & Powell, K.E. (1990). Distance between homes and exercise facilities related to the frequency of exercise among San Diego residents. *Public Health Reports, 105,* 179–185.

Sallis, J.F., Hovell, M.F., Hofstetter, C.R., Elder, J.P., Faucher, P., Spry, V.M., Barrington, E., & Hackley, M. (1990). Lifetime history of relapse from exercise. *Addictive Behaviors, 15,* 573–579.

Sallis, J.F., Hovell, M.F., Hofstetter, C.R., & Barrington, E. (1992). Explanation of vigorous physical activity during two years using social learning variables. *Social Science and Medicine, 34,* 25–32.

Sallis, J.F., Nader, P.R., Broyles, S.L., Berry, C.C., Elder, J.P., McKenzie, T.L., & Nelson, J.A. (1993). Correlates of physical activity at home in Mexican-American and Anglo-American preschool children. *Health Psychology, 12,* 390–398.

Sallis, J.F., & Owen, N. (1998). *Physical activity and behavioral medicine.* Newbury Park, CA: Sage.

Shea, S., Stein, A.D., Basch, C.E., Lantigua, R., Maylahn, C., Strogatz, D.S., & Novick, L. (1991). Independent associations of educational attainment and ethnicity with behavioral risk factors for cardiovascular disease. *American Journal of Epidemiology, 134,* 567–582.

Stucky-Ropp, R.C., & DiLorenzo, T.M. (1993). Determinants of exercise in children. *Preventive Medicine, 22,* 880–889.

Tappe, M.K., Duda, J.L., & Ehrnwald, P.M. (1989). Perceived barriers to exercise among adolescents. *Journal of School Health, 59,* 153–155.

U.S. Department of Health and Human Services. (1990). *Healthy people 2000.* Washington, DC: U.S. Government Printing Office.

U.S. Department of Health and Human Services. (1996). *Physical activity and health: A report of the Surgeon General.* Atlanta, GA: Centers for Disease Control and Prevention.

Whitehead, J.R. (1993). Physical activity and intrinsic motivation. *Physical Activity and Fitness Research Digest, 1(2),* 1–6.

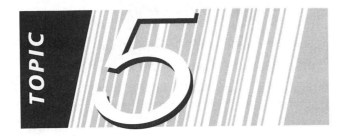

Physical Activity and Intrinsic Motivation

James R. Whitehead
UNIVERSITY OF NORTH DAKOTA

INTRODUCTION: THEORY DEVELOPMENT

Over the past 20 plus years, we have accumulated considerable evidence to document the health benefits of physical activity. Researchers have established with a fair degree of confidence just how much physical activity is necessary to produce fitness improvement and benefits to health (ACSM, 1990; Pate et al., 1995; DHHS, 1990). Given this rather clear picture of how to obtain desirable benefits, an obvious question is why do less than one quarter of the population engage in light-to-moderate physical activity? The answer to this question is found largely in the realm of psychology—specifically in the area of motivation. The task of this topic is to review current knowledge and to translate it into suggestions for enhancing physical activity. Specific guidelines for fostering intrinsic motivation toward physical activity are outlined.

Motivational studies have long focused on factors that initiate, influence, and modify behavior. Early theories dealt essentially with the *deterministic* aspects of those factors; focusing on instinctual drives (e.g., Freud, 1923/1962), physiological drives (e.g., Hull, 1943), or environmental influences (e.g., Skinner, 1953, 1971). Although these theories had (and

still have) considerable value, their apparent view of people as passive beings that are pushed and pulled around by their physiology or environment has given rise to concern and criticism. A different point of view was published as a monograph by White (1959), who proposed that people are driven by a need to be *competent,* or *effective* in mastering all aspects of our environment. He suggested that when attempts to master the challenges of our surroundings were successful, the result was positive—a "feeling of efficacy" (p. 329)—which, in turn, served intrinsically to motivate further behavior. White's monograph led to a wealth of study on intrinsic motivation, and in that respect it can be seen as the foundation of subsequent studies that are described below.

REFINEMENTS OF THE THEORY

A major development of White's (1959) monograph is represented by the addition of a formal statement of *cognitive evaluation theory* (Deci, 1975; Deci & Ryan, 1985). Cognitive evaluation theory states that intrinsic motivation is driven by an innate need for competence and self-determination in dealing with

ORIGINALLY PUBLISHED AS SERIES 1, NUMBER 2, OF THE PCPFS *RESEARCH DIGEST.*

HIGHLIGHT ||▊| ||▊▊▊▊ ▊▊ ▊▊▊▊|| ▊▊|| ▊▊| ▊ ▊▊▊▊▊ ▊▊▊▊▊▊▊▊| ▊ ▊ ▊▊▊ ▊▊ ▊▊ ||▊ ▊▊▊▊▊▊ ▊▊ ▊▊▊ ||| ▊

"Children are born intrinsically motivated to be physically active. That motivation—if kept alive by physical success, freedom, and fun—will do more than promote the fitness behaviors that add years to life. It will maintain the physical zest that adds life to the years."

one's surroundings. The intrinsic rewards for the behaviors motivated by this need are satisfying feelings of competence and autonomy, positive emotions such as enjoyment and excitement, and possibly the sensation of flow (complete absorption in the activity). These feelings, in turn, serve to maintain or increase a person's intrinsic motivation for the particular behavior.

In a nutshell (according to the theory), an individual's desire to pursue a particular activity depends upon whether his or her feelings of competence, autonomy, and positive affect persist over time. Conversely, if an individual begins to perceive him or herself as incompetent at the activity and/or under external control to do it, then his or her intrinsic motivation is undermined. The outcome is then either a state of *extrinsic motivation* (the activity might continue dependent on the continuance of external rewards and/or coercion), or a state of *amotivation* (further activity unlikely because the perceptions of incompetence lead to a sense of futility).

A wealth of studies in general psychology have supported the validity of cognitive evaluation theory Many studies have clearly shown that when individuals receive information that undermines their sense of competence and/or perception of self-determined choice, their intrinsic motivation declines. Readers who wish to review that research comprehensively are referred to Deci and Ryan (1985). However, of immediate interest to this paper is an overview of the ways in which intrinsic motivation is enhanced—or undermined—in the field of sport, exercise, and other physical activities.

INTRINSIC MOTIVATION IN SPORTS AND EXERCISE

Common sense alone tells us that participation in many sports and physical activities can lead to feelings of autonomy and competence and may produce joy, excitement, thrills, and other satisfying emotions. In that respect it is easy to see that physical activities may be inherently intrinsically motivating. On the other hand, some people say that they would not participate unless there was a material payoff, or unless they were coerced. Others declare that attempting physical challenges leaves them feeling incompetent and humiliated, anxious or pressured. Thus, if we wish to help people reap the benefits of participation and avoid the motivational pitfalls, it is necessary to understand the processes that may lead to specific perceptual outcomes.

Persistence at exercise is related to the motivational constructs described above and has research support. For example, young athletes cite "fun" as a primary reason for participating in sports (Gill, Gross, & Huddleston, 1983; Scanlan & Lewthwaite, 1986). Further examination has shown that this feeling of fun depends on experiencing the intrinsic satisfactions of skill improvement, personal accomplishment, and excitement—rather than being a result of extrinsic factors such as winning, getting rewards, or pleasing others (Wankel & Kreisel, 1985; Wankel & Sefton, 1989). Similar findings have also been related by Gould (1987) in a review of the reasons why children drop out of sports, and by Brustad (1988) from a study of affective outcomes of competitive youth sport.

However, as researchers know well, circumstantial support for the use of a theory of motivation to a particular area (in this case physical activity) is not enough to make a case for its value. The theory should also hold up under experimental testing. In particular, manipulations of people's perceptions of competence and control should produce changes in their intrinsic motivation. Unfortunately, there is not the volume of evidence in the physical activity setting as there is in general and educational psychology, but several studies do show support for the hypotheses predicted by intrinsic motivation theory.

For example, Orlick and Mosher (1978) hypothesized that an extrinsic reward (a trophy) for performance on a stabilometer (balance board) would be perceived by children as controlling—and thus their intrinsic motivation for what is generally

Applying Theory to Practice

The following recommendations represent an attempt to translate logically the theoretical exposition into guidelines for promoting motivation in practical situations. Note that although these guidelines are presented as a series of DOs and DON'Ts, they are not meant to be coercing or controlling. The reader has the choice of which to accept!

■ DO try to emphasize individual mastery.

Since the foundation of intrinsic motivation is said to stem from a need to be effective it makes sense to begin with a recommendation for promoting competence perceptions. For example, when giving feedback to an exerciser or sport participant in a coaching or teaching situation, try to reinforce the personal progress that has been made (e.g., "You're really starting to get the hang of that backhand stroke."). Also, sweeten bitter medicine by prefacing comments with a competence-promoting introduction (e.g., "If you want to make that good shot great—why not try to . . .").

■ DON'T overemphasize peer comparisons of performance.

This is an alternative form of the previous recommendation. Peer comparisons inevitably do the greatest motivational damage to those who need encouragement the most—those with low ability. Teachers, coaches, and fitness leaders should consider the perceptions that are created by their grading plans, or other evaluation procedures. In particular, since children's fitness test *scores* are determined to a considerable degree by genetics and level of maturation, the use of rankings, curves, or percentile tables for evaluation is questionable. What counts is an active lifestyle—so why not find a plan that reinforces mastery of the learning and participation *process?* (See Fox & Biddle, 1988, for an exposition on this point.)

A footnote to this part: Since comments (like those above) about the use of percentiles have sometimes been interpreted as a blanket castigation, a clarification is merited. Although the use of percentiles for *individual* evaluation is questioned, this is because (by definition) it forces peer comparison—and, consequently, it promotes competitive competence-seeking orientations. In contrast, the calculation of percentile scores to follow national fitness changes over time would be an example of a highly appropriate use of comparative data.

■ DO promote perceptions of choice.

A second conceptual area for recommendations is concerned with the other fundamental aspect of intrinsic motivation—perceptions of control. In many ways translating this guideline into action involves awareness of the connotations of words and phrases. For example, consider the meaning of the term "exercise *prescription.*" This language certainly doesn't suggest choice. On the other hand, this does not mean that exercise leaders and teachers have to let participants do whatever they want! A perception of choice can be fostered—even within fairly narrow guidelines—providing reasons are given for constraints. Thus an exercise leader might be advised to explain which activities, equipment, facilities, etc., are appropriate for a client's current fitness level—but then a choice should be allowed from within that range.

■ DON'T undermine an intrinsic focus by misusing extrinsic rewards.

This guideline is a different way of expressing recommendations concerning perceptions of control. If the answer to the question: "Why are we doing this exercise, skill, fitness test, sport, etc.?"—is "Because it's for a payment/trophy/reward," or "Because you have to do it," then the focus is moved to external regulation. In that case the behavior will most likely cease when the extrinsic motivator is won, lost, or removed. This does not mean all forms of awards are harmful. It depends on how they are

(continued)

perceived. Because of a growing appreciation of this point, recently disseminated youth fitness programs have emphasized individual competence attainment by using *recognition* (of exercise participation and mastery) schemes, rather than employing the extrinsically focused traditional awards that are solely dependent on fitness test results (Fitness Canada, 1992; Prudential FITNESSGRAM, 1992).

■ DO promote the intrinsic fun and excitement of exercise.

Fortunately, this is easy to do because many physical activities are naturally intrinsically motivating—so long as we keep them that way by attention to the other guidelines.

■ DON'T turn exercise into a bore or a chore.

To use an analogy: Rather than a bland repetitive "diet" of a physical activity, think of a "menu" in which taste is enhanced by variety, new "recipes," and the "sugar and spice" of fun, excitement, and thrills (Whitehead, 1989). In the same vein, it should be remembered that health-related fitness is a construct that is adult-oriented (Malina, 1991). This is not meant as a criticism of health-related fitness itself. The point (particularly when dealing with children) is that we should not overshadow the *play* value inherent in physical activity with an overbearing view of its potential as a "medicine."

■ DO promote a sense of purpose by teaching the value of physical activity to health, optimal function, and quality of life.

This recommendation is designed to highlight the motivational value of cognitive learning. Even if many forms of exercise do not produce the intrinsic rewards of excitement, pleasure, etc., knowledge of the benefits of exercise may promote a sense of purpose for choosing to do it. It may also require the development of cognitive skills such as fitness self-evaluation and problem solving (Corbin, 1987). Research on the outcomes of conceptually based fitness classes does support the premise that learning fitness knowledge and skills promotes activity in the future (Slava, Laurie, & Corbin, 1984).

■ DON'T create amotivation by spreading fitness misinformation.

While this might seem painfully obvious, the sobering reality is that many people believe in ineffective or dangerous methods of weight management (e.g., fad diets, spot reducing, sauna suits), and many others are hoodwinked into paying for quack methods of fitness improvement such as passive exercise or unproven dietary supplements (Gauthier, 1987; Jarvis, 1992; Lightsey & Attaway, 1992). Unfortunately, the likely motivational penalty for the continued failure that results from the use of ineffective or useless products and methods is amotivation. True fitness professionals are thus urged to make every effort to disseminate knowledge that is derived from good science and experience.

an interesting and challenging physical task would be undermined. The hypothesis was supported: When given a free-choice period, the children whose earlier participation was for a trophy showed a decrease in the time they spent voluntarily playing on the stabilometer compared to the children who had no expectation of a reward.

In another study of performance at a stabilometer task, Rudisill (1989) hypothesized that training children to understand that their performance improvement was personally controllable (i.e., dependent on practice and effort) would improve their subsequent performance—and would also lead them to persist longer at mastery attempts—even in the face of perceived failure. Again, the results of the experimental manipulation supported the hypothesis that perceptions of personal control enhance intrinsic motivation.

Taking research outside the laboratory, Thompson and Wankel (1980) manipulated the perception of exercise choice of adult women who had recently enrolled in a health club. After an initial meeting to discuss activity preferences, the women were randomly allocated to either a perceived choice or a perceived no-choice condition. The initial activity preferences were actually used as the basis for all of the women's programs. However, the women in the no-choice group were led to believe that they had been assigned a standard program determined by the instructor. Six weeks later the attendance of the women in the perceived choice group was higher, and they also expressed a greater intention to continue exercising at the health club.

Experimental manipulations designed to affect perceptions of competence at physical activities have also been shown to change intrinsic motivation in line with the predictions of the theory. As before, some studies have employed a stabilometer. For example, Weinberg and Jackson (1979) gave subjects bogus success or failure feedback for their balancing ability by telling them that they had either exceeded the 82nd percentile ("...very good..."), or they had fallen below the 18th percentile ("...not very good..."). In line with intrinsic motivation theory, success feedback enhanced interest and enjoyment, and reduced boredom with the task—and failure feedback had the opposite effect.

Using a similar type of protocol and a stabilometer task, Vallerand and Reid (1984, 1988) manipulated feedback by making verbal comments to subjects suggesting that they were doing either well or poorly. Like Weinberg and Jackson (1979) the results showed that success feedback led to enhanced intrinsic motivation while lack of success feedback reduced it. Additionally, a more in-depth analysis of the results allowed the experimenters to show that it was not the effect of the feedback per se, but rather it was the effect of feedback on the subjects' perceptions of competence that moderated changes in intrinsic motivation. In other words, this study showed that it was not the feedback itself so much as the *meaning* of the feedback to the subjects that produced the motivational outcome.

Wishing to see if similar results would be obtained from manipulations of feedback in a youth physical fitness testing situation, Whitehead and Corbin (1991) set up an experiment in a junior high school using a shuttle run-type fitness test (the Illinois Agility Run). Bogus high or low percentile feedback was given to randomly determined groups, and the results replicated the Vallerand and Reid (1984,1988) findings. Again, apparently high percentile scores raised intrinsic motivation and low percentile scores lowered it—and as before, the motivational outcomes were mediated by the subjects' *perceptions* of competence at the task rather than directly changed by the feedback itself.

THE INDIVIDUALITY OF PERCEPTIONS

So far, and in its simplest form, the theoretical model of motivation has been presented as follows: Our intrinsic need to be competent or effective motivates mastery behaviors. If the attempts are self-determined and successful, then intrinsic motivation is maintained or enhanced. If not, intrinsic motivation is undermined and may be replaced by extrinsic motivation or amotivation. However, as several of the studies above have shown (e.g., Thompson & Wankel, 1980; Vallerand & Reid, 1984; Whitehead & Corbin, 1991) this is an oversimplification. It is a person's *perception* of events that counts. A person's motivation will depend on his or her personal *cognitive evaluation* (through intuition and appraisal) of success and autonomy in any particular situation. Given that point, it is obviously important to try to understand factors that lead to individual differences before the theory can be translated into guidelines for motivational enhancement (see the box earlier in this topic).

A primary concern is the need for an understanding of differences in the ways in which individuals form perceptions of competence. There appear to be three main ways (or orientations) in which individuals judge their competence. Those with a *competitive* orientation tend to compare their abilities or performance to those of their peers. Those with a *cooperative* orientation tend to look for social approval while involved in group activities. Those with an *individualistic* orientation tend to focus more on their individual improvement and task mastery (Ames & Ames, 1984). Logically, an obvious potential problem with a competitive orientation is that it leads to perceptions of winning and losing that are dependent on who beats whom, or where a person ranks in a hierarchy (e.g., a percentile table). In contrast, a cooperative, or more particularly, an individualistic orientation would seem to hold more hope of personal success because improvement under those conditions almost inevitably results from effort and practice.

This logic has been supported by research in sport and fitness settings. For example, Marsh and

Peart (1988) randomly assigned eighth-grade girls to fitness classes that either stressed competition or cooperation. Results showed that the cooperative program led to enhanced perceptions of physical competence. Similarly, Lloyd and Fox (1992) studied adolescent girls in a fitness program. They found that putting the focus on an individualistic orientation led to improvements in enjoyment and motivation compared to the outcomes of a competitively focused environment. The logic also held in a sport setting: Seifriz, Duda, and Chi (1992) found that when high school basketball players perceived an individual mastery-oriented climate in their practice sessions they experienced more enjoyment and had higher intrinsic motivation compared to those players who perceived practice as a more competitive performance-oriented environment.

Also of immediate concern is the need to appreciate how events may be perceived as controlling. The previously mentioned Thompson and Wankel (1980) study showed that the perception of choice can be modified and other studies have revealed that the context in which potentially controlling events occur makes a difference. For example, Ryan (1980) found some sport specificity in whether athletes perceived sport scholarships as affirmations of their competence (thus supporting intrinsic motivation), or as extrinsically controlling (thus undermining intrinsic motivation). Specifically, athletes in the sport of football (where scholarships were common at that time) were more likely to perceive the scholarships as controlling than were wrestlers or female athletes (for whom scholarships were rare in the late 1970s).

Other research has shown several other factors that may or may not be perceived as controlling depending on the social context and informational emphasis. For example, competition, performance awards, and coaching styles can produce alternative outcomes. Unfortunately, space limitations preclude a detailed citation of individual studies here, but it may be sufficient to say that a common determining factor of an extrinsic focus is whether an individual senses an external pressure to perform or behave in a particular way. Readers who wish to look further at research on those topics are encouraged to read the review by Vallerand, Deci, and Ryan (1987). Suggestions for practitioners may be found earlier in this paper.

SUMMARY

This paper argues that intrinsic motivation is one key element in promoting active healthy lifestyles. Figure 5.1, "The Stairway to Intrinsic Motivation,"

FIGURE 5.1
The stairway to intrinsic motivation.*

Threshold of Intrinsic Rewards

INTRINSIC MOTIVATION
"I do this behavior for its own sake and because I want to. I like the feelings of success and enjoyment that come from doing it right."

INTEGRATED REGULATION
"I do this behavior because it symbolizes who and what I am."

Threshold of Autonomy

IDENTIFIED REGULATION
"I purposely choose to do this behavior because it's a means to an end that I value."

INTROJECTED REGULATION
"I do this behavior because I feel a tension inside me (e.g., guilt) that pressures me into doing it."

Threshold of Motivation

EXTERNAL REGULATION
"I do this behavior for pay or a reward—or because I am coerced into it."

AMOTIVATION
"It's futile for me to even attempt this behavior because I don't see much chance of success at it— or of receiving any other type of payoff."

*The different types of motivation are from Vallerand and Reid (1990) and Vallerand and Bissonnette (1992). The examples of cognitive self-statements in the figure are based upon their descriptions. The arrangement of the types into a stairway, and the inclusion of the three thresholds is the work of the author of this paper.

provides a visual summary of the various stages of personal motivation. The wise use of the guidelines presented in the preceding pages will help people avoid the constraints of amotivation, and may help them to move beyond externally controlled forms of motivation to self-determined and intrinsic motivation. Well-tested theory suggests that personal competence and control are the essential foundations of intrinsic motivation. Fortunately, a wide variety of sports and physical activities are available, and these provide many opportunities for self-chosen optimal challenges that can help *all people* to enjoy the sense of autonomy and mastery that underpins intrinsic motivation. By their very nature, most physical activities are intrinsically appealing because of their benefits to personal wellness, and because of the fun, excitement, and thrills that can result from participation in them.

REFERENCES

American College of Sports Medicine. (1990). The recommended quantity and quality of exercise for developing and maintaining cardiorespiratory and muscular fitness in healthy adults. *Medicine and Science in Sports and Exercise, 22,* 265–274.

Ames, A., & Ames, R. (1984). Goal structures and motivation. *The Elementary School Journal, 85(1),* 40–52.

Brustad, R.J. (1988). Affective outcomes in competitive youth sport: The influence of intrapersonal and socialization factors. *Journal of Sport and Exercise Psychology, 10,* 307–321.

Corbin, C.B. (1987). Physical fitness in the K–12 curriculum: Some defensible solutions to perennial problems. *Journal of Physical Education, Recreation, and Dance, 58(7),* 49–54.

Deci, E.L. (1975). *Intrinsic motivation.* New York: Plenum Press.

Deci, E.L., & Ryan, R.M. (1985). *Intrinsic motivation and self-determination in human behavior.* New York: Plenum Press.

Fitness Canada. (1992). *The Canadian Active Living Challenge.* Ottawa: Government of Canada.

Fox, K.R., & Biddle, S.J.H. (1988). The use of fitness tests: Educational and psychological considerations. *Journal of Physical Education, Recreation, and Dance, 59(2),* 47–53.

Freud, S. (1923/62). *The ego and the id.* New York: Norton.

Gauthier, M.M. (1987). Continuous passive motion: The no-exercise exercise. *The Physician and Sportsmedicine, 15(8),* 142–148.

Gill, D.L., Gross, J.B., & Huddleston, S. (1985). Participation motivation in youth sports. *International Journal of Sport Psychology. 14,* 1–14.

Gould, D. (1987). Understanding attrition in children's sport. In D. Gould & M. R. Weiss (Eds.), *Advances in pediatric sport sciences* (Vol. 2, pp. 61–85). Champaign, IL: Human Kinetics Publishers.

Hull, C.L. (1943). *Principles of behavior.* New York: Appleton-Century-Crofts.

Jarvis, W.T. (1992). Quackery: A national scandal. *Clinical Chemistry, 38,* 1574–1586.

Lightsey, D.M., & Attaway, J.R. (1992). Deceptive tactics used in marketing purported ergogenic aids. *National Strength and Conditioning Association Journal, 14(2),* 26–31.

Lloyd, J., & Fox, K.R. (1992). Achievement goals and motivation to exercise in adolescent girls: A preliminary intervention study. *British Journal of Physical Education Research Supplement, II(Summer),* 12–16.

Malinal, R.M. (1991). Fitness and performance: Adult health and the culture of youth. In R.J. Park & H.M. Eckert (Eds.), *The Academy Papers: Vol. 24. New possibilities, new paradigms* (pp. 30–38). Champaign, IL: Human Kinetics Publishers.

Marsh, H.W., & Peart, N.D. (1988). Competitive and cooperative physical fitness training programs for girls: Effects on physical fitness and multidimensional self-concepts. *Journal of Sport and Exercise Psychology, 10,* 390–407.

Orlick, T.D., & Mosher, R. (1978). Extrinsic rewards and participant motivation in a sport-related task. *International Journal of Sport Psychology, 9,* 27–39.

Pate, R.R., Pratt, M., Blair, S.N., Haskell, W.L., Macera, C.A., Bouchard, C., Buchner, D., Ettinger, W., Heath, G.W., King, A.C., Kriska, A., Leon, A.S., Marcus, B.H., Morris, J., Paffenbarger, R.S., Patrick, K., Pollock, M.L., Rippe, J.M., Sallis, J., & Wilmore, J.H. (1995). Physical activity and public health. *Journal of the American Medical Association, 273,* 402–407.

Prudential FITNESSGRAM. (1992 flier). *The Prudential FITNESSGRAM recognition system & program materials.* Dallas, TX: Cooper Institute for Aerobics Research.

Rudisill, M.E. (1989). Influence of perceived competence and causal dimension orientation on expectations, persistence, and performance during perceived failure. *Research Quarterly for Exercise and Sport, 60,* 166–175.

Ryan, E.D. (1980). Attribution, intrinsic motivation, and athletics: A replication and extension. In C.H. Nadeau, W.R. Halliwell, K.M. Newell, & G.C. Roberts (Eds.), *Psychology of motor behavior and sport* (pp. 19–26). Champaign, IL: Human Kinetics Publishers.

Scanlan, T.K., & Lewthwaite, R. (1986). Social psychological aspects of competition for male youth sport participants: IV. Predictors of enjoyment. *Journal of Sport Psychology, 8,* 25–35.

Seifriz, J.J., Duda, J.L., & Chi, L. (1992). The relationship of perceived motivational climate to intrinsic motivation and beliefs about success in basketball. *Journal of Sport and Exercise Psychology, 14,* 375–391 .

Skinner, B.F. (1953). *Science and human behavior.* New York: Macmillan.

Skinner, B.F. (1971). *Beyond freedom and dignity.* New York: Penguin.

Slava, S., Laurie, D.R., & Corbin, C.B. (1984). Long-term effects of a conceptual physical education program. *Research Quarterly for Exercise and Sport, 55,* 161–168.

Thompson, C.E., & Wankel, L.M. (1980). The effects of perceived activity choice upon frequency of exercise behavior. *Journal of Applied Social Psychology, 10,* 436–443.

U.S. Department of Health and Human Services. (1990). *Healthy people 2000. National health promotion and disease prevention objectives.* Washington, DC: U.S. Government Printing Office.

Vallerand, R. J., & Bissonnette, R. (1992). Intrinsic, extrinsic, and amotivational styles as predictors of behavior: A prospective study. *Journal of Personality, 60,* 599–620.

Vallerand, R. J., & Reid, G. (1984). On the causal effects of perceived competence on intrinsic motivation: A test of cognitive evaluation theory. *Journal of Sport Psychology, 6,* 94–102.

Vallerand, R.M., & Reid, G. (1988). On the relative effects of positive and negative verbal feedback on males' and females' intrinsic motivation. *Canadian Journal of Behavioral Sciences, 20,* 239–250.

Vallerand, R.J., & Reid, G. (1990). Motivation and special populations: Theory, research, and implications regarding motor behavior. In G. Reid (Ed.), *Problems in movement control* (pp. 159–197). Elsevier Science Publishers.

Vallerand, R.J., Deci, E.L., & Ryan, R.M. (1987). Intrinsic motivation in sport. In K.B. Pandolt (Ed.), *Exercise and sport science reviews* (Vol. 15, pp. 387–425). New York: Macmillan.

Wankel, L.M., & Kreisel, P.S.J. (1985). Factors underlying enjoyment of youth sports: Sport and age group comparisons. *Journal of Sport Psychology, 7,* 51–64.

Wankel, L.M., & Sefton, J.M. (1989). A season-long investigation of fun in youth sports. *Journal of Sport and Exercise Psychology, 11,* 355–366.

Weinberg, R.S., & Jackson, A. (1979). Competition and extrinsic rewards: Effect on intrinsic motivation and attribution. *Research Quarterly, 50,* 494–502.

Weiss, M.R., Bredemeier, B.J., & Shewchuk, R.M. (1985). An intrinsic/extrinsic motivation scale for the youth sport setting: A confirmatory factor analysis. *Journal of Sport Psychology, 7,* 75–91.

White, R.W. (1959). Motivation reconsidered: The concept of competence. *Psychological Review, 66,* 279–333.

Whitehead, J.R. (1989). Fitness assessment results—some concepts and analogies. *Journal of Physical Education, Recreation, and Dance, 60(6),* 39–43.

Whitehead, J.R., & Corbin, C.B. (1991). Youth fitness testing: The effect of percentile-based evaluative feedback on intrinsic motivation. *Research Quarterly for Exercise and Sport, 62,* 225–231.

General Health Benefits of Physical Activity

This section contains three papers. The first paper, published here as Topic 6, was the first issue of the first volume of the resurrected *Digest,* published in 1993. Topic 6, unlike the paper that follows it, does not provide the most recent findings on physical activity; however, it does give the reader a historical perspective on the state of the knowledge prior to that reflected in the second paper. That paper, Topic 7, is a summary of the landmark Surgeon General's Report on Physical Activity. The third paper in this section, by Christine Wells, discusses physical activity and women's health.

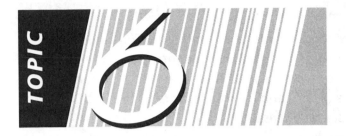

The Health Benefits of Physical Activity

Charles B. Corbin
Robert P. Pangrazi
ARIZONA STATE UNIVERSITY

In 1990, *Healthy People 2000* was released by Dr. Louis Sullivan, Secretary, Department of Health and Human Services. The document elaborated national health promotion and disease prevention goals for the year 2000. A central goal of the document is to increase the span of healthy life for Americans. While improved treatment of disease to prevent premature death is an important concern, *Healthy People 2000* emphasizes the importance of prevention of illness/disease, especially lifestyle or chronic illnesses that have become the leading sources of death in our society. But perhaps most important of all, the goals focus on efforts to promote a quality of life and a sense of well-being associated with good health. Dr. Michael McGinnis, Director of the Office of Disease Prevention and Health Promotion, made the following statement.

> . . . it is not through happenstance that the physical activity category is the first priority area of the *Healthy People 2000* effort. Physical activity is related to the health of all Americans. It has the ability to reduce directly the risk of several major chronic diseases as well as to catalyze positive changes with respect to other risk factors of these diseases. Dr. William Foege, former Director of

the Centers for Disease Control, suggests that physical activity may provide the shortcut we in public health have been seeking for the control of chronic diseases, much like immunization has facilitated progress against infectious diseases (McGinnis, 1992, p. S196).

The inclusion of physical activity as an important lifestyle for promoting good health is now clear. But for those interested in the health benefits of physical activity, it is not easy to find a single source that summarizes these benefits. For this reason, we have attempted to provide a simple summary of the benefits in three sections: disease prevention and treatment; health promotion; and physical fitness development. Six principal sources are used for this summary. Readers are encouraged to consult these references and their sources for more complete details.

DISEASE PREVENTION AND TREATMENT

Prior to 1940, the leading killers in the United States were infectious diseases. Improvement in public health practices, implementation of personal and

ORIGINALLY PUBLISHED AS SERIES 1, NUMBER 1, OF THE PCPFS *RESEARCH DIGEST.*

"It is clear that moderate levels of fitness offer considerable health benefits. The key is moving from the unfit category—some 30 to 40 million people in this country—to the moderately fit category. By beginning programs of moderate, regular exercise—half an hour each day, three times a week—anyone can join this group, and markedly lower their death rates from all-cause mortality, cancer, and cardiovascular disease."

Dr. Steven Blair, The Cooper Institute for Aerobics Research

public health education, and vaccines have greatly reduced the incidence of these diseases. As indicated in the early statement by Dr. Foege, "chronic diseases" are now our major health concerns. These chronic diseases are often referred to as "lifestyle diseases" because changes in lifestyle, including increased activity and fitness, can reduce the threat of early death and the incidence of disease. Figure 6.1 lists several of the diseases for which regular physical activity can reduce risk, either of getting the disease or of dying from it. Also illustrated in Figure 6.1 are some of the possible reasons why exercise reduces risk of these diseases.

In spite of the fact that deaths from heart disease have decreased in recent years, it is still the leading cause of death. Studies by Paffenbarger and colleagues (1989) as well as others have clearly shown that those who do regular physical activity are at less risk of dying from this major killer. Physically inactive people have almost twice the risk of developing heart disease as active people (Powell et al., 1987). In fact, the American Heart Association (Fletcher et al., 1992) has recently classified inactivity (sedentary living) as a primary risk factor for heart disease comparable to high blood pressure, high blood cholesterol, and cigarette smoking. Both stroke (lack of blood flow and oxygen to the brain) and peripheral vascular disease (lack of blood flow and oxygen to the limbs) have been shown (Haskell et al., 1992) to be associated with sedentary living for many of the same reasons why inactivity is related to heart disease (see Figure 6.1). High blood pressure or hypertension is a condition that predisposes people to other health risks such as heart disease and diabetes. Regular exercise has been shown to reduce blood pressure among those who have high levels though, by itself, exercise cannot normalize high blood pressure for most people (Haskell et al., 1992).

In the introduction of the Physical Activity and Fitness section of *Healthy People 2000* (Public Health Service, p. 94), it is noted that physical activity can help to prevent and manage non-insulin-dependent diabetes and osteoporosis. Recent evidence also has shown that inactive people have a higher incidence of colon and breast cancer than active people. While the evidence is less than complete, one researcher reached the following conclusion based on a review of recent research.

> Given the consistency in the direction and magnitude of the findings regarding colon cancer . . . the evidence supports the conclusion that activity is protective against colon cancer. Although that protective effect may be small, the attributable risk of colon cancer associated with inactivity may be quite high given the prevalence of inactivity in Western societies. (Sternfeld, 1992, p. 1195)

It is generally conceded that regular muscle fitness and flexibility exercise can aid in improving posture. Together, exercise and good posture can have a positive effect on back problems as evidenced by less risk of back pain. In a recent review, Plowman (1992) noted that while we do not yet know the exact amounts of muscle strength, muscle endurance, and flexibility necessary to reduce the risk of back pain, there is support for the notion that poor scores on these fitness measures are predictive of low back pain.

The potential benefits of regular physical activity in reducing obesity are well documented. Regular exercise expends calories that can result in reduced fat storage in the body's fat cells. At the same time, exercise designed to build muscle fitness increases lean body tissue (muscle), which can result in a lesser relative percentage of fat in the body and a higher resting metabolism. Getting obese Americans to adopt regular exercise that would help them achieve normal levels of body fatness is not as successful as we might hope. Nevertheless, physical activity has great potential for

FIGURE 6.1

Physical activity and major lifestyle diseases.

Disease	Physical Activity Benefit
Heart Disease	Healthy heart muscle
	■ lower resting heart rate
	■ more blood pumped with each beat
	■ reduced blood pressure in submaximal work
	Healthy arteries
	■ less atherosclerosis (deposits in arteries)
	■ higher HDL ("good" cholesterol)
	■ better blood fat profile (fewer "bad" fats)
	■ decreased platelet and less fibrin (related to atherosclerosis)
	■ better blood flow
	Better working capacity
	■ fewer demands during work
	■ greater ability to meet work demands
Stroke	Healthy arteries (see above)
	■ lower blood pressure
Peripheral Vascular Disease	Improved working capacity
	Higher HDL
	Better blood fat profile
High Blood Pressure	Reduction in blood pressure among those with high levels
	Reduction in body fatness (associated with high blood pressure)
Diabetes (non-insulin)	Reduced body fatness (may relieve symptoms of adult onset diabetes)
	Better carbohydrate metabolism (improved insulin sensitivity)
Cancer	Less risk of colon cancer (better transit time of food?)
Obesity	Increases lean body mass
	Decreases body fat percentage
	Less central fat distribution
Depression	Relief from some symptoms
Back Pain	Increased muscle strength and endurance
	Improved flexibility
	Improved posture
Osteoporosis	Greater bone density as a result of stressing long bones

reducing the incidence of obesity in our society (Epstein et al., 1990).

Depression is a major medical problem that causes much pain and suffering. The number of bed days and disabilities associated with depression is greater than that for the eight major chronic health conditions (Public Health Service, 1990). A recent position statement of the International Society of Sport Psychology (1992) states that studies on depressed patients reveal that aerobic exercises are as effective as different forms of psychotherapy. In addition, the Society summarizes by saying: "Exercise can have beneficial emotional effects across all ages and for both sexes."

HEALTH PROMOTION

The previous section dealt primarily with disease. Of course, disease treatment and prevention are critical to good health in our society. Nevertheless, it is widely acknowledged that optimal health is much more than freedom from disease. The challenge of *Healthy People 2000* (Public Health Service, 1990) illustrates this point.

> The health of people is measured by more than death rates. Good health comes from reducing unnecessary suffering, illness, and disability. It comes as well from an improved quality of life. Health is thus best measured by citizens' sense of well-being. (p. 6)

Prevention of disease is a high priority and regular physical activity has been shown to help prevent the conditions discussed in the preceding sections. But what of high-quality living and a sense of well-being? Many of these are quite subjective. Corbin and Lindsey (1990) summarize some of the perceived benefits of exercise based on subjective feelings of people responding to national surveys. Some of the reported benefits are supported by scientific evidence, including a reduction in stress levels and in symptoms of depression (International Society of Sport Psychology, 1992), improved appearance, and increased working capacity. Other benefits such as improved sleep habits, greater ability to enjoy leisure, improved general sense of well-being, and improved self-esteem are less easy to document. Nevertheless, what people think is true influences their quality of life and the results of national opinion polls show that many

Americans have positive feelings about the benefits they receive from regular exercise (Corbin and Lindsey, 1990). Among older adults, regular physical activity has been shown to increase independent functioning, increase the ability to drive a car, and improve social interactions (Corbin and Lindsey, 1990). There is similar evidence to show that physical activity can positively influence other health-related behaviors (Blair, 1985). One survey, for example, showed that regular exercisers were 50% more likely to quit smoking; 40% more likely to eat less red meat; 30% more likely to cut down on caffeine; 250% more likely to eat low calorie foods and drinks; 200% more likely to lose weight, and 25% more likely to cut down on salt and sugar than non-exercisers (Harris & Gurin, 1985).

Physical activity's contribution to quality of life and a personal sense of well-being is more difficult to document than its contribution to prevention and treatment of disease. In the long run, however, it may be equally important if the national goal of lengthening healthy life is to be achieved. It is doubtful that most Americans would favor an extended life if "quality of life" was lacking. The evidence suggests that humans were designed to be physically active and that physical activity has great potential for enhancing quality of life and sense of well-being. Additional research is necessary to determine the full extent of activity's contribution to these important variables.

PHYSICAL FITNESS

There is no doubt that regular physical activity builds physical fitness. What has become increasingly clear in recent years is that physical activity and physical fitness, as evidenced by performance on fitness tests, are independent but related phenomena. Likewise, physical fitness is associated with good health. For example, Blair et al. (1989) have shown that those with "good" levels of fitness have less heart disease risk than those with "low" levels of fitness. The previously cited review by Plowman (1992) suggests that muscle fitness is necessary to prevent back pain. Others have pointed out the importance of fitness to injury prevention (McGinnis, 1992). Body fatness, often considered a health-related component of physical fitness, is associated with medical problems of various kinds.

Fitness, as measured by fitness tests, is NOT solely related to regular physical activity. As noted in Figure 6.2, there are many other factors that contribute to physical fitness. Among children, fitness scores are influenced by chronological age and maturation (physiological age). In some cases, children and adolescents who are inactive have higher fitness scores than younger or more active peers (Pangrazi & Corbin, 1990; Pate, Dowda, & Ross, 1990). Bouchard and colleagues (1992) have demonstrated that heredity plays a significant role in a person's ability to improve fitness as a result of exercise. Some people respond to training more favorably than others, so it is possible that regular exercisers could sometimes have lower fitness performance levels than those who are sedentary. Of course, other factors such as nutrition, learned skills, and environment also play a role in fitness performances.

There is little doubt that good physical fitness is associated with reduced risk of disease. Further, it can be stated that good fitness helps people function effectively, look better, and have the ability to enjoy their free time. But evidence exists to support other important statements about physical fitness.

- Physical fitness, as measured by fitness tests, is not as meaningful to good health as physical fitness that results from regular physical activity as part of the normal lifestyle.

- Physical fitness, as measured by fitness tests, will ultimately improve as the result of regular exercise to the extent that hereditary predispositions allow. The amount and rate of change in fitness will take longer for some to achieve than for others.

- Physical fitness is associated with good health but is not the same as good health. Regular physical activity has positive benefits for both good health and adequate physical fitness.

FIGURE 6.2
Factors affecting physical fitness performances.

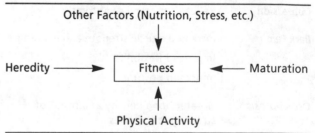

■ For good health benefits to result, it is important NOT to be in a low fit category. On the other hand, high levels of fitness test performance do NOT seem to be necessary for attaining health benefits. All people with regular physical activity have the potential to achieve adequate levels of fitness that are associated with good health.

SUMMARY

In recent years, much has been learned about regular physical activity and physical fitness. Many of the health benefits of exercise and physical fitness are now well documented. Other potential benefits require much more research. In the meantime, the following quotes seem to best summarize our knowledge. From leading researchers Paffenbarger and Hyde (1980):

> Evidence mounts that the relationship between exercise and good health is more than circumstantial. If some questions are not yet answered, they are far less important than those that have been.

From Edward Cooper during a news conference for the American Heart Association, July 1, 1992:

> Now I'd like to say to those who are not engaged in "exercise training" that *any* physical activity is better than none. According to our panel, housework, gardening, shuffleboard—anything that causes us to move—is beneficial. Maybe you don't have time or ability to attain "cardiovascular fitness," that is, to enable your heart to function at its most efficient level . . . maybe you don't have the money to join a health club or buy a bicycle . . . still there are activities you can perform as a part of your daily life that will benefit your heart. I encourage you to make activity a part of your routine every day—just as much a part of your day as brushing your teeth or enjoying breakfast.

From John Dryden, spoken several hundred years ago, as cited by Paffenbarger and Hyde (1980):

> Better to hunt in fields, for health unbought, than fee the doctor for nauseous draught; the wise, for cure, on exercise depend; God never made his work for man to mend.

REFERENCES

Blair, S.N. (1985). Relationship between exercise or physical activity and other health behaviors. *Public Health Reports, 100,* 172–180.

Blair, S.N., Kohl, H.W., Paffenbarger, R.S., Clarke, D.G., Cooper, K.H., & Gibbons, L.W. (1989). *Journal of the American Medical Association, 262,* 2395–2401.

Bouchard, C., Dionne, F.T., Simoneau, J., & Boulay, M.R. (1992). Genetics of aerobic performances. In J.O. Holloszy (Ed.), *Exercise and sport sciences reviews:* Vol. 20 (pp. 27–58). Baltimore: Williams and Wilkins.

Corbin, C.B., & Lindsey, R. (1990). *Concepts of physical fitness.* (7th ed.). Dubuque, IA: Wm. C. Brown Co.

Epstein, L.H., McCurley, M., Wing, R.R., Valoski, A. (1990). Five-year follow-up of family-based behavioral treatments for childhood obesity. *Journal of Consulting Clinical Psychology, 58,* 661–664.

Fletcher, G.F., Blair, S.N., Blumenthal, J., Caspersen, C., Chaitman, B., Epstein, S., Falls, H., Froelicher, E., Froelicher, V., & Pina, I. (1992). Statement on exercise: Benefits and recommendations for physical activity for all Americans. *Circulation, 86,* 2726–2730.

Harris, T.G., & Gurin, J. (1985). Look who's getting it all together. *American Health, 4 (2),* 42–47.

Haskell, W.L., Leon, A.S., Caspersen, C., Froelicher, V.F., Hagberg, J.M., Harlan, W., Holloszy, J.O., Regensteiner, J.G., Thompson, P.D., Washburn, R.A., & Wilson, P.W.F. (1992). Cardiovascular benefits and assessment of physical activity and physical fitness in adults. *Medicine and Science in Sports and Exercise, 24,* S201–S220.

International Society of Sport Psychology. (1992). Physical activity and psychological benefits. *Physician and Sportsmedicine, 20,* 179–184.

McGinnis, J.M. (1992). The public health burden of a sedentary lifestyle. *Medicine and Science in Sports and Exercise, 24,* S196–S200.

Paffenbarger, R.S., & Hyde, R.T. (1980). Exercise as protection against heart attack. *New England Journal of Medicine, 302,* 1026–1027.

Paffenbarger, R.S., Hyde, R.T., Wing, A.L., & Hsieh, C. (1986). Physical activity, all-cause mortality, and longevity of college alumni. *New England Journal of Medicine, 314,* 605–614.

Pangrazi, R.P., & Corbin, C. B. (1990). Age as a factor relating to physical fitness test performance. *Research Quarterly for Exercise and Sport, 61,* 410–414.

Pate, R.R., Dowda, M., & Ross, J.G. (1990). Association between physical activity and physical fitness of children. *American Journal of Diseases in Children, 144,* 1123–1129.

Powell, K.E., Thompson, K.D., Caspersen, C.J., & Kendrick, J.S. (1987). Physical activity and the incidence of coronary heart disease. *Annual Review of Public Health, 8,* 253–287.

Public Health Service. (1990). *Healthy People 2000.* Washington, DC: U.S. Government Printing Office.

Sternfeld, B. (1992). Cancer and the protective effect of physical activity: The epidemiological evidence. *Medicine and Science in Sports and Exercise, 24,* 1195–1209.

What you need to know about the . . .
Surgeon General's Report on Physical Activity and Health

Charles B. Corbin, Robert P. Pangrazi
ARIZONA STATE UNIVERSITY

WHAT IS THE SURGEON GENERAL'S REPORT ON PHYSICAL ACTIVITY AND HEALTH?

In 1964, the Surgeon General began alerting the nation to the hazards of smoking. Subsequently, several other reports addressing tobacco's effects on health were released. In 1988, the *Surgeon General's Report on Nutrition and Health* was released. These reports have had a great impact on the behaviors of American citizens. The reports on tobacco did much to change the social norm concerning smoking. Similarly, the report on nutrition and health focused national attention on the need for sound nutrition. Now, under the leadership of Department of Health and Human Services Secretary Donna E. Shalala, the Office of the Surgeon General has released a report on physical activity and health. **The main purpose of the *Surgeon General's Report on Physical Activity and Health* is to summarize existing research showing the benefits of physical activity in preventing disease and to draw conclusions that can be useful to Americans who are interested in improving their health.** This hallmark report will provide impetus for an active lifestyle just as other health-related behaviors were encouraged through previous Surgeon Generals' reports.

WHY WAS THE REPORT DONE NOW?

In recent years, scientific evidence linking physical activity and health and organizational statements supporting the value of regular physical activity have increased. The American Heart Association (AHA) in 1992 identified physical inactivity as a major risk factor for coronary heart disease. The 1995 National Institutes of Health (NIH) Consensus Development Conference on Physical Activity and Cardiovascular Health confirmed the importance of physical activity for cardiovascular health. In 1995, the American College of Sports Medicine (ACSM) and the Centers for Disease Control and Prevention

---

ORIGINALLY PUBLISHED AS SERIES 2, NUMBER 6, OF THE PCPFS *RESEARCH DIGEST*.

Note: Portions of this material, including the conclusions, have been taken from the *Surgeon General's Report on Physical Activity and Health.*

HIGHLIGHT

"By making the relatively small change from an inactive lifestyle to one that includes moderate but regular physical activity, even the most sedentary Americans can prevent disease and premature death and improve their quality of life."

Florence Griffith Joyner and Tom McMillen,
Co-Chairs, President's Council on Physical Fitness & Sports

(CDC) recommended that all Americans accumulate at least 30 minutes of moderate-intensity physical activity on most, preferably all, days of the week. These actions and others like them are based on a growing body of research showing the health benefits of regular physical activity.

"This landmark review of the research on physical activity—the most comprehensive ever—has the potential to catalyze a new physical activity and fitness movement in the United States."

Donna E. Shalala,
Secretary of Health and
Human Services

WHO PREPARED THE REPORT?

In July 1994, the Office of the Surgeon General authorized the CDC to serve as lead agency in preparing the first *Surgeon General's Report on Physical Activity and Health*. The CDC was joined in this effort by the President's Council on Physical Fitness and Sports (PCPFS) as a collaborative partner representing the Office of the Surgeon General. Because of the wide interest in the health effects of physical activity, the report was planned collaboratively with representatives from the Office of the Surgeon General, the Office of Public Health and Science (Office of the Secretary), the NIH, and many other government agencies. CDC's nonfederal partners—including the American Alliance for Health, Physical Education, Recreation, and Dance; the ACSM; and the AHA—provided consultation throughout the developmental process. Dr. Steven Blair served as the Senior Scientific Editor, and Dr. Adele Franks served as Scientific Editor. Each chapter was written and reviewed by top scholars in exercise science.

WHAT DOES THE REPORT INCLUDE?

The report's main purpose is to summarize existing literature on the role of physical activity in preventing disease and on the status of attempts to increase physical activity among Americans of all ages. Any report on a topic this broad must restrict its scope to keep the message clear. The report concentrates on endurance-type physical activity (activity involving repeated use of large muscles, such as walking or bicycling) because the health benefits of this type of activity have been studied extensively. While the report acknowledges the importance of other types of activities (strength training, activities for special populations), it does not emphasize these. The content is presented as follows:

1. Introduction, Summary, and Chapter Conclusions
2. Historical Background and Evolution of Physical Activity Recommendations
3. Physiologic Responses and Long-Term Adaptations to Exercise
4. The Effects of Physical Activity on Health and Disease
5. Patterns and Trends in Physical Activity
6. Understanding and Promoting Physical Activity

WHAT DOES THE REPORT CONCLUDE?
(Chapter 1)

The main message is that Americans can substantially improve their health and quality of life by including moderate amounts of physical activity in their daily lives. The report emphasizes that most Americans can achieve health benefits from physical activity even if they dislike vigorous exercise or previously were discouraged because of the difficulty in adhering to a program of vigorous exercise.

Major Conclusions of the Surgeon General's Report

- People of all ages, both male and female, benefit from regular physical activity.

- Significant health benefits can be obtained by including a moderate amount of physical activity (e.g., 30 minutes of brisk walking or raking leaves, 15 minutes of running, or 45 minutes of playing volleyball) on most, if not all, days of the week. Through a modest increase in daily activity, most Americans can improve their health and quality of life.

- Additional health benefits can be gained through greater amounts of physical activity. People who can maintain a regular regimen of activity that is of longer duration or of more vigorous intensity are likely to derive the greater benefit.

- Physical activity reduces the risk of premature mortality in general and of coronary heart disease, hypertension, colon cancer, and diabetes mellitus, in particular. Physical activity also improves mental health and is important for the health of muscles, bones, and joints.

- More than 60% of American adults are not regularly physically active. In fact, 25% of all adults are not active at all.

- Nearly half of American youths 12–21 years of age are not vigorously active on a regular basis. Moreover, physical activity declines dramatically during adolescence.

- Daily enrollment in physical education classes has declined among high school students from 42% in 1991 to 25% in 1995.

- Research on understanding and promoting physical activity is at an early stage, but some interventions to promote physical activity through schools, worksites, and health care settings have been evaluated and found to be successful.

There is increasing agreement from the ACSM/CDC statement, the NIH Consensus Conference, and now the *Surgeon General's Report* concerning what physical activity should be recommended to

---

"Many Americans may be surprised at the extent and strength of the evidence linking physical activity to numerous health improvements. Most significantly, regular physical activity greatly reduces the risk of dying from coronary heart disease, the leading cause of death in the United States. Physical activity also reduces the risk of developing diabetes, hypertension, and colon cancer, enhances mental health, fosters healthy muscles, bones and joints, and helps maintain function and preserves independence in older adults."

Philip R. Lee,
Assistant Secretary for Health

David Satcher, Director,
Centers for Disease Control and Prevention

---

enhance health and fitness. It is a two-level recommendation. First, *sedentary* individuals can realize major health gains by including regular, moderate activity in their lives. Next, individuals who already include moderate activity in their daily lives can see additional health and fitness improvement if they increase the duration of their moderate activity and/or include vigorous activities 3–5 days per week.

WHAT DOES THE REPORT SAY ABOUT THE EVOLUTION OF THE STUDY OF PHYSICAL ACTIVITY AS IT RELATES TO HEALTH?
(Chapter 2)

Chapter 2 offers a historical perspective tracing the importance of physical health from Greco-Roman times to the present, including the role of physical activity in Eastern countries. From the 16th century to the early 1900s, concepts were developed in Europe that formed the basis for early American beliefs about exercise and health. Postwar research by prominent physical educators and physicians led to the current epidemiological, descriptive, and experimental research that provides the foundation for this report. This chapter defines terms, describes measurement techniques, and summarizes previous recommendations on physical activity and health.

WHAT DOES THE REPORT SAY ABOUT HOW THE BODY RESPONDS TO PHYSICAL ACTIVITY, BOTH OVER THE SHORT AND THE LONG TERM? *(Chapter 3)*

This chapter provides an overview of how the body responds to an episode of exercise and adapts to exercise training and detraining. The discussion focuses on aerobic or cardiorespiratory endurance exercise (e.g., walking, jogging, running, cycling, swimming, dancing, and in-line skating) and resistance exercise (e.g., strength-developing exercises). It does not address training for speed, agility, or flexibility. In discussing the multiple effects of exercise, this overview orients the reader to the physiologic basis for the relationship between physical activity and health.

WHAT DOES THE REPORT SAY ABOUT THE EFFECTS OF PHYSICAL ACTIVITY ON SPECIFIC HEALTH CONCERNS? *(Chapter 4)*

This chapter examines how physical activity and cardiorespiratory fitness relate to a variety of health problems. The primary focus is on diseases and conditions for which sufficient data exist to evaluate an association with physical activity, the strength of

Conclusions of Chapter 2: Historical Background and Evolution of Physical Activity Recommendations

- Physical activity for better health and well-being has been an important theme throughout much of Western history.

- Public health recommendations have evolved from emphasizing vigorous activity for cardiorespiratory fitness to including the option of moderate levels of activity for numerous health benefits.

- Recommendations from experts agree that for better health, physical activity should be performed regularly. The most recent recommendations advise people of all ages to include a minimum of 30 minutes of physical activity of moderate intensity (such as brisk walking) on most, if not all, days of the week. It is also acknowledged that for most people, greater health benefits can be obtained by engaging in physical activity of more vigorous intensity or of longer duration.

- Experts advise previously sedentary people embarking on a physical activity program to start with short durations of moderate-intensity activity and gradually increase the duration or intensity until the goal is reached.

- Experts advise consulting with a physician before beginning a new physical activity program for people with chronic diseases, such as cardiovascular disease and diabetes mellitus, or for those who are at high risk for these diseases. Experts also advise men over age 40 and women over age 50 to consult a physician before they begin a vigorous activity program.

- Recent recommendations from experts also suggest that cardiorespiratory endurance activity should be supplemented with strength-developing exercises at least twice per week for adults, in order to improve musculoskeletal health, maintain independence in performing the activities of daily life, and reduce the risk of falling.

Conclusions of Chapter 3: Physiologic Responses and Long-Term Adaptations to Exercise

- Physical activity has numerous beneficial physiologic effects. Most widely appreciated are its effects on the cardiovascular and musculoskeletal systems, but benefits on the functioning of metabolic, endocrine, and immune systems are also considerable.

- Many of the beneficial effects of exercise training—from both endurance and resistance activities—diminish within two weeks if physical activity is substantially reduced, and effects disappear within two to eight months if physical activity is not resumed.

- People of all ages, both male and female, undergo beneficial physiologic adaptations to physical activity.

such relationships, and their potential biologic mechanisms. Much of the research summarized is based on studies that had only white men as participants. It remains to be clarified whether the relationships described here are the same for women, racial and ethnic minorities, and people with disabilities.

The findings are based on studies comparing activity levels of people who have or develop diseases and those who do not; studies that follow populations forward in time to observe how physical activity habits affect disease occurrence or death; case-control studies that compare groups of people who have a disease with those who do not; cross-sectional studies that assess the association between physical activity and disease at the same point in time; and clinical trials that attempt to alter physical activity patterns and assess whether disease occurrence is modified as a result.

Many of these topics are discussed in other papers in this book including health benefits of activity related to children, adolescents and women, obesity and weight control, low back function, cancer, and osteoporosis, to name a few.

Conclusions of Chapter 4: The Effects of Physical Activity on Health and Disease

Overall Mortality

1. Higher levels of regular physical activity are associated with lower mortality rates for both older and younger adults.

2. Even those who are moderately active on a regular basis have lower mortality rates than those who are least active.

Cardiovascular Diseases

1. Regular physical activity or cardiorespiratory fitness decreases the risk of cardiovascular disease mortality in general and of coronary heart disease mortality in particular. Existing data are not conclusive regarding a relationship between physical activity and stroke.

2. The level of decreased risk of coronary heart disease attributable to regular physical activity is similar to that of other lifestyle factors, such as keeping free from cigarette smoking.

3. Regular physical activity prevents or delays the development of high blood pressure, and exercise reduces blood pressure in people with hypertension.

Cancer

1. Regular physical activity is associated with a decreased risk of colon cancer.   *(continued)*

2. There is no association between physical activity and rectal cancer. Data are too sparse to draw conclusions regarding a relationship between physical activity and endometrial, ovarian, or testicular cancers.

3. Despite numerous studies on the subject, existing data are inconsistent regarding an association between physical activity and breast or prostate cancers.

Non–Insulin-Dependent Diabetes Mellitus

1. Regular physical activity lowers the risk of developing non-insulin-dependent diabetes mellitus.

Osteoarthritis

1. Regular physical activity is necessary for maintaining normal muscle strength, joint structure, and joint function. In the range recommended for health, physical activity is not associated with joint damage or development of osteoarthritis and may be beneficial for many people with arthritis.

2. Competitive athletics may be associated with the development of osteoarthritis later in life, but sports-related injuries are the likely cause.

Osteoporosis

1. Weight-bearing physical activity is essential for normal skeletal development during childhood and adolescence and for achieving and maintaining peak bone mass in young adults.

2. It is unclear whether resistance- or endurance-type physical activity can reduce the accelerated rate of bone loss in postmenopausal women in the absence of estrogen replacement therapy.

Falling

1. There is promising evidence that strength training and other forms of exercise in older adults preserve the ability to maintain independent living status and reduce the risk of falling.

Obesity

1. Low levels of activity, resulting in fewer kilocalories used than consumed, contribute to the high prevalence of obesity in the United States.

2. Physical activity may favorably affect body fat distribution.

Mental Health

1. Physical activity appears to relieve symptoms of depression and anxiety and improve mood.

2. Regular physical activity may reduce the risk of developing depression, although further research is needed on this topic.

Health-Related Quality of Life

1. Physical activity appears to improve health-related quality of life by enhancing psychological well-being and by improving physical functioning in persons compromised by poor health.

Adverse Effects

1. Most musculoskeletal injuries related to physical activity are believed to be preventable by gradually working up to a desired level of activity and by avoiding excessive amounts of activity.

2. Serious cardiovascular events can occur with physical exertion, but the net effect of regular physical activity is a lower risk of mortality from cardiovascular disease.

"Because physical activity is so directly related to preventing disease and premature death and to maintaining a high quality of life, we must accord it the same level of attention that we give other public health practices that affect the entire nation."

Audrey F. Manley, Surgeon General (Acting)

WHAT DOES THE REPORT SAY ABOUT PATTERNS AND TRENDS IN ACTIVITY AMONG AMERICANS? *(Chapter 5)*

This chapter documents patterns and trends of reported leisure-time physical activity of adults and adolescents in the United States and compares the findings to the goals set by *Healthy People 2000,* the national goals for disease prevention and health promotion. The information is based on cross-sectional data from national- and state-based surveillance systems sponsored by CDC that track health behaviors, including leisure-time physical activity.

WHAT DOES THE REPORT SAY ABOUT PROMOTING PHYSICAL ACTIVITY AND UNDERSTANDING WHY PEOPLE ARE ACTIVE OR SEDENTARY? *(Chapter 6)*

As the benefits of moderate, regular physical activity have become more widely recognized, the need to find ways to promote this healthful behavior has become increasingly important. Because theories and models of human behavior can guide the development and refinement of intervention efforts, various behavioral and social science theories and

Conclusions of Chapter 5: Patterns and Trends in Physical Activity

Adults

1. Approximately 15% of U.S. adults engage regularly (3 times a week for at least 20 minutes) in vigorous physical activity during leisure time.
2. Approximately 22% of adults engage regularly (5 times a week for at least 30 minutes) in sustained physical activity of any intensity during leisure time.
3. About 25% of adults report no physical activity at all in their leisure time.
4. Physical inactivity is more prevalent among women than men, among blacks and Hispanics than whites, among older than younger adults, and among the less affluent than the more affluent.
5. The most popular leisure-time physical activities among adults are walking and gardening or yardwork.

Adolescents and Young Adults

1. Only about one-half of U.S. young people (ages 12–21 years) regularly participate in vigorous physical activity. One-fourth report no vigorous physical activity.
2. Approximately one-fourth of young people walk or bicycle (i.e., engage in light to moderate activity) nearly every day.
3. About 14% of young people report no recent vigorous or light-to-moderate physical activity. This indicator of inactivity is higher among females than males and among black females than white females.
4. Males are more likely than females to participate in vigorous physical activity, strengthening activities, and walking or bicycling.
5. Participation in all types of physical activity declines strikingly as age or grade in school increases.
6. Among high school students, enrollment in physical education remained unchanged during the first half of the 1990s. However, daily attendance in physical education declined from approximately 42% to 25%.
7. The percentage of high school students who were enrolled in physical education and who reported being physically active for at least 20 minutes in physical education classes declined from approximately 81% to 70% during the first half of this decade.
8. Only 19% of all high school students report being physically active for 20 minutes or more in daily physical education classes.

Conclusions of Chapter 6: Understanding and Promoting Physical Activity

1. Consistent influences on physical activity patterns among adults and young people include confidence in one's ability to engage in regular physical activity (e.g., self-efficacy), enjoyment of physical activity, support from others, positive beliefs concerning the benefits of physical activity, and lack of perceived barriers to being physically active.

2. For adults, some interventions have been successful in increasing physical activity in communities, worksites, and health care settings, and at home.

3. Interventions targeting physical education in elementary school can substantially increase the amount of time students spend being physically active in physical education class.

models that have been used to guide much of the research on physical activity are described. This chapter reviews factors influencing physical activity and describes research methods to improve participation in regular physical activity among children, adolescents, and adults. To put in perspective the difficulty of increasing individual participation in physical activity, the chapter examines societal barriers to engaging in physical activities and describes existing resources that can increase opportunities for activity.

The *Surgeon General's Report* clearly states that a moderate amount of physical activity on a regular basis can improve one's health and quality of life. A moderate amount of physical activity is roughly equivalent to physical activity that uses approximately 150 calories of energy per day or 1,000 calories per week.

Fortunately, as the following table shows, moderate physical activity can be achieved in a variety of ways. Individuals can select activities that they can fit into their daily routine and enjoy throughout their lives.

COMMENTS FROM THE PRESIDENT'S COUNCIL ON PHYSICAL FITNESS AND SPORTS

Since its establishment in 1956, the PCPFS has promoted physical activity, fitness, and sports for all Americans. The President's Council has held physical activity and fitness clinics, implemented programs that reach millions of individuals each year, conducted extensive public service advertising campaigns, and provided grassroots support for educators, parents, and community leaders. Based on this history and experience in helping our nation become more physically active, the PCPFS offers the following:

Parents. What children do when they are young greatly influences what they do when they grow older. Be active with your children. Be active yourself—children model what they see. Be involved in school and community programs that promote activity. Maintain your interest when your children become teens. Encourage children and teens to do active work around home, to walk more, and to be active as part of their normal lifestyle. Plan special family events that involve physical activity.

School boards and superintendents. Just as many employers now recognize the importance of corporate fitness and wellness programs, school officials are beginning to realize that *their* teachers, staff, and students all can benefit from physical activity. Schools need scheduled time in which employees and students can be active. As worksite programs have demonstrated, giving workers time off for physical activity results in fewer absences, increased productivity, and reduced health care costs. *Support daily, quality physical education in all schools.* Recess in elementary schools, physical activity breaks in schools, fitness facilities in schools, and activity opportunities before or after school are essential if lifetime activity is to become a reality. School administrators and school board officials must monitor programs to ensure quality programs.

Examples of Activities Expending 150 Calories

LESS VIGOROUS, MORE TIME

Washing and waxing a car for 45–60 minutes

Washing windows or floors for 45–60 minutes

Playing volleyball for 45 minutes

Playing touch football for 30–45 minutes

Gardening for 30–45 minutes

Wheeling self in wheelchair for 30–40 minutes

Walking 1³/₄ miles in 35 minutes (20 min/mile)

Basketball (shooting baskets) for 30 minutes

Bicycling 5 miles in 30 minutes

Dancing fast (social) for 30 minutes

Pushing a stroller 1¹/₂ miles in 30 minutes

Raking leaves for 30 minutes

Walking 2 miles in 30 minutes (15 min/mile)

Water aerobics for 30 minutes

Swimming laps for 20 minutes

Wheelchair basketball for 20 minutes

Basketball (playing a game) for 15–20 minutes

Bicycling 4 miles in 15 minutes

Jumping rope for 15 minutes

Running 1¹/₂ miles in 15 minutes (10 min/mile)

Shoveling snow for 15 minutes

Stairwalking for 15 minutes

MORE VIGOROUS, LESS TIME

For people who are unable to set aside a block of time as listed with the activities above, shorter episodes are clearly better than no activity. Both the CDC/ACSM recommendation and the NIH Consensus Conference Statement encourage the accumulation of short bouts of activity throughout the day when longer bouts are not possible.

Youth sport coaches and recreation workers. Youth sports provide children with regular activity and enjoyment. It is important for those who work in these programs to understand that how children are treated today can affect whether they will stay active later in life. Avoid using exercise as punishment—help young people to enjoy physical activity! Make participation fun—not a situation in which criticism is common. Enjoyment and personal success are the keys to a lifetime of activity. Many children drop out of sports in their teens because they lack success or do not enjoy the activities. Modify or create new programs to involve more teens.

Physical education teachers. Develop programs that focus on teaching lifetime activities and self-management skills necessary for an active lifestyle. Programs such as those outlined in the *Surgeon General's Report* are encouraged. Physical education classes should provide for lifetime activity needs for students and be guided by the following points:

1. education need not be a physical training class where students are forced to do regimented activities;
2. classes should encourage out-of-school as well as in-class activity, and
3. at the secondary level, physical education concepts should be taught in a classroom as well as in a gymnasium.

Employers. Worksite fitness and health programs provide benefits for employees and employers. It is to the employers' benefit to find ways they can help employees become more physically active. Quality personnel, activity options, accessibility, and social support are important aspects of motivation to begin and continue activity.

Public officials. There can never be too many public opportunities for physical activity. Biking trails, parks, fitness courses, sidewalks, and swimming pools are facilities that can be provided to promote active lifestyles. Support legislation to promote activity in schools and in the workplace and funding for preventive programs including research related to activity and health.

Physicians and health professionals. Physicians and allied health professionals can play a major role in encouraging patients to become more physically active. All health care givers are encouraged to make activity promotion a part of their regular practice.

Insurance companies. Insurance companies have a unique opportunity to play a major role in improving Americans' health by rewarding active behavior. Offer preventive programs that promote active behavior and consider reducing premiums for physically active individuals.

All Americans. Most of us know that physical activity is good for our health. But many may not know just *how* important regular physical activity is to preventing the development of chronic diseases and improving our quality of life. The *Surgeon General's Report on Physical Activity and Health* makes it clear that some physical activity is better than none—even if it is a moderate amount. We encourage each person to perform daily activity that expends about 150 calories of energy. Find an activity that you enjoy and make it part of your daily plan. If this is too much, start with less activity and do it each day or do the activity several days a week as a starter. *Remember—participating in some activity is better than doing nothing at all—and more is even better!*

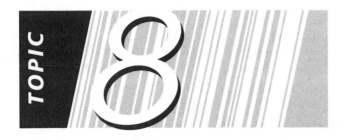

Physical Activity and Women's Health

Christine L. Wells
ARIZONA STATE UNIVERSITY

A NOTE FROM THE EDITORS

Many more women are active today compared to when the first studies of activity in America were conducted. However, as a group, girls and women are still less active than boys and men. Some of this difference in activity between males and females can be explained by the historical disparity in opportunities for females. Since 1972, when Title IX was implemented, more females have become involved in organized sport. We have yet to discover the effects of this increased participation on lifetime activity among females.

Much of the literature concerning health benefits of physical activity is based on studies done primarily with men. Only recently have large-scale studies been initiated to investigate the effects of physical activity on women's health and wellness. Chris Wells, the author of this paper, has been a pioneer in the study of physical activity for women. As you will see, much more research studying girls and women is necessary, but much has been accomplished in recent years. Diseases often thought to be "diseases of men" affect women as well as men.

The evidence now suggests there are many health benefits for females who become regularly involved in physical activity.

This article clearly shows that women, especially women of color, are more likely to be sedentary. Sedentary living increases risk of heart disease, various cancers, hypertension, stroke, and non-insulin diabetes. Controlling body fatness, another factor that is related to increased risk of chronic diseases, is also associated with inactivity. Continued efforts that focus on increasing physical activity among girls and women will reduce the risk of chronic diseases and death.

INTRODUCTION

Healthy People 2000 sets forth the nation's health goals for the next decade (Public Health Service, 1990). One of three primary goals is to reduce health disparities among Americans. This goal addresses reducing preventable disease and death from chronic diseases among racial and ethnic minorities in the United States. Also of importance is

ORIGINALLY PUBLISHED AS SERIES 2, NUMBER 5, OF THE PCPFS *RESEARCH DIGEST.*

"We have failed—in physical education and medicine—to clarify for women the importance of habitual physical activity, physical fitness, and maintenance of 'normal' body weight. We must mount new educational efforts to develop culturally sensitive and ethnic-specific health messages and programs."

the disparity that exists among women as compared to men and among women of different racial and ethnic groups. It is significant that of eight priorities for health promotion and disease prevention, increased physical activity and fitness leads the list. If we could *increase* physical activity and *decrease* obesity, the reasoning goes, much of the premature death, disease, and disability of high-risk populations could be virtually eliminated. But, what is the relationship between physical activity and health in women? Can a strong case be made for increasing physical activity in women as a primary preventive measure for major chronic disease? Will increasing physical activity reduce risk of disease and improve the health and wellness of women? Is physical activity as beneficial for women as research has shown it to be for men?

This paper will address this issue by presenting the growing body of evidence for the beneficial relationships between physical activity (including exercise and physical fitness) and the major chronic diseases in women, with special reference to race and ethnicity. It will be evident that American women need to make significant lifestyle modifications to alter their health risks, and that health and educational professionals must mount new efforts to develop culturally appropriate and sensitive health programs and educational materials.

But, first, how physically active are American women?

HOW PHYSICALLY ACTIVE ARE AMERICAN WOMEN?

The most current data on habitual physical activity are from the Behavioral Risk Factor Surveillance System (BRFSS), a state-based, random-digit-dialed telephone survey that collects self-reported information from a representative sample of people 18 years of age and older. In 1992, BRFSS data were available from 55,506 women from 48 states and the Dis-

trict of Columbia (Prevalence of recommended levels . . . , 1995). These women were asked about the frequency, duration, and intensity of their leisuretime physical activity (LTPA) during the preceding month. Respondents were categorized as having (1) no LTPA, (2) irregular activity that did *not* meet the recommended criteria for either vigorous physical activity ($\geq$20 minutes per day of vigorous physical activity on $\geq$3 days per week) or the newer moderate activity recommendation (accumulation of >30 minutes per day of moderate activity on $\geq$5 days per week) (Summary Statement, CDC and ACSM, 1993). Only 27.1 % of these women reported participation in recommended activity levels, and 30.2% reported no leisuretime physical activity whatsoever. The prevalence of no LTPA increased with age from 25.6% among women 18 to 34 years to 42.1 % among women over age 65. Racial/ethnic disparity was clearly evident. Black non-Hispanic women were less likely to be active (43.6%) than Hispanic women (40.2%) or white non-Hispanic women (27.6%). Physical inactivity was inversely related to income. Women with $\leq$\$14,999 annual household income were most likely to have no LTPA (40.2%), and women with $\geq$\$50,000 annual income were least likely to have no LTPA (21.2%).

BRFSS data from 1991 and 1992 were combined to increase precision of prevalence estimates for minority populations (Prevalence of selected . . . , 1994). Sedentary lifestyle was defined as reported participation in fewer than three 20-minute sessions of LTPA per week excluding usual job-related physical activity. A sedentary lifestyle was reported most frequently among black women (68%) and least frequently among white women (56%). When racial/ethnic data were further stratified by level of education, the prevalence of sedentary lifestyle varied inversely with education within all five population groups. These data are shown in Table 8.1.

Other estimates of physical activity among American women have been equally low. Caspersen et al. (1986) estimated that 30.2% of American

TABLE 8.1 |||||||| |||||||||||| || ||| ||| || ||||||||||||||||| ||

Prevalence of sedentary lifestyle in U.S. women, by race, ethnicity, and education level. Behavioral risk factor surveillance system, United States, 1991–1992.

Women	White	Black	Hispanic	Native American/ Alaskan Native	Asian/ Pacific Islander
Sedentary Lifestyle	56.4	67.7	61.9	64.1	64.7
Education Level					
<12 years	72.0	78.2	73.6	76.6	68.5
12 years	63.3	70.0	58.2	70.5	70.0
>12 years	48.8	59.5	53.4	49.9	62.4

Adapted from: Prevalence of selected risk factors for chronic disease by education level in racial/ethnic populations—United States, 1991–1992. *Morbidity and Mortality Weekly Report, 43(48),* pp. 895, 897. December 9, 1994.

women were sedentary, 31.3% were irregularly active, 31.5% were regularly active at low levels of intensity, and that only 7% of women were sufficiently active to achieve the 1990 physical activity objectives for the nation. Ford et al. (1991) reported that women of higher socioeconomic status (SES) living in Pittsburgh spent significantly more time per week in LTPA, job-related physical activity, and household physical activity than did lower SES women. They estimated that only 7% of lower SES women expended ≥2,000 kcal/week, the energy expenditure linked to lower allcause mortality in college alumni (Paffenbarger et al., 1986), compared to 16.8% of higher SES women.

Under the general assumption that low habitual energy expenditure results in obesity (excessive body fat), another way to estimate population specific physical activity is to assess body weight relative to height. BRFSS data on prevalence of overweight using body mass index (BMI = weight in kilograms divided by height in meters squared) ≥27.3 as the definition of overweight, indicates that black women have the highest prevalence of overweight (37.7%), followed by American Indian/ Alaskan Native women (30.3%), Hispanic women (26.5%), white women (21.7%), and Asian/Pacific Islander women (10.1%) (Prevalence of selected . . . , 1994). In addition, the prevalence of overweight varied inversely with level of education with all five population groups. Except for the low prevalence of overweight in Asian/Pa-

cific Islander women, these values correspond to those of Table 8.1 for sedentary lifestyle.

LEADING CAUSES OF MORTALITY IN AMERICAN WOMEN

In 1990, four of the ten leading causes of death in American women were chronic diseases directly associated with modifiable behavioral factors including physical inactivity or sedentary lifestyle. They were heart disease, certain forms of cancer (specifically, breast and colon cancers), cerebrovascular disease (hypertension and stroke), and non-insulin-dependent diabetes mellitus (NIDDM) (National Center for Health Statistics, 1993). McGinnis and Foege (1993) summarized reports that attributed dietary factors and sedentary lifestyles with 22 to 30% of cardiovascular deaths, 20 to 60% of cancer deaths, and 30% of diabetes deaths. The only more prominent behavioral contributor to mortality than diet and physical inactivity was use of tobacco.

Table 8.2 presents age-adjusted mortality rates for chronic diseases associated with sedentary lifestyle in U.S. women by race and ethnicity. Coronary heart disease (CHD) and cerebrovascular disease (stroke) are the two leading causes of death in all five population groups. Diabetes ranks as the third leading cause of death from chronic disease in black, Hispanic, Native American/Alaskan Native,

TABLE 8.2 |||||||| |||||||||||| || ||| ||| || ||||||||||||||||| ||

Age-adjusted mortality rates*, U.S. women, 1990.

	White	Black	Hispanic	Native American/ Alaskan Native	Asian/ Pacific Islander
CHD	130.2	148.3	147.1	74.5	73.7
Stroke	45.8	68.7	45.4	31.4	43.7
Breast Cancer	29.1	33.4	25.0	12.1	11.9
Colorectal Cancer	17.0	22.9	15.0	9.7	9.9
Diabetes	14.8	37.1	27.6	1.0	11.8

*Rate per 100,000 persons adjusted to the 1980 standard U.S. population.

Adapted from: Centers for Disease Control and Prevention (1994). *Chronic Disease in Minority Populations,* pp. C-3–C-4, Atlanta, GA: Centers for Disease Control and Prevention.

TABLE 8.3 ▌▌▐▐▐▌▌ ▐▐▌▌▌▌▐▌ ▌▐ ▌▌▐▌ ▐▌▐ ▌▌ ▌▐▐▌▐▐▌▐▐▌▐▐▌ ▐▌
Age-adjusted prevalence* of chronic disease, U.S. women, 1986–1990.

	White	Black	Hispanic	Native American/ Alaskan Native	Asian/ Pacific Islander
Hypertension	10.96	19.73	10.55	13.82	8.35
Diabetes	2.36	4.89	3.53	5.04	2.38
Coronary Heart Disease	1.83	1.42	3.53	n.a.	n.a.
Stroke	0.98	1.20	1.10	n.a.	n.a.

*Per 100,000.

Adapted from: Centers for Disease Control and Prevention (1994). *Chronic Disease in Minority Populations*, Atlanta, GA: Centers for Disease Control and Prevention.

and Asian/Pacific Islander women (exceeding death rates from lung cancer, breast cancer, chronic obstructive pulmonary disease, and colorectal cancer) (Centers for Disease Control, 1994).

Morbidity data correspond closely to mortality data. Table 8.3 provides age-adjusted prevalence of chronic disease in U.S. women between 1986 and 1990. Health disparities among racial/ethnic groups are evident with exceedingly high morbidity from chronic diseases that are major causes of death among black, Hispanic, and Native American/Alaskan Native women compared to white and Asian/Pacific Islander women.

The remainder of this paper will describe evidence linking sedentary lifestyle/physical inactivity with diseases of the heart, hypertension and stroke, breast and colorectal cancer, and non-insulin-dependent diabetes mellitus.

PHYSICAL INACTIVITY AND DISEASES OF THE HEART IN WOMEN

According to the American Heart Association, in 1991, 51.8% of all deaths from "total cardiovascular diseases" occurred in women (American Heart Association, 1994). The National Heart, Lung, and Blood Institute (Public Health Service, 1992) reports that one in ten women 45 to 64 years of age has some form of heart disease, and that this increases to one in four in women over age 65. Major modifiable risk factors include smoking, high blood cholesterol,

high blood pressure, and physical inactivity. The following discussion will exclude smoking.

Physical activity and blood cholesterol in women. A blood lipid profile that places an individual at risk consists of elevated total cholesterol (TC), elevated low-density lipoprotein-cholesterol (LDL-C), and elevated triglycerides (TG). High levels of high-density lipoprotein-cholesterol (HDL-C) are considered protective from CHD. Women generally have higher HDL-C and lower LDL-C values than men prior to menopause. This is attributed to estrogen, which interferes with the uptake of LDL-C in arterial walls. Following menopause, HDL-C values decline, LDL-C values increase, and TC values increase, sometimes well above those of age-matched men.

Following a meta-analysis to examine the effect of exercise training on serum lipids in women, Lokey and Tran (1989) concluded that training was associated with lower TC, TG, and TC/HDL-C, but not to changes in HDL-C or LDL-C. The average age of the subjects was 29.5 years, and the women with the most atherogenic lipid profiles benefited the most. In 20- to 40-year-old women, 24 weeks of walking yielded an increase in HDL-C independent of walking intensity (Duncan et al., 1991). In the Healthy Women's Study, a longitudinal study that is following originally premenopausal women through menopause, women with higher physical activity had the least age-related weight gain and the least decline in HDL-C (Owens et al., 1992). At the beginning of the study, only women reporting >2000 kcal/week energy expenditure had significantly better profiles for TC, TG, LDL-C, and HDL_2-C (Owens et al., 1990).

In their review, Shoenhair and Wells (1995) concluded that cross-sectional data strongly support an inverse relationship between current physical fitness and TC, TG, TC/HDL-C, and HDL-C/LDL-C. HDL-C values appear to be elevated in only the most highly fit women. Pre- and postmenopausal athletes have less atherogenic lipid profiles than sedentary or less active women matched for age and menopausal status (Rainville & Vaccaro, 1984; Harting et al., 1984; Stevenson et al., 1995).

Physical activity and blood pressure in women. In the Healthy Women's Study, systolic blood pressure was lower in women expending >500 kcal per week, and diastolic blood pressure was lower in those expending >1000 kcal/week compared to sedentary women (Owens et al., 1990). In the Stanford Community Health Survey, lower diastolic blood pressure was associated with both vigorous exercise (Sallis et al., 1986a) and moderate intensity exercise (Sallis et al., 1986b). In 1991, Reaven et al. reported a significant inverse relationship between physical activity and blood pressure in women. They reported that the most active women had systolic blood pressures 9–24 mmHg lower and diastolic blood pressures 3–13 mmHg lower than the least active women after accounting for differences in body mass index.

A strong relationship also appears to exist between physical fitness and blood pressure in women. In the Aerobics Center Longitudinal Study, Gibbons et al. (1983) reported that cardiovascular fitness was independently associated with lower blood pressure. In Canadian women, blood pressure was significantly lower in subjects with the highest fitness classification (Jette et al., 1992).

Physical inactivity and cardiovascular disease in women.

Very few studies have been completed on physical inactivity and CVD in American women (for an extensive review including international literature, see Schoenhair & Wells, 1995). In a homogeneous population of 17,000 Seventh-Day Adventist women, a population at relatively low risk for CVD, occupational and leisuretime activity was combined and subjects were grouped into three activity classifications. A strong inverse relationship was found between physical activity and CHD mortality. Relative risk ratios for the "high," "moderate," and "low" activity groups were .41, .61, and 1.0, respectively (Fraser et al., 1992). After 24 years of observation, an active lifestyle lowered the age-adjusted incidence of CHD and myocardial infarction in Framingham women by a factor of 2.5 (Kannel & Sorlie, 1979).

In a classic prospective study of allcause mortality in the predominantly white, upper SES population of the Aerobics Center Longitudinal Study, Blair et al. (1989) reported a strong inverse relationship between cardiorespiratory fitness and death from cardiovascular disease. Women in the lowest quintile of physical fitness had an age-adjusted death rate from cardiovascular disease of 7.4 (per 10,000 person-years) compared to 2.9 and 0.8 for women in fitness groups 2–3 and 4–5. Women in the lowest fitness category had an age-adjusted relative risk of 8.0 when compared with women in fitness quintiles 4 and 5.

In summary, there is strong observational and experimental evidence that physical inactivity plays a significant role in the development of cardiovascular disease in women, and that habitual physical activity and at least a moderate level of cardiorespiratory fitness offers protection from these diseases in women as well as in men.

PHYSICAL INACTIVITY, HYPERTENSION AND STROKE IN WOMEN

Nonfatal stroke is the leading cause of disability among American women. Risk factors for stroke include hypertension, heart disease, and smoking. Approximately two-thirds of all stroke victims have hypertension (HT). Until age 64, HT is more prevalent in men, and thereafter is more prevalent in women (Cowley et al., 1992). There is increasing prevalence of HT with age, and wide disparity among race/ethnic groups ranging from 2% in young white women to 83% in black women over 65 (Public Health Service, 1990, p. 392).

In the subjects originally studied by Gibbons et al. (1983), and followed for one to 12 years, Blair et al. (1984) reported that low physical fitness was an independent contributor to the risk of developing hypertension (RR = 1.52) after controlling for sex, age, baseline blood pressure, baseline body mass index, and follow-up interval. In a related study, lower fitness was significantly related to the increased incidence of nonfatal stroke (Blair et al., 1989).

A strong inverse relationship between LTPA and death from stroke was observed in postmenopausal women (Paganini-Hill et al., 1988). Those who were physically active less than 30 minutes per day had twice the age-adjusted mortality from stroke as women who were active at least one hour per day.

Although there is less research available, it seems clear that habitual physical activity reduces the risk of hypertension in women, and consequently, is a primary preventive measure against stroke.

PHYSICAL INACTIVITY AND BREAST AND COLORECTAL CANCERS IN WOMEN

Data on cancer relative to physical activity have been inconsistent and difficult to interpret because cancer represents not one disease, but many distinct, site-specific diseases. To further complicate the situation, risk factors are specific to each disease. Nevertheless, over the past decade, increasing evidence indicates that physical activity is associated with decreased overall cancer mortality and decreased incidence of specific types of cancers (Sternfeld, 1992; Lee, 1995). The cancer site most frequently studied in relation to physical activity is colon cancer, and findings overwhelmingly support an inverse relationship. The two most likely potential mechanisms by which physical activity may be protective of colon cancer are (1) shortened intestinal transit time, and (2) decreased levels of body fat. Shortened intestinal transit time is thought to decrease the amount of contact between possible carcinogenic substances and intestinal mucosa, but evidence remains controversial on this matter. For several cancers (including colon and breast cancers), high levels of body fat are associated with increased risk.

Most research on physical activity and colon cancer has focused on occupational physical activity in men. Clearly, men with sedentary jobs have increased risk of colon cancer (Sternfeld, 1992). One of the most comprehensive studies that included women was a case-control study of Utah residents that took into account differences in dietary patterns and body weight, confounding factors not usually controlled (Slattery et al., 1988). Comparing both occupational and leisuretime activities, the sedentary individuals of both sexes were at nearly two-fold increased risk for colon cancer.

The relationship between physical activity and breast cancer is less clear, but several studies in American women suggest that risk may be lowered in those who are habitually active. An extensive review of this subject is now available including international studies (Kramer & Wells, 1996). Only studies utilizing American subjects are reviewed here. In 1985, Frisch et al. assessed prevalence of breast cancer in 5,398 former collegiate women athletes and nonathletes from 10 colleges and universities from classes spanning 56 years. A higher percentage of former athletes reported they were currently exercising than nonathletes. Comparing the prevalence of breast cancer between the two groups, the nonathletes had 1.85 times the risk of the former athletes, strong evidence for an inverse

relationship between lifetime physical activity and breast cancer.

From the National Health and Nutrition Examination Survey database (NHANES I), Albanes et al. (1989) examined breast cancer incidence relative to baseline recreational and nonrecreational physical activity levels. After 10 years of follow-up, premenopausal women with high levels of activity were associated with slightly *increased* risk of breast cancer. Among postmenopausal women, however, high physical activity conferred a protective effect.

More recently, Bernstein et al. (1994) studied the *timing* of physical activity relative to estrogen exposure in premenopausal women from Los Angeles County. Using a case-control study design, they report a strong dose response relationship between leisuretime exercise since menarche and decreased risk of breast cancer. Women reporting 3.8 or more hours per week of exercise since menarche had a 50% reduction in breast cancer risk. A 30% reduction was observed in women reporting one to three hours per week of exercise since menarche. A slightly weaker relationship was observed among nulliparous women. The observed benefit of exercise was attributed to reduced exposure to endogenous estrogen subsequent to shorter luteal phases and higher incidence of anovulatory menstrual cycles. An even more recent study (Thune et al., 1996) confirmed the beneficial relationship between physical activity and breast cancer and reported the largest benefits in premenopausal women, the period when age-specific mortality rates for breast cancer are highest.

High to moderate levels of habitual physical activity may decrease lifetime exposure to endogenous sex hormones in two ways: (1) prior to menopause, high levels of physical activity may delay menarche, decrease the number of ovulatory cycles, and hence reduce exposure to endogenous estrogen (Frisch et al., 1980; Bernstein et al., 1987), and (2) following menopause, maintenance of low levels of adipose tissue may mediate the conversion of androgenic compounds to extraglandular estrogen (Siiteri, 1987; Hershcopf & Bradlow, 1987).

In summary, lifetime physical activity appears to reduce the risk of colon cancer and breast cancer in white women, but there is an obvious need to incorporate minority women into future research on these topics.

PHYSICAL INACTIVITY AND NON–INSULIN-DEPENDENT DIABETES MELLITUS IN WOMEN

About 14 million Americans have diabetes, with 95% having non–insulin-dependent diabetes mellitus (NIDDM). Tables 8.2 and 8.3 indicate that certain minority women have exceedingly high mortality and prevalence rates from this adult-onset chronic disease. Diabetes is a leading cause of death in women, and a leading cause of adult blindness, leg and foot amputations, circulatory disease, kidney failure, and birth defects. In NIDDM, the pancreas may secrete insulin, but cells and tissues of the body are insulin resistant, and consequently, patients are characterized by high levels of insulin (hyperinsulinemia) and blood glucose (hyperglycemia). Those at highest risk for NIDDM include the overweight or obese, and particularly, those over 40 years of age (American Diabetes Association, 1992).

According to the American Diabetes Association (1990), an appropriate exercise program should be an adjunct to diet and/or drug therapy to improve glycemic control, reduce cardiovascular risk factors, and increase psychological wellbeing in women with NIDDM. Individuals who are most likely to respond favorably are those with moderate glucose intolerance and hyperinsulinemia. Unfortunately, findings from the 1990 National Health Interview Survey (Ford & Herman, 1995) indicate that women with diabetes are less likely to report exercising regularly than women without diabetes. A comparison of the effects of exercise on insulin sensitivity in women with NIDDM recently revealed that low intensity exercise was as effective as high intensity exercise in enhancing insulin sensitivity (Braun et al., 1995). Duration of the two exercise regimes was adjusted so that energy expenditure was equal. This is important because obesity, diabetic complications, and general lack of physical fitness are common in women with glucose intolerance or NIDDM. Prescription of low intensity exercise is no doubt safer and more practicable, especially for older women with NIDDM. A recent community-based study (San Luis Valley Diabetes Study) also demonstrated this. Higher levels of physical activity were associated with improved insulin action in individuals with impaired glucose tolerance (Regensteiner et

al., 1995), further supporting the concept that habitual physical activity reduces incidence of impaired glucose tolerance and lowers morbidity from NIDDM.

Two studies directly indicate that habitual physical activity in women is a promising approach to the primary prevention of NIDDM. In one, Frisch and colleagues (1986) report a significantly lower prevalence of diabetes among every age group (20 to more than 70 years) in 5,398 women who engaged in long-term athletic activity compared to their nonathletic classmates. In the other investigation, reduced incidence of NIDDM among women who exercised regularly was observed in a prospective cohort of 87,253 women 34 to 59 years (Manson et al., 1991).

In summary, regular physical activity has an important role in both treatment and prevention of NIDDM through its association with reduced body weight, and its independent effects on insulin sensitivity and glucose tolerance.

OBESITY, MORBIDITY, AND MORTALITY IN WOMEN

Data from nationally representative cross-sectional surveys reveal that prevalence of overweight in U.S. women has increased in all age groups since the 1960s (Kuczmarski et al., 1994). These data also indicate that the prevalence of obesity is substantially higher in black, Hispanic, Pacific Islander, and Native American and Alaskan Native women than in white women (Kuczmarski et al., 1994; Kumanyika, 1993). Altogether, about 32 million American women are overweight or obese. In addition, the particularly high-risk upper-body fat distribution (central adiposity) occurs to a greater extent in some minority populations than in whites (Kumanyika, 1993).

High body weight or weight gain since age 18 in women has been associated with coronary heart disease (Willett et al., 1995), allcause mortality (Manson et al., 1995), and hyperinsulinemia (fasting insulin and insulin following glucose load) (Wing et al., 1992). Lowest mortality among U.S. women was observed in those who weighed at least 15% less than the U.S. average for women of similar age and whose weight had been stable since early adulthood (Manson et al., 1995).

Clearly, high body weight and body fat in women is related to increased incidence of coronary heart disease, hypertension, NIDDM, breast cancer, and allcause mortality. Greater attention to prevention and treatment of obesity in minority populations may help to address critical health issues in American women (St Jeor, 1993).

CONCLUSION

There is an obvious national shortfall in closing the gap in health disparities among Americans— especially, American women. We have failed—in physical education and sport, and in medicine—to clarify the importance of habitual physical activity, physical fitness, and maintenance of "normal" body weight to good health. One major reason is that we have attempted to use health messages, programs, and approaches based on white, middle-class values and culture, and then wondered why they were not enthusiastically embraced. Research and educational efforts must focus on conceptually based programs in schools and communities that are culturally sensitive and ethnic-specific.

REFERENCES

Albanes, D., Blair, A., and Taylor, P.R. (1989). Physical activity and risk of cancer in the NHANES I population. *American Journal of Public Health, 79,* 744–750.

American Diabetes Association. (1992). Alexandria, VA.

American Diabetes Association. (1990). Diabetes mellitus and exercise. Position statement of the American Diabetes Association. *Diabetes Care, 13,* 804–805.

American Heart Association. (1994). *Heart and stroke facts: 1995 statistical supplement.* Dallas, TX: American Health Association.

Bernstein, L., Henderson, B.E., Hanisch, R., Sullivan-Halley, J., & Ross, R.K. (1994). Physical exercise and risk of breast cancer in young women. *Journal of the National Cancer Institute, 86,* 1403–1408.

Bernstein., L., Ross, R.K., Lobo, R.A., Hanisch, R., Krailo, M.D., & Henderson, B.E. (1987). The effects of moderate physical activity on menstrual cycle patterns in adolescence: Implications for breast cancer prevention. *British Journal of Cancer, 55,* 681–685.

Blair, S.N., Goodyear, N.N., Cooper, K.H., & Smith, M. (1984). Physical fitness and incidence of hypertension in healthy normotensive men and women. *Journal of the American Medical Association, 252,* 487–490.

Blair, S.N., Kohl, H.W., Paffenbarger, R.S., Clark, D.G., Cooper, K.H., & Gibbons, L.W. (1989). Physical fitness and all-cause mortality: A prospective study of healthy men and women. *Journal of the American Medical Association, 262,* 2395–2401.

Braun, B., Zimmermann, M.B., & Kretchmer, N. (1995). Effects of exercise intensity on insulin sensitivity in women with non-insulin-dependent diabetes mellitus. *Journal of Applied Physiology, 78,* 3000–3036.

Caspersen, C.J., Christenson, G.M., & Pollard, R.A. (1986). Status of the 1990 physical fitness and exercise objectives—evidence from NHIS 1995. *Public Health Reports, 101,* 587–592.

Centers for Disease Control and Prevention. (1994). *Chronic disease in minority populations.* Atlanta: Centers for Disease Control and Prevention.

Cowley, A.W., Jr., Dzau, V., Buttrick, P., Cooke, J., Devereux, R.B., Grines, C.L., Haidet, G.C., & Thames, M.C. (1992). Working group on noncoronary cardiovascular disease and exercise in women. *Medicine and Science in Sports and Exercise, 24,* S277–S287.

Duncan, J.J., Gordon, N.F., & Scott, C.B. (1991). Women walking for health and fitness: How much is enough? *Journal of the American Medical Association, 266,* 3295–3299.

Ford, E.S., & Herman, W.H. (1995). Leisure-time physical activity patterns in the U.S. diabetic population. *Diabetes Care, 18,* 27–33.

Ford, E.S., Merritt, R.K., Heath, G.W., Rowell, K.E., Washburn, R.A., Kriska, A., & Heile, G. (1991). Physical activity behaviors in lower and higher socioeconomic status populations. *American Journal of Epidemiology, 133,* 1246–1256.

Fraser, G.E., Strahan, T.M., Sabate, J., Beeson, W.L., & Kissinger, D. (1992). Effects of traditional coronary risk factors on rates of incident coronary events in a low-risk population: The Adventist Health Study. *Circulation, 86,* 406–413.

Frisch, R.E., Wyshak, G., Albright, N.L., Albright, T.E., Schiff, I., Jones, K.P., Witschi, J., Shiang, E., Koff, E., & Marguglio, M. (1985). Lower prevalence of breast cancer and cancers of the reproductive system among former college athletes compared to nonathletes. *British Journal of Cancer, 52,* 885–891.

Frisch, R.E., Wyshak, G., Albright T.E., Albright, N.L., & Schiff, I. (1986). Lower prevalence of diabetes in female former college athletes compared with nonathletes. *Diabetes, 35,* 1101–1105.

Frisch, R.E., Wyshak, G., & Vincent, L. (1980). Delayed menarche and amenorrhea in ballet dancers. *New England Journal of Medicine, 303,* 17–19.

Gibbons, L.W., Blair, S.N., Cooper, K.H., & Smith, M. (1983). Association between coronary heart disease risk factors and physical fitness in healthy adult women. *Circulation, 67,* 977–983.

Harting, G.H., Moore, C.E., Mitchell, R., & Kappus, C.M. (1984). Relationship of menopausal status and exercise level to HDL cholesterol in women. *Experimental and Aging Research, 10,* 13–18.

Hershcopf, R.J., & Bradlow, H.L. (1987). Obesity, diet, endogenous estrogens, and the risk of hormone-sensitive cancer. *American Journal of Clinical Nutrition, 45,* 283–289.

Jette, M., Sidney, K., Quenneville, J., & Landry, F. (1992). Relation between cardiorespiratory fitness and selected risk factors for coronary heart disease in a population of Canadian men and women. *Canadian Medical Association Journal, 146,* 1353–1360.

Kannel, W.B., & Sodie, R. (1979). Some health benefits of physical activity: The Framingham study. *Archives of Internal Medicine, 139,* 857–861.

Kramer, M.M., & Wells, C.L. (1996). Does physical activity reduce risk of estrogen-dependent cancer in women? A review. *Medicine and Science in Sports and Exercise, 28,* 322–334.

Kuczmarski, R J., Flegal, K.M., Campbell, S.M., & Johnson, C.L. (1994). Increasing prevalence of overweight among US adults: The National Health and Nutrition Examination Surveys, 1960 to 1991. *Journal of the American Medical Association, 272,* 205–211.

Kumanyika, S.K. (1993). Special issues regarding obesity in minority populations. *Annals of Internal Medicine, 119,* 650–654.

Lee, I. (1995). Physical activity and cancer. *PCPFS Physical Activity and Fitness Research Digest, 2(2).* Washington, DC: PCPFS.

Lokey, E.A., & Tran, Z.V. (1989). Effects of exercise training on serum lipid and lipoprotein concentrations in women: A meta-analysis. *International Journal of Sports Medicine, 10,* 424–429.

Manson, J.E., Rimm, E.B., Stampfer, M.J., Colditz, G.A., Willett, W.C., Krolemki, A.S., Rosner, B., Hennekens, C.H., & Speizer, F.E. (1991). Physical activity and incidence of non-insulin-dependent diabetes mellitus in women. *The Lancet, 338,* 774–778.

Manson, J.E., Willett, W.C., Stampfer, M.J., Colditz, G.A., Hunter, D.J., Hankinson, S.E., Hennekens, C.H., & Speizer, F.E. (1995). Body weight and mortality among women. *New England Journal of Medicine, 333,* 677–685.

McGinnis, J.M., & Foege, W.H. (1993). Actual causes of death in the United States. *Journal of the American Medical Association, 270,* 2207–2212.

National Center for Health Statistics. (1990). Advance Report of Final Mortality Statistics, 1990. Hyattsville, MD: Department of Health and Human Services, 1993. *Monthly Vital Statistics Report, 41(7).*

Owens, J.F., Matthews, K.A., Wing, R.R., & Kuller, L.H. (1990). Physical activity and cardiovascular risk: A cross-sectional study of middle-aged premenopausal women. *Preventive Medicine, 19,* 147–157.

Owens, J.F., Matthews, K.A., Wing, R.R., & Kuller, L.H. (1992). Can physical activity mitigate the effects of aging in middle age women? *Circulation, 85,* 1265–1270.

Paffenbarger, R.S., Jr., Hyde, R.T., Wing, A.K., & Hsieh, C.C. (1986). Physical activity, allcause mortality and longevity of college alumni. *New England Journal of Medicine, 314,* 605–613.

Pagagini-Hill, A., Ross, R.K., & Henderson, B.E. (1988). Postmenopausal estrogen treatment and stroke: A prospective study. *British Medical Journal, 297,* 519–522.

Prevalence of recommended levels of physical activity among women—Behavioral Risk Factor Surveillance System, 1992 (1995). *Morbidity and Mortality Weekly Report, 44(6),* 105–108.

Prevalence of selected risk factors for chronic disease by education level in racial/ethnic populations, United States, 1991–1992 (1994). *Morbidity and Mortality Weekly Report, 43(48),* 894–899.

Public Health Service. (1990) *Healthy people 2000: National heath promotion and disease prevention objectives.* Washington, DC: Department of Health and Human Services. Publication PHS 91-50212.

Public Health Service. (1992). *The healthy heart handbook for women.* National Heart, Lung and Blood Institute, National Institutes of Health, Washington, DC: NIH publication no. 92-2720.

Rainville, S., & Vaccaro, P. (1984). The effects of menopause and training on serum lipids. *International Journal of Sports Medicine, 5,* 137–141.

Reaven, R.D., Barrett-Connor, E., & Edelstein, S. (1991). Relation between leisure-time physical activity and blood pressure in older women. *Circulation, 83,* 559–565.

Regensteiner, J.G., Shetterly, S.M., Mayer, E.J., Eckel, R.H., Haskell, W.L., Baxter, J., & Hamman, R.F. (1995). Relationship between habitual physical activity and insulin area among individuals with impaired glucose tolerance: The San Luis Valley Diabetes Study. *Diabetes Care, 18,* 490–497.

Sallis, J.F., Haskell, W.L., Wood, P.D., Fortmann, S.P., & Vranizan, K.M. (1986a). Vigorous physical activity and cardiovascular risk factors in young adults. *Journal of Chronic Diseases, 39,* 115–120.

Sallis, J.F., Haskell, W.L., Fortmann, S.P., Wood, P.D., & Vranizan, K.M. (1986b). Moderate-intensity physical activity and cardiovascular risk factors: The Stanford Five-City Project. *Preventive Medicine, 15,* 561–568.

Shoenhair, C.L., & Wells, C.L. (1995). Women, physical activity, and coronary heart disease: A review. *Medicine, Exercise, Nutrition, Health, 4(4),* 200.

Siiteri, P.K. (1987). Adipose tissue as a source of hormones. *American Journal of Clinical Nutrition, 45,* 277–282.

Slattery, M.L., Schumacher, M.C., Smith, K.R., West, D.W., & Abd-Elghany, N. (1988). Physical activity, diet and risk of colon cancer in Utah. *American Journal of Epidemiology, 128,* 989–999.

St Jeor, S.T. (1993). The role of weight management in the health of women. *Journal of the American Dietetic Association, 93,* 1007–1012.

Sternfeld, B. (1992). Cancer and the protective effect of physical activity: The epidemiological evidence. *Medicine and Science in Sports and Exercise, 24,* 1195–1209.

Stevenson, E.T., Davy, K.P., & Seals, D.R. (1995). Hemostatic, metabolic, and androgenic risk factors for coronary heart disease in physically active and less active postmenopausal women. *Arteriosclerosis, Thrombosis, and Vascular Biology, 15,* 23–31.

Summary Statement Workshop on Physical Activity and Public Health. (1993). Centers for Disease Control and Prevention and American College of Sports Medicine. *Sports Medicine Bulletin, 24(4),* 7.

Thune, I., Brenn, T., Lund, E., & Gaard, M. (1996). Physical activity and the risk of breast cancer. *New England Journal of Medicine, 336,* 1269–1275.

Willett, W.C., Manson, J.E., Stampfer, M.J., Colditz, G.A., Rosner, B., Speizer, F.E., & Hennekens, C.H. (1995). Weight, weight change, and coronary heart disease in women: Risk within the "normal" weight range. *Journal of the American Medical Association, 273,* 461–465.

Wing, R.R., Matthews, K.A., Kulter, L.H., Smith, D., Becker, D., Plantinga, P.L., & Meilahn, E.N. (1992). Environmental and familial contributions to insulin levels and change in insulin levels in middle-aged women. *Journal of the American Medical Association, 268,* 1890–1985.

Physical Activity and the Reduction of Risk for Chronic Health Problems

This section covers many of the chronic illnesses and health conditions that are related to a sedentary lifestyle. Unlike the previous section that outlines the general health benefits of activity, this section gives in-depth coverage to specific health problems. William Haskell discusses the role of physical activity in the management of our nation's leading killer, heart disease. Noted epidemiologist, I-Min Lee, discusses the second leading cause of death, cancer. Andrea Kriska provides information about Type II diabetes, while Janet Shaw and Christine Snow review activity and its effect on osteoporosis. Sharon Plowman considers the relationship of physical activity to low back pain, one of the nation's leading medical complaints.

Physical Activity in the Prevention and Management of Coronary Heart Disease

William L. Haskell
STANFORD UNIVERSITY

INTRODUCTION

The concept that a sedentary lifestyle leads to an increase in the clinical manifestations of coronary heart disease (CHD), especially myocardial infarction and sudden death, has become generally accepted by the public and many health professionals. Most often, the idea has been expressed that regular exercise, in conjunction with other risk-reducing behaviors, will help protect against an initial cardiac episode (primary prevention); will aid in the recovery of patients following myocardial infarction, coronary artery bypass surgery, or coronary angioplasty (cardiac rehabilitation); and will reduce the risk of recurrent cardiac events (secondary prevention).

Evidence relating level of habitual exercise to risk of CHD has been derived from a variety of sources including animal studies, clinical impressions, observational surveys of the general population or special groups, and experimental studies in which the exercise of subjects assigned to "treatment" was increased in relation to sedentary control subjects. No one of these studies provides irrefutable evidence of a causal relationship between exercise status and CHD pathology, even

though many sources of information do generally support such a contention. This situation is not unique to our understanding of the preventive role of exercise as it relates to CHD since a similar situation exists for all other "lifestyle" risk factors.

The presentation of information here is designed to provide the scientific basis for making decisions regarding the potential value of exercise in the primary and secondary prevention of CHD. Data on the relationship of exercise to CHD are reviewed, the possible biologic mechanisms by which beneficial effects may occur are summarized, the risks of developing cardiac complications during exercise are briefly discussed, and physical activity guidelines for promoting cardiovascular health are provided.

PHYSICAL ACTIVITY AND THE PRIMARY PREVENTION OF CORONARY HEART DISEASE

During the past half century more than 50 studies have been published reporting on the association between habitual level of physical activity and the

ORIGINALLY PUBLISHED AS SERIES 2, NUMBER 1, OF THE PCPFS *RESEARCH DIGEST*.

> *"Along with stopping smoking, maintaining a physically active lifestyle is one of the least expensive and most productive health behaviors available to the public."*

prevalence or incidence of initial clinical manifestations of CHD, especially myocardial infarction and sudden cardiac death (Berlin & Colditz, 1990; Powell et al., 1987). These studies have included the determination of on-the-job or leisure-time activity in free-living populations of many men and relatively few women with activity classifications based on job category, self-report questionnaires, or interviewer determinations. Manifestations of CHD were established by examination of death certificates, hospital or physician records, questionnaires completed by the subjects or physicians, and medical evaluations conducted by the investigators. Reported activity levels range from daily caloric expenditures exceeding 6,000 kilocalories (kcal) per day in Finnish lumberjacks at one extreme to very sedentary civil servant managers and postal clerks at the other. Studies have been conducted in major industrial environments as well as rural and primate living areas.

As a result of the diverse protocols used in the various studies, including sample-selection procedures, physical activity classification methods, clinical event determination criteria, and statistical treatment of the data, it is not possible to collate the results into a single summary statement or interpretation. However, certain findings, although not universally obtained, occur sufficiently frequently to warrant the formulation of preliminary conclusions to use as a basis for program recommendations and planning future research.

More Active Persons Appear to Be at Lower Risk

The general impression obtained as the result of a comprehensive review of the scientific reports containing data on the primary preventive effect of physical activity is that more active people develop less CHD than their inactive counterparts, and when they do develop CHD, it occurs at a later age and tends to be less severe (Berlin & Colditz, 1990; Powell et al., 1987). The results of the numerous reports are quite variable, with some studies demon-

strating a highly significant beneficial effect of exercise (Lakka et al., 1994; Morris et al., 1980; Paffenbarger, Wing, & Hyde, 1978; Shapiro et al., 1969; Shaper & Wannamethee, 1991), others showing a favorable but nonsignificant trend in favor of the more active (Costas et al., 1978; Salonen, Puska, & Tuomilehto, 1982), and a few early studies showing no difference in CHD rates (Chapman & Massey, 1964; Paul, 1969). Of major importance is the consistent finding that being physically active *does not increase* an individual's overall risk of CHD.

No specific study characteristics can be identified that explain the differences in results among the various studies, but in some cases the physical activity measure is not very accurate or reliable and the activity gradient among the population is quite small (Shapiro et al., 1969). Also, with populations in whom CHD mortality is exceptionally high and in whom major risk factors such as hypercholesterolemia, hypertension, and cigarette smoking are prevalent, even very high levels of physical activity do not appear to exert a major protective effect. Finnish lumberjacks are an example of very physically active individuals in whom CHD risk remains high (Karvonen et al., 1961). It appears that in observational studies that are well designed, the inverse association between activity and CHD mortality is stronger than reported in scientifically less rigorous studies (Powell et al., 1987).

Moderate Amounts of Exercise May Be Protective

A striking feature of many studies demonstrating a reduced CHD risk for more active individuals is that the greatest difference in risk is achieved between those people who do almost nothing and those who perform a moderate amount of exercise on a regular basis. Much smaller differentials in risk are observed when moderately active individuals are compared with the most active persons (Leon et al., 1987; Lakka et al., 1994; Paffenbarger et al., 1993).

The amount of activity, in both intensity and duration, that is associated with a decrease in CHD clinical manifestations varies substantially among the different reports. Several studies have observed significant differences in CHD indicators with quite small differences in habitual activity level at a relatively low intensity (Leon et al., 1987; Kahn, 1963; Shapiro et al., 1969), whereas other authors interpret their data to indicate that a "threshold" of higher intensity or amount of activity is needed in order to obtain a benefit (Cassel et al., 1971; Morris et al., 1980; Paffenbarger, Wing, & Hyde, 1978). The types of activity performed by the more active groups include brisk walking on level or hilly ground, climbing stairs, lifting and carrying light objects, lifting heavy objects, operating machinery or appliances, light and heavy gardening, performing home maintenance or repairs, and participating in active games and sports. The results of several studies, however, indicate that an intensity threshold of approximately 7 kcal/min (e.g., brisk walking, heavy gardening) may exist, with exercise more vigorous than this providing greater protection than a similar amount of less vigorous activity (Cassel et al., 1971; Morris et al., 1990). Of greatest benefit seems to be large muscle dynamic or "aerobic" activity that substantially increases cardiac output with rather small increases in mean arterial blood pressure. Such activity is in contrast to heavy resistance or isometric exercise that substantially increases arterial blood pressure with a relatively small increase in cardiac output. Participation in "physical fitness" or "athletic conditioning" programs contributes little to the more active classification in most observational studies so far reported.

On-the-Job Activity

Most of the initial observations establishing an association between physical activity status and CHD manifestations used on-the-job activity. It is much easier (but likely less accurate) to classify individuals as inactive or active according to their job title or description than it is to obtain self-assessments by interview, questionnaire, or direct observation of job-related or leisure-time activity. The early studies that obtained a difference in CHD rates between inactive and active classifications, such as the reports by Morris on London busmen (Morris et al., 1953), Kahn's observation on Washington, D.C., postal workers (Kahn, 1963) or Taylor's studies on U.S. railroad workers (Taylor et al., 1970) included

job situations in which the major exercise of the more active groups was walking on flat ground, up stairs, or up and down hills. If the more physically active status is responsible for the lower CHD rates in these populations, the intensity threshold for an activity-related benefit is not high. Other on-the-job studies, however, have not found any protective association with activity level until a classification of "heavy work" was obtained (Cassel et al., 1971; Morris et al., 1953; Morris et al., 1990).

The estimated net energy expenditure (above the energy expenditure of the inactive group) associated with a decrease in CHD mortality in the various occupational studies ranges from 300 to 800 kcal/day. The intensity of the activity contributing to this increased energy expenditure includes walking, lifting and carrying objects, farming, and laboring-type jobs. In most cases, the higher-intensity activities (i.e., heavy lifting or carrying) are performed in relatively short bursts throughout the workday with the lower intensities (i.e., walking) being carried out for longer durations.

Leisure-Time Activity

Accurate quantitative assessments of leisure time or non-job activity status are difficult to obtain on samples of the size needed to evaluate the relationship of habitual activity status and CHD clinical events. Various diary and recall techniques have been used, and they all present significant administration and scoring difficulties. However, in the studies that have attempted to quantitate various aspects of non-job activities, several have identified an inverse association between activity status and CHD similar to the relationship reported in the earlier occupational-based studies.

Evidence of some protection possibly being provided by non-job, low-intensity activity on a regular basis was first reported by Rose (1969). He observed that the prevalence of "ischemic-type" resting electrocardiographic (ECG) abnormalities was inversely associated with duration of walking to work among 8,948 executive grade civil service workers in London. Those employees who walked 20 or more minutes to work on a regular basis had one third fewer ECG abnormalities than their counterparts who rode to work. This association could not be accounted for as a result of differences in age, grade of employment, smoking habits, serum cholesterol, or glucose tolerance. Those who walked regularly, however, tended to be a little less overweight.

The relationship of leisure-time activity to CHD mortality among middle-aged male civil servant workers in Britain has been studied using a two-day activity recall procedure (Morris et al., 1980; Morris et al., 1990). Morris and coworkers reported that non-job activity, as assessed by a self-administered 48-hour recall questionnaire completed on a Monday for the preceding Friday and Saturday, was significantly associated with CHD mortality only when activities requiring a peak energy expenditure of 7.5 kcal/min for 30 minutes or longer each day were performed ("vigorous activity"). Lesser amounts of activity appeared to carry no protective benefit. This apparent protective action of "vigorous activity" was not related to plasma total cholesterol, blood pressure, cigarette smoking, or adiposity, and it occurred at all ages from 40 to 69 years.

Paffenbarger and colleagues (1986, 1993) have continued to evaluate the relationship between past and recent physical activity habits and cardiovascular health in Harvard University alumni. Analyses of 572 first heart attacks among 16,936 men between 1962 and 1972 and 1,413 total deaths between 1962 and 1978 showed that it was habitual post-college exercise, not student sports play, that predicted low coronary heart disease risk. They have shown that sedentary alumni who were ex-varsity athletes had high risk while sedentary students who became active in later life seemed to acquire a low risk. These results are similar to several reports of job-related activity and heart disease risk where more physically active jobs early in a career followed by years of sedentary work resulted in higher risk than when the active job was continued throughout a person's career.

The relationship of self-selected leisure-time physical activity (LTPA) to first major CHD events and overall mortality was studied in 12,138 middle-aged men participating in the Multiple Risk Factor Intervention Trial (Leon et al., 1987). Total LTPA over the preceding year was quantitated in mean minutes per day at baseline by questionnaire, with subjects classified into tertiles (low, moderate, and high) based on LTPA distribution. During seven years of follow-up, moderate LTPA was associated with 64% as many fatal CHD events and sudden

deaths, and 73% as many total deaths as low LTPA (p<.01). Mortality rates with high LTPA were similar to those in moderate LTPA; however, combined fatal and nonfatal major CHD events were 20% lower with high as compared with low LTPA (p<.05). These risk differentials persisted after statistical adjustments for possible confounding variables, including other baseline risk factors.

Physical activity at work and in leisure time was studied by questionnaire in a random sample of residents living in Eastern Finland (Salonen, Puska, & Tuomilehto, 1982). The study population consisted of 3,978 men aged 30–59 years and 3,688 women aged 35–59 years. During a seven-year follow-up, low physical activity at work was associated with an increased risk of myocardial infarction, cerebral stroke, and death due to any disease in both men and women, even after controlling for age, cholesterol, diastolic blood pressure, weight and smoking status using a multiple logistic model. The relative risk for myocardial infarction was 1.5 (95% confidence interval = 1.2–2.0) for men and 2.4 (95% confidence interval = 1.5–3.7) for women. Men and women at highest risk were those who reported no vigorous exercise during either work or leisure time while those at lowest risk reported vigorous exercise during both times.

Recently Lakka and colleagues (1994) reported the results of following 1,453 men aged 42 to 60 years for about five years. In the more active third of the men (>2.2 hours per week of activity) the relative risk of a myocardial infarction was 0.31 (95% confidence interval = 0.12 to 0.85; p = 0.02) compared to the least active third. Similar results were obtained when aerobic capacity as determined by maximal oxygen uptake was related to risk of myocardial infarction.

A major criticism of the observational studies that demonstrate a protective effect of exercise is that the differences in CHD rates between active and inactive individuals may be due to less healthy people selecting a less active lifestyle, not that increased activity prevents disease. Such self-selection may account for some of the differences reported; but in several reports, the investigators considered this problem in their data analyses and still found that being physically active was of significant benefit (Kahn, 1963; Paffenbarger, Wing, & Hyde, 1978). Also, Paffenbarger and colleagues (1993) recently reported that an increase in activity from one examination to the next was associated with a lower CHD mortality rate. These results strengthen the argument that it is an increase in activity that causes the reduction in mortality.

PHYSICAL FITNESS AND PRIMARY PREVENTION

Only in the past decade have studies been published that have adequately measured cardiovascular functional capacity or physical fitness on a sample of sufficient size and then followed their clinical status long enough to be able effectively to evaluate the relationship of physical fitness to future CHD or total mortality. If a higher level of habitual activity causes a reduction in cardiovascular morbidity and mortality, then a similar association should be observed with an accurate and reliable measure of fitness.

This issue was examined in a study of 4,276 men, 30 to 69 years of age, who were screened as part of the Lipid Research Clinic's prevalence survey and followed for an average of 8.5 years (Ekelund et al., 1988). Examination at baseline included assessment of conventional coronary risk factors and treadmill exercise testing. The heart rate during submaximal exercise (stage 2 of the Bruce exercise test) and the duration of exercise were used as measures of physical fitness. After adjustment for age and cardiovascular risk factors, a lower level of physical fitness was associated with a higher risk of death from CVD and CHD. The relative risk for death due to CVD for the least fit healthy men versus the most fit healthy men was 3.6 (95% confidence interval = 1.6 to 5.6; p = 0.0004) and for death due to CHD it was 2.8 (95% confidence interval = 1.3 to 6.1; p = 0.007). Highly significant associations were also seen for men who had CVD at their initial evaluation and for all-cause mortality. Thus, a low level of physical fitness is associated with a higher risk of death, especially from CVD and CHD, in men independent of conventional risk factors.

The relationship of physical fitness, as measured by maximal treadmill performance, to all-cause and cause-specific mortality was evaluated in 10,224 men and 3,120 women who had completed comprehensive medical examinations at the Cooper Clinic (Blair et al., 1989). Average follow-up was slightly more than eight years, for a total of 110,482 person-years of observation. There were 240 deaths

in men and 43 deaths in women. Age adjusted all-cause mortality rates declined across physical fitness quintiles from 64.0 per 10,000 person-years in the least-fit men to 18.6 per 10,000 person-years in the most-fit men. Corresponding values for women were 39.5 per 10,000 person-years to 8.5 per 10,000 person-years. These trends remained after statistical adjustments for age, smoking habit, cholesterol level, systolic blood pressure, fasting blood glucose level, parental history of coronary heart disease, and follow-up interval. Higher levels of physical fitness appeared to delay all-cause mortality primarily due to lowered rates of cardiovascular disease and cancer.

The relationship of maximal oxygen uptake measured during a maximal test on a cycle ergometer to CVD mortality during a 16-year follow-up was reported for 2,014 Norwegian men initially aged 40 to 59 years (Sandvick et al., 1993). The relative risk of death from any cause in fitness quartile 4 (highest) as compared with quartile 1 (lowest) was 0.54 after adjustment for age, smoking status, serum lipids, blood pressure, resting heart rate, vital capacity, body mass index, level of physical activity, and glucose tolerance. The adjusted relative risk of death from CVD in fitness quartile 4 as compared with quartile 1 was 0.41 (p = 0.013). The corresponding relative risks for quartile 3 and 2 (as compared to quartile 1) were 0.45 (p = 0.026) and 0.59 (p = 0.15), respectively.

The results of these three physical fitness studies and the data reported by Sobolski, Kornitzer, and De Backer (1987) and Lakka and colleagues (1994) are highly consistent with the observational data on physical activity and cardiovascular mortality: the least fit and active have the highest rate of disease with only moderate increases in fitness and activity associated with a significant reduction in risk. There is a continued dose-response relationship at higher levels of fitness, but the magnitude of the benefit tends to decline as fitness levels increase, with the most fit generally having the lowest CHD mortality rate.

SECONDARY PREVENTION OF CORONARY HEART DISEASE

As with primary prevention, there is no definitive study demonstrating a significant reduction in new cardiac events as a result of exercise training in patients with established CHD. But in addition to studies that have simply compared morbidity or mortality rates in active with inactive cardiac patients, controlled experimental trials have been conducted in which myocardial infarction patients have been randomly assigned to exercise and control groups.

Here again, the trend in mortality favors the more physically active patients, with benefits apparently derived from an increase in caloric expenditure of no more than 300 to 400 kcal per session three to four times per week at a moderate intensity (60 to 75% of maximal exertion or aerobic capacity). All of the studies published, which show either no differences or lower mortality rates in the active population, have either design or implementation flaws that prohibit definitive conclusions regarding the hypothesis, "Does an increase in exercise reduce the future likelihood of recurrent myocardial infarction, cardiac arrest, or sudden cardiac death?"

Randomized clinical trials of cardiac rehabilitation following hospitalization for myocardial infarction usually have demonstrated a tendency for lower mortality in treated patients, but a statistically significant reduction occurred in only one trial (Wilhelmsen et al., 1975; Rechnitzer et al., 1983; Shaw, 1981). To overcome the problem of inadequate power of any one study to detect small but clinically important benefits on cardiovascular morbidity and mortality in randomized trials of rehabilitation, a meta-analysis was performed on the combined results of ten clinical trials (Oldridge et al., 1988). All of the trials had to have good documentation of myocardial infarction, randomization of patients, a rehabilitation program lasting at least six weeks, follow-up for 24 months or longer, and comprehensive documentation of outcome. Data on a total of 4,347 patients were analyzed. The pooled odds ratio of 0.76 (95% confidence interval, 0.63 to 0.92) for all-cause deaths and of 0.75 (95% confidence intervals, 0.62 to 0.93) for cardiovascular death were significantly lower for the rehabilitation group than the control group, with no significant difference for recurrent myocardial infarction. A similar review, but evaluating a total of 22 randomized trials of rehabilitation after myocardial infarction reached a very similar conclusion (O'Conner et al., 1989).

BIOLOGIC MECHANISMS PROTECTING AGAINST CORONARY HEART DISEASE

A variety of biologic changes or mechanisms have been proposed to explain how physical activity might decrease the development of CHD clinical manifestations or improve the clinical status of patients with CHD. Most of these changes either decrease myocardial oxygen demand or increase myocardial oxygen supply and thus decrease the likelihood of myocardial ischemia at rest or during exercise. These mechanisms can be classified as either those that contribute to the maintenance or increase of oxygen supply to the myocardium or those that contribute to a decrease in myocardial work and oxygen demands. Also, it is possible that exercise training enhances the intrinsic mechanical or metabolic functioning of the myo-cardium or increases its electrical stability. It is these very same mechanisms through which all preventive and therapeutic measures for reducing clinical manifestations of CHD work. The specific data supporting the possible existence of these mechanisms have been extensively reviewed recently (Bouchard, Shephard, & Stephens, 1994).

CARDIOVASCULAR RISKS DURING EXERCISE

When someone dies suddenly due to a "heart attack" during vigorous recreational or sporting activities the event receives much more publicity than if the same individual had died while at home or work. Because of this publicity, the percentage of all sudden cardiac deaths (SCD) that occur during sporting activities in the general population probably is lower than it would seem based on casual observation. However, if an individual has underlying cardiac disease that significantly reduces myocardial perfusion, the increased myocardial oxygen demand imposed by either vigorous static or dynamic exercise can precipitate sudden cardiac arrest or sudden death (Thompson & Mitchell, 1984).

Adults in the general population who participate in vigorous activities such as jogging, long-distance running, cross-country skiing, cycling, or vigorous sports may be at greater risk of SCD during exercise than when not exercising (Siscovick et al., 1984; Thompson et al., 1982; Vuori,

Makarainen, & Jaaselainen, 1978). For example, in a study of 133 men who died suddenly of cardiac arrest without known prior heart disease, Siscovick et al. (1984) reported that while the overall risk of cardiac arrest was lower in men performing habitual physical activity, the risk of primary cardiac arrest was transiently increased during vigorous exercise compared to that at other times. Among men who performed vigorous activity very infrequently the risk of cardiac arrest during that activity was 56 times greater (95% confidence limits = 23 to 131) than at other times, but this risk decreased to a factor of 5 (95% confidence limits = 2 to 14) among men at the highest level of vigorous activity. Based on the circumstances surrounding 2,606 sudden deaths in Finland during one year, Vuori and colleagues (1978) concluded that SCD in connection with sporting activities in the general population are quite rare; instantaneous deaths were even rarer (<1% of all incidences of SCD) and occurred only with coexisting activity. Of the deaths associated with exercise, 73% were caused by acute or chronic ischemic heart disease and most of the subjects had serious cardiovascular risk factors that were known in advance or could have been identified easily.

In adults who have had a recent medical evaluation, the risk for SCD during exercise is extremely small. Gibbons and colleagues (1980) documented only two nonfatal cardiac arrests and no deaths in 374,798 person-hours of vigorous exercise. In a very large experience obtained by Vander and associates (Vander et al., 1982) from 40 exercise facilities over five years, the fatality rate associated with exercise in the general population was quite low. In 33,726,000 participant-hours of exercise, only 38 fatal cardiovascular complications occurred for a fatality rate of one death every 887,526 hours of participation. This means one could expect one death per year if 3,400 adults were exercising five hours per week each. Also, the mortality rate while exercising in this group is about one percent per year, nearly the same as the annual CHD mortality rate for middle-aged men in the United States.

PHYSICAL ACTIVITY TO PROMOTE CARDIOVASCULAR HEALTH

Recently a consensus was reached by an expert panel working under the auspices of the Centers for

FIGURE 9.1

Biological mechanisms by which exercise may contribute to the primary or secondary prevention of coronary heart disease.*

Maintain or increase myocardial oxygen supply

Delay progression of coronary atherosclerosis (possible)

Improve lipoprotein profile (increase HDL-C/LDL-C ratio) (probable)

Improve carbohydrate metabolism (increase insulin sensitivity) (probable)

Decrease platelet aggregation and increase fibrinolysis (probable)

Decrease adiposity (usually)

Increase coronary collateral vascularization (unlikely)

Increase epicardial artery diameter by dilitation or remodeling (possible)

Increase coronary blood flow (myocardial perfusion) or distribution (possible)

Decrease myocardial work and oxygen demand

Decrease heart rate at rest and during submaximal exercise (usually)

Decrease systolic and mean arterial pressure during submaximal exercise (usually) and at rest (possible)

Decrease cardiac output during submaximal exercise (possible)

Decrease circulating plasma catecholamine levels (decrease sympathetic tone) at rest (probable) and at submaximal exercise (usually)

Increase myocardial function

Increase stroke volume at rest and in submaximal and maximal exercise (likely)

Increase ejection fraction at rest and during exercise (likely)

Increase intrinsic myocardial contractility (possible)

Increase myocardial function resulting from decreased "afterload" (probable)

Increase myocardial hypertrophy (probable); but this may not reduce CHD risk

Increase electrical stability of myocardium

Decrease regional ischemia at rest or at submaximal exercise (possible)

Decrease catecholamines in myocardium at rest (possible) and at submaximal exercise (probable)

Increase ventricular fibrillation threshold due to reduction of cyclic AMP (possible)

---

*Expression of likelihood that effect will occur for an individual participating in endurance-type training program for 16 weeks or longer at 65% to 80% of functional capacity for 25 minutes or longer per session (300 kilocalories) for three or more sessions per week ranges from unlikely, possible, likely, probable, to usually.

Abbreviations: HDL-C = high-density lipoprotein cholesterol; LDL-C = low-density lipoprotein cholesterol; CHD = coronary heart disease; AMP = adenosine monophosphate.

Disease Control and Prevention and the American College of Sports Medicine on a "public health recommendation" for promoting physical activity (Pate et al., 1995). While these recommendations were made on the basis that improvement in overall health of the person was the primary goal, much of the data supporting these recommendations were derived from the favorable relationship between physical activity and improved CHD risk factor status and lower CHD mortality. Thus, these guidelines provide a useful framework for recommending a program of physical activity to promote cardiovascular health. The essence of these recommendations is that all adults will benefit by performing at least 30 minutes of physical activity at a moderate intensity or higher on most days. For maximum cardiovascular benefits, this exercise should be of the endurance or aerobic type using the larger muscles of the legs or trunk including brisk walking, jogging, hiking, cycling, swimming, rowing, aerobic and active social dancing, selected calisthenics, and a variety of active games or sports.

A new twist in these recommendations as compared to those issued previously by various organizations is that the 30 minutes of activity can be achieved by performing short bouts of moderate intensity activity throughout the day in addition to performing a single bout of activity for 30 minutes or longer. These recommendations are not precise on the issue of how long these short bouts of activity need to be to warrant credit as time exercising. My suggestion, until more scientific data are available, is to assign credit to only those bouts of activity that last for five minutes or longer. The activity during these bouts needs to be of at least moderate intensity (defined as activity equivalent in intensity to that of brisk walking). These guidelines emphasize that prior guidelines by the President's Council on Physical Fitness and Sports, the American College of Sports Medicine, and the American Heart Association are still valid and that these new recommendations are an attempt to expand the opportunity for adults to exercise for health benefits. These guidelines do not change either the recommended intensity or amount of activity to be performed. Similar guidelines for children and youth were recently published (Sallis et al., 1994).

Existing scientific data strongly support the value of frequently performed activity of moderate intensity as part of a comprehensive program of heart disease prevention and cardiac rehabilitation. Physical activity and endurance fitness make contributions to decreased risk independent of other established heart disease risk factors and can provide substantial health benefits beyond cardiovascular health (Bouchard, Shephard, & Stephens, 1994). Along with stopping smoking, maintaining a physically active lifestyle is one of the least expensive and most productive health behaviors available to the public.

REFERENCES

Berlin, J.A., & Colditz, G.A. (1990). A meta-analysis of physical activity in the prevention of coronary heart disease. *American Journal of Epidemiology, 132,* 612–628.

Blair, S.N., Kohl, H.W., Paffenbarger, R.S., Clark, D.G., Cooper, K.H., & Gibbons, L.W. (1989). Physical fitness and all-cause mortality: A prospective study in healthy men and women. *Journal of the American Medical Association, 262,* 2395–2399.

Bouchard, C., Shephard, R.J., Stephens, T. (Eds.) (1994). *Physical Activity, Fitness and Health. International Proceedings and Consensus Statement.* Champaign, IL: Human Kinetics Publishers.

Cassel, J., Heyden, S., Bartel, A.G., et al. (1971). Occupation and physical activity and coronary heart disease. *Archives of Internal Medicine, 128,* 920–926.

Chapman, J.M., & Massey, F.J. (1964). The interrelationship of serum cholesterol, hypertension, body weight and risk of coronary disease. *Journal of Chronic Diseases, 17,* 933–941.

Costas, R., Garcia-Palmieri, M.R., Nazario, E., & Sorlie, P. (1978). Relation of lipids, weight and physical activity to incidence of coronary heart disease: The Puerto Rico Heart Study. *American Journal of Cardiology, 42,* 653–660.

Ekelund, L.G., Haskell, W.L., Johnson, J.L., Wholey, F.S., Criqui, M.H., & Sheps, D.S. (1988), Physical fitness as a prevention of cardiovascular mortality in asymptomatic North American men. *New England Journal of Medicine, 319,* 1379–1384.

Gibbons, L.W., Cooper, K.H., Myer, B., & Ellison, C. (1980). The acute cardiac risk of strenuous exercise. *Journal of the American Medical Association, 244,* 1799–1804.

Kahn, H.A. (1963). The relationship of reported coronary heart disease mortality to physical activity of work. *American Journal of Public Health, 53,* 1058–1063.

Karvonen, M.J., Rautaharju, P. M., Orma, E., et al. (1961). Heart disease and employment: Cardiovascular studies on lumberjacks. *Journal of Occupational Medicine, 3,* 49–57.

Lakka, T.A., Venalainen, J.M., Rauramaa, R., et al. (1994). Relation of leisure-time activity and cardiorespiratory fitness to the risk of acute myocardial infarction in men. *New England Journal of Medicine, 330,* 1549–1554.

Leon, A.S., Cornett, J., Jacobs, D.R., & Rauramaa, R. (1987). Leisure-time physical activity levels and risk of coronary heart disease and death: The multiple risk factor intervention on trial. *Journal of the American Medical Association, 258,* 2388–2395.

Morris, J.N., Clayton, D.G., Everitt, M.G., Semmence, A.M., & Burgess, E.H. (1990). Exercise in leisure time: Coronary attack and death rates. *British Heart Journal, 63,* 325–334.

Morris, J.N., Heady, J.A., Raffle, P.A.B., et al. (1953). Coronary heart disease and physical activity of work. *Lancet, 1053,* 1111–1120.

Morris, J.N., Pollard, R., Everitt, M.G., & Chave, S.P.W. (1980). Vigorous exercise in leisure time: Protection against coronary heart disease. *Lancet, 8206,* 1207–1210.

O'Conner, G.T, Boving, J.E., Yusuf, S., et al. (1989). An overview of randomized trials of rehabilitation with exercise after myocardial infarction. *Circulation, 80,* 234–244.

Oldridge, N.B., Guyatt, G.H., Fisher, M.E., & Rimm, A.A. (1988). Cardiac rehabilitation after myocardial infarction: Combined exercise of randomized clinical trials. *Journal of the American Medical Association, 260,* 945–950.

Paffenbarger, R.S., Hyde, R.T., Wing, A.L., & Hsieh, C. (1986). Physical activity, all-cause mortality, and longevity of college alumni. *New England Journal of Medicine, 314,* 605–613.

Paffenbarger, R.S., Hyde, R.T., Wing, A.L., Lee, I-M., Jung, D.L., & Kampert, J.B. (1993). The association of changes in physical activity level and other lifestyle characteristics with mortality among men. *New England Journal of Medicine, 328,* 538–545.

Paffenbarger, R.S., Wing, A.L., & Hyde, R.T. (1978). Physical activity as an index of heart attack in college alumni. *American Journal of Epidemiology, 108,* 161–167.

Pate, R.R., Pratt, M., Blair, S.N., Haskell, W.L., et al. (1995). Physical activity and public health: A recommendation from the Centers for Disease Control and Prevention and the American College of Sports Medicine. *Journal of the American Medical Association, 273,* 402–407.

Paul, O. (1969). Physical activity and coronary heart disease, Part II. *American Journal of Cardiology, 23,* 303–318.

Powell, K.E., Thompson, P.D., Caspersen, C.J., & Kendrech, J.S. (1987). Physical activity and incidence of coronary heart disease. *Annual Review of Public Health, 8,* 253–287.

Rechnitzer, P.A., Cunningham, D.A., Andre, G.M., et al. (1983). Relation of exercise to the recurrence rate of my-

ocardial infarction in men. *American Journal of Cardiology, 51,* 65–69.

Rose, G. (1969). Physical activity and coronary heart disease. *Proceedings of the Royal Society of Medicine, 62,* 1183–1187.

Sallis, J.F. (Ed.) (1994). Physical activity guidelines for adolescents. *Pediatric Exercise Science, 6,* 299–465.

Salonen, J.T., Puska, P., & Tuomilehto, J. (1982). Physical activity and risk of myocardial infarction, cerebral stroke and death: A longitudinal study in Eastern Finland. *American Journal of Epidemiology, 115,* 526–537.

Sandvick, L., Erikssen, J., Thaulow, E., et al. (1993). Physical fitness as a predictor of mortality among healthy middle-aged Norwegian men. *New England Journal of Medicine, 328,* 533–537.

Shaper, A.G., & Wannamethee, G. (1991). Physical activity and ischemic heart disease in middle-aged British men. *British Heart Journal, 66,* 384–394.

Shapiro, S., Weinblatt, E., Frank, C.W., & Sager, R.V. (1969). Incidence of coronary heart disease in a population insured for medical care (HIP). *American Journal of Public Health (suppl.), 59,* 1–101.

Shaw, L. (1981). Effects of a prescribed supervised exercise program on mortality and cardiovascular morbidity in patients after myocardial infarction. *American Journal of Cardiology, 48,* 39–46.

Siscovick, D.S., Weiss, N.S., Fletcher, R.H., & Lasky, T. (1984). The incidence of primary cardiac arrest during vigorous exercise. *New England Journal of Medicine, 311,* 874–877.

Sobolski, J., Kornitzer, M., & De Backer, G. (1987). Protection against ischemic heart disease in the Belgian Physical Fitness Study: Physical fitness rather than physical activity. *American Journal of Epidemiology, 125,* 601–610.

Taylor, H.L., Blackburn, H., Keys, A., Parlin, R.W., Vasquez, C., & Pucher, T. (1970). Five-year follow-up of employees of selected U.S. railroad companies. *Circulation, 41 (Suppl. 1),* 20–39.

Thompson, P., Funk, E., Carleton, R., & Sturner, W. (1982). Incidence of death during jogging in Rhode Island from 1975 through 1980. *Journal of the American Medical Association, 247,* 2535–2538.

Thompson, P.D., & Mitchell, J.H. (1984). Exercise and sudden cardiac death. Protection or provocation? *New England Journal of Medicine, 311,* 914–915.

Vander, L., Franklin, B., & Rubenfire, M. (1982). Cardiovascular complications of recreational physical activity. *The Physician and Sports Medicine, 10,* 89–95.

Vuori, I., Makarainen, M., & Jaaselainen, A. (1978). Sudden death and physical activity. *Cardiology, 63,* 287–304.

Wilhelmsen, L., Sanne, H., Elmfeldt, D., et al. (1975). A controlled trial of physical training after myocardial infarction: Effects on risk factors, nonfatal reinfarction and death. *Preventive Medicine, 4,* 491–508.

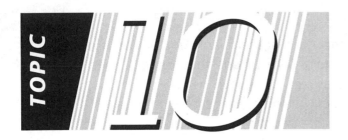

Physical Activity and Cancer

I-Min Lee
HARVARD MEDICAL SCHOOL

INTRODUCTION

Cancer is the second leading cause of death, after heart disease, in the United States today (Boring et al., 1994). In 1994, the American Cancer Society estimated that 540,000 Americans died from cancer, while 1,210,000 new cases of this disease occurred that same year (Boring et al., 1994).

Two of the important avoidable causes of cancer are cigarette smoking and alcohol consumption. If we totally eliminated these two factors, perhaps one-third of all cancers might be avoided (Doll & Peto, 1981). In the search for other modifiable aspects of human behavior that potentially may reduce risk of developing cancer, physical activity emerges as a promising candidate. Higher levels of exercise have been shown to be associated with numerous health benefits, including decreased incidence of coronary heart disease (Berlin & Colditz, 1990), hypertension (Hagberg, 1990), non-insulin-dependent diabetes mellitus (Helmrich et al., 1991) and increased longevity (Paffenbarger et al., 1993). Is there also an association between physical activity and reduced rates of cancer occurrence? This hypothesis—that exercise can reduce cancer risk—is

not new; in fact, in the early twentieth century, Cherry (1922) observed that men involved in physically active occupations experienced lower cancer mortality rates than their fellow men engaged in less strenuous jobs.

In this review, we first will discuss potential biologic mechanisms whereby exercise might be expected to reduce cancer risk, then proceed to explore the epidemiologic data on the relation between physical activity and cancer of various sites.

POTENTIAL BIOLOGIC MECHANISMS UNDERLYING AN EXERCISE–CANCER ASSOCIATION

Among the many complex functions of the human immune system is the regulation of susceptibility to cancer. Thus, if exercise can enhance the immune system, it is plausible for physical activity to reduce cancer risk.

As far back as 1902, investigators observed that vigorous exercise (i.e., running a marathon) could influence certain components of the immune system

ORIGINALLY PUBLISHED AS SERIES 2, NUMBER 2, OF THE PCPFS *RESEARCH DIGEST*.

HIGHLIGHT

> "Two of the important avoidable causes of cancer are cigarette smoking and alcohol consumption. If we totally eliminated these two factors, perhaps one-third of all cancers might be avoided. In the search for other modifiable aspects of human behavior that potentially may reduce risk of developing cancer, physical activity emerges as a promising candidate."

(Larrabee, 1902). Today, investigators have attempted to study the effects of exercise on the immune system in several ways. Markers of immune function examined have included susceptibility to upper respiratory infections and the function of cells (e.g., cells of the monocyte-macrophage system and natural killer or NK cells) that serve as the body's first line of defense against the development and spread of cancer (Mackinnon, 1989; Roitt et al., 1989; Shephard, 1991). Upper respiratory infections have been studied because the human immune system also is responsible for regulating susceptibility to infection.

Available evidence suggests that increasing levels of physical activity, up to a certain point, enhance the immune function; beyond this, immune system function appears instead to decrease (Nieman, 1994; Pedersen & Ullum, 1994; Woods & Davis, 1994). What this cut-point is remains unclear. Moderate amounts of physical activity (e.g., brisk walking) have been shown to reduce risk of upper respiratory infection (Nieman, 1994), as well as enhance the function of cells of the monocyte-macrophage system (Woods & Davis, 1994) and NK cells (Pedersen & Ullum, 1994). At more intense levels of exercise, however, immune suppression appears to occur instead. For example, following marathon-type races, runners appear to have increased rates of upper respiratory tract infections for a one- to two-week period (Nieman, 1994). Also, elite athletes (e.g., cyclists) have increased NK cell activity at rest, but depressed function following intense activity (Pedersen & Ullum, 1994).

To summarize, then, it appears plausible for exercise—at least, in moderate amounts—to reduce cancer risk by enhancing the function of the human immune system.

For site-specific cancers, other mechanisms may operate. With colon cancer, it has long been postulated that a shortened intestinal transit time may reduce cancer incidence by decreasing the amount of contact between potential carcinogens, co-carcinogens or promoters in the fecal stream and colonic mucosa (Burkitt et al., 1971, 1972). Thus, if exercise can reduce transit time within the colon, risk of this cancer may be decreased. However, whether exercise does or does not reduce transit time within the intestine is unclear. Several investigators have shown that exercise does indeed decrease transit time (Holdstock et al., 1970; Cordain et al., 1986; Oettlé, 1991); others have not (Bingham & Cummings, 1989; Lampe et al., 1991; Coenen et al., 1992). Apart from the methodologic limitations of these studies, it is possible that the inconsistent findings resulted because exercise may shorten transit time within certain segments of the gut without affecting total (i.e., oral-anal) transit time (Lupton & Meacher, 1988).

Turning to cancers of the reproductive system, various hormones are necessary for their development. Thus, if exercise can alter the levels of these hormones, this represents another plausible mechanism for physical activity to decrease cancer risk. In females, estrogen, as well as the combination of estrogen and progesterone, stimulate cell proliferation in the breast and so have been implicated in the development of breast cancer (Henderson et al., 1993). Studies of female athletes have shown that training can lower estrogen and progesterone levels (Shangold, 1984). Further, in young girls, strenuous training also can delay the onset of menarche (Warren, 1980), thus reducing a woman's total lifetime exposure to these hormones. In males, testosterone appears to be important in the development of prostate cancer (Gittes, 1991). Strenuous exercise may lower basal testosterone levels, potentially reducing risk of this cancer (Lee et al., 1992).

Finally, exercise may influence cancer risk via its effect on decreasing body weight and reducing body fat. For certain cancers such as colon cancer (Lew & Garfinkel, 1979) and breast cancer (Kelsey & Gammon, 1991), obesity is associated with increased risk.

Physical Activity and Reduced Cancer Risk: Potential Biologic Mechanisms	
Cancer Type	*Potential Mechanisms*
Most cancer types	Enhanced immune system
Colon cancer	Shortened intestinal transit time
	Decreased body fat
Breast cancer	Hormone level changes
	Decreased body fat
Prostate cancer	Hormone level changes

PHYSICAL ACTIVITY AND COLON CANCER

Of the various site-specific cancers, colon cancer has been the most commonly studied cancer. The first detailed epidemiologic study was conducted by Garabrant et al. (1984). They examined the occupation of men, aged 20–64 years, who had developed colon cancer. Based on the estimated amount of physical activity required on the job, men were classified as sedentary, moderately active, or highly active. Investigators also examined occupational data among similarly aged men with cancers other than colon cancer. Using this comparison, investigators reported that sedentary men had 1.6 times the risk of developing colon cancer, when compared with highly active men.

It could be argued that the increased risk observed by Garabrant et al. may have been due to higher consumption of fat in the diet among sedentary men, since dietary fat is associated with increased colon cancer risk (Willett et al., 1990). However, another study by Slattery et al., conducted in Utah, did take into account differences in dietary patterns, as well as differences in body weight (1988). When investigators compared the occupational and leisure-time activities of men and women with colon cancer against the activity patterns of a random sample of the population without this disease, they also found sedentary individuals to be at increased risk. The magnitude of this increased risk was approximately twofold.

In their study of over 17,000 men, followed for up to 26 years, Lee et al. observed that physical activity, assessed at one point in time, did not predict risk of subsequent colon cancer (1991). However, men who were sedentary (expending <1,000 kcal/week) at two time points, separated by 11 to 15 years, had twice the risk of those active (expending >2,500 kcal/week) at both times. This led investigators to postulate that for physical activity to protect against colon cancer, it may be necessary for the activity to be sustained over time. Investigators also put forward an alternate hypothesis: In this study, men were asked, on questionnaires, how much walking and stair climbing they did, the kinds of leisure-time sports and recreational activities they engaged in, and the frequency and time spent on these activities. Investigators then calculated the energy expenditure for each subject, based on these data. Thus, two assessments of physical activity may have increased the precision of activity measurement and allowed investigators to better distinguish between the sedentary and the active men.

To date, 33 publications on the relation between physical activity and colon cancer have resulted (reviewed in Lee, 1994; Markowitz et al., 1992; Vetter et al., 1992; Arbman et al., 1993; Chow et al., 1993; Dosemeci et al., 1993; Fraser & Pearce, 1993; Vineis et al., 1993). The majority—25 publications—have shown that individuals who exercise have a lower incidence of colon cancer than their sedentary counterparts. This relation has been described in the United States, Europe, the Far East, and Australia. The magnitude of increased risk experienced by sedentary persons has been reported to be 1.2 to 3.6 times, with most studies describing the magnitude of increased risk to be between one-and-a-half to twofold. From currently available data, it is unclear whether a gradient relation, i.e., increasing protection with increasing activity, exists (Lee, 1994).

PHYSICAL ACTIVITY AND RECTAL CANCER

Many of the studies of colon cancer above also examined rectal cancer (reviewed in Lee, 1994). In contrast to colon cancer, most studies in which rectal cancer was studied separately (as opposed to those that grouped colorectal cancers into a single category) found no significant relation between increased physical activity and risk of this cancer. Where colorectal cancer was studied as a single entity, investigators tended to report a protective effect of physical activity, perhaps reflecting the relation with colon cancer instead.

PHYSICAL ACTIVITY AND BREAST CANCER

While it is attractive to postulate that exercise can decrease risk of breast cancer as few modifiable risk factors for this cancer exist, available data do not consistently support this hypothesis. Frisch et al. first described an inverse relation between physical activity and breast cancer in 1985. They contacted 5,398 surviving alumnae of the classes of 1925–1981 from 10 colleges or universities by questionnaire and asked them to report whether they had developed breast cancer. These women represented 2,622 former athletes from the institutions and a random sample of nonathletes. A total of 69 breast cancers had developed among these surviving alumnae. When investigators compared the prevalence of breast cancer among athletes with nonathletes, they found that the latter had 1.9 times the risk of the former, after taking into account differences in reproductive characteristics between the two groups.

Subsequent studies did not consistently reproduce these findings (reviewed in Lee, 1994; Pukkala et al., 1993; Zheng et al., 1993; Bernstein et al., 1994; Dorgan et al., 1994). Of eight other publications, three described an inverse relation between physical activity and breast cancer risk; four, no relation; and one, a suggestion of a *direct* association, i.e., risk increased with increasing physical activity.

This last publication used data from the Framingham Heart Study, a study ongoing since 1948 (Dorgan et al., 1994). Subjects in this study are brought in every two years to be examined. In this analysis of physical activity and breast cancer, 2,307 women reported their physical activity to physicians in 1954–1956. They then were followed for the development of breast cancer until 1984. A total of 117 women were diagnosed with breast cancer during follow-up. Investigators divided women into quartiles, based on their level of physical activity. They found that women in the highest

quartile of physical activity had 1.6 times the breast cancer risk of those in the least active quartile, and this finding was of borderline statistical significance.

Recently, Bernstein et al. (1994) hypothesized that the timing of physical activity is pertinent with respect to risk for breast cancer. They studied 545 women, aged 40 years or younger, with breast cancer, and compared their physical activity patterns to those of 545 women without breast cancer, who were from the same neighborhood and of the same age, race, and parity. Investigators divided subjects into five categories, depending on the number of hours per week that a woman spent in physical activity, after she had reached menarche. Women who did not spend any time in physical activity had 2.4 times the breast cancer risk of their colleagues who exercised for ≥ 3.8 hours per week. There was a strong gradient of increasing risk with decreasing hours of physical activity. Investigators did take into account differences in reproductive history, use of oral contraceptives, a family history of breast cancer, and obesity in their analysis. The protective effect of physical activity during young adulthood appeared stronger for women having borne children than for women never having borne children.

PHYSICAL ACTIVITY AND PROSTATE CANCER

As with breast cancer, the epidemiologic data do not consistently support an association between physical activity and risk of this cancer, even though a plausible hypothesis has been put forward to explain the biologic basis for an inverse association (Lee et al., 1992). Of 10 epidemiologic studies on this topic, five observed inverse relations between physical activity and risk of this cancer (reviewed in Lee, 1994). For example, Lee et al. (1992) followed 17,719 men, initially aged 30–79 years, for up to 26 years for the development of prostate cancer. For men aged ≥ 70 years, those who expended <1,000 kcal/week in walking, climbing stairs, and leisure-time sports and recreational activities had 1.9 times the risk of their more active colleagues who expended >4,000 kcal/week. For younger men, there was no significant association between level of exercise and risk of this cancer.

Another three studies found significant direct associations between level of physical activity and prostate cancer risk. That is, these studies observed risk of this cancer to increase with increasing levels of physical activity. For example, Le Marchand et al. (1991) examined the lifetime occupational physical activity of 452 Hawaiian men with prostate cancer and compared this with the lifetime occupational activity of 899 men without such cancer. Men were classified into five categories of activity, depending on the proportion of their life that they had spent in sedentary jobs or jobs involving only light work. Among men aged ≥70 years, the most sedentary fifth of men had only half the risk of prostate cancer of the least sedentary fifth of men. There also was a gradient relation, with risk decreasing as sedentariness increased. For men aged younger than 70 years old, no clear pattern emerged.

Two other indices of lifetime occupational activity also were created: the proportion of life spent in moderately active jobs and the proportion of life spent in heavy or very heavy work. Neither of these two indices was significantly related to prostate cancer risk. The remaining two studies reported no significant relation between the amount of exercise in men and risk of prostate cancer.

PHYSICAL ACTIVITY AND OTHER SITE-SPECIFIC CANCERS

Because of the potential for physical activity to influence levels of reproductive hormones, investigators have postulated that active individuals may experience lower risks of other reproductive cancers, in addition to breast and prostate cancers. In their study of college alumnae, Frisch et al. (1985) also examined the relation between college athleticism and all reproductive cancers (i.e., cancers of the breast, uterus, cervix, vagina, and ovary). Women who had been nonathletes had 2.5 times the risk of these cancers, compared with women who had been college athletes. In another study conducted in Italy and Switzerland, the most sedentary women, based on self-reported physical activity, had 2.4 to 8.6 times the risk (for physical activity at different ages) of endometrial cancer, compared with the most active women (Levi et al., 1993). However, a study from China did not find risk of cancers of the corpus uteri or ovary to differ between women who were inactive or active on the job (Zheng et al., 1993).

Meanwhile, among men, investigators from the United Kingdom have reported that physical activity is inversely related to risk of testicular cancer in those aged 15–49 years. Men who did not exercise experienced a doubling of risk of this cancer, compared with those who spent ≥15 hours a week in exercise (United Kingdom Testicular Cancer Study Group, 1994). Using a different measure of physical activity, men who spent ≥10 hours a day sitting had 1.7 times the risk of testicular cancer of those who spent only 0–2 hours sitting.

Other site-specific cancers that have been studied in relation to physical activity include lung and pancreatic cancers (reviewed in Lee, 1994). Currently, the data are insufficient to conclude whether any association exists. For the remaining site-specific cancers, the data have been even more sparse (reviewed in Lee, 1994).

PHYSICAL ACTIVITY AND PATIENTS WITH CANCER

There is little information on whether patients who already have developed cancer do or do not benefit from physical activity. In animal experiments, investigators found that among tumor-bearing rats that were allowed to feed freely, those rats allowed to exercise spontaneously experienced delayed onset of appetite loss when compared with nonexercised rats (Daneryd et al., 1990). In addition, exercised animals were found to have reduced tumor weights. In humans, exercise has a mood-elevating effect and, thus, may improve the quality of life of cancer patients. In a study of 24 women with breast cancer, investigators developed a moderate exercise program for each patient and followed women for six months (Peters et al., 1994). After five weeks, but not at six months, satisfaction with life was significantly enhanced when compared with baseline attitude. Investigators postulated that this may have been due to decreased adherence to the exercise protocol between five weeks and six months. Further, at the end of the six months, these women were found to have increased NK cell activity at rest compared with baseline NK cell activity, indicating enhancement of this aspect of the immune system.

SUMMARY

Exercise has been shown to be inversely related to risk of developing a whole host of chronic diseases in humans, including coronary heart disease, hypertension and non-insulin-dependent diabetes mellitus. Since 1985, there has been accumulating epidemiologic data suggesting that exercise also may decrease risk of cancer, in particular colon cancer. However, exercise appears to be unrelated to rectal cancer risk. With regard to other cancers, because physical activity can alter levels of reproductive hormones, investigators have hypothesized that active individuals should experience decreased incidence of breast or prostate cancer. However, the epidemiologic data do not consistently support this hypothesis. Data on other site-specific cancers have been sparse. Finally, preliminary data suggest that exercise also may be beneficial for cancer patients by improving the quality of life and enhancing immune function; while promising, this needs more careful research.

REFERENCES

Arbman, G., Axelson, O., Fredriksson, M., Nilsson, E., & Sjidahl, R. (1993). Do occupational factors influence the risk of colon and rectal cancer in different ways? *Cancer, 72,* 2543–2549.

Berlin, J.A., & Golditz, G.A. (1990). A meta-analysis of physical activity in the prevention of coronary heart disease. *American Journal of Epidemiology, 132,* 612–628.

Bernstein, L., Henderson, B.E., Hanisch, R., Sullivan-Halley, J., & Ross, R.K. (1994). Physical exercise and reduced risk of breast cancer in young women. *Journal of the National Cancer Institute, 86,* 1403–1408.

Bingham, S.A., & Cummings, J.H. (1989). Effect of exercise and physical fitness on large intestinal function. *Gastroenterology, 97,* 1389–1399.

Boring, C.C., Squires, T.S., Tong, T., & Montgomery, S. (1994). Cancer statistics, 1994. *Cancer, 44,* 7–26

Burkitt, D.P. (1971). Epidemiology of cancer of the colon and rectum. *Cancer, 28,* 3–13.

Burkitt, D.P., Walker, A.R.P., & Painter, N.S. (1972). Effect of dietary fibre on stools and transit-times and its role in the causation of disease. *Lancet, ii,* 1408–1411.

Cherry, T. (1922). A theory of cancer. *Medical Journal of Australia, 1,* 425–438.

Chow, W-H., Dosemeci, M., Zheng, W., Vetter, R., McLaughlin, J.K., Gao, Y-T. & Blot, W.J. (1993). Physical activity and occupational risk of colon cancer in Shanghai, China. *International Journal of Epidemiology, 22,* 23–29.

Coenen, C., Wegener, M., Wedmann, B., Schmidt, G., & Hoffmann, S. (1992). Does physical exercise influence bowel transit time in healthy young men? *American Journal of Gastroenterology, 87,* 292–295.

Cordain, L., Latin, R.W., & Behnke, J.J. (1986). The effects of an aerobic running program on bowel transit time. *Journal of Sports Medicine, 26,* 101–104.

Daneryd, P.L.E., Hafstrim, L.R., & Karlberg, I.H. (1990). Effects of spontaneous physical exercise on experimental cancer anorexia and cachexia. *European Journal of Cancer, 10,* 1083–1088.

Doll, R., & Peto, R. (1981). *The causes of cancer: Quantitative estimates of the avoidable risks of cancer in the United States today* (pp. 1220–1256). New York: Oxford University Press.

Dorgan, J.F., Brown, C., Barrett, M., Splansky, G.L., Kreger, B.E., D'Agostino, R.B., Albanes, D., & Schatzkin, A. (1994). Physical activity and risk of breast cancer in the Framingham Heart Study. *American Journal of Epidemiology, 139,* 662–669.

Dosemeci, M., Hayes, R.B., Vetter, R., Hoover, R.N., Tucker, M., Engin, K., Unsal, M., & Blair, A. (1993). Occupational physical activity, socioeconomic status, and risks of 15 cancer sites in Turkey. *Cancer Causes Control, 4,* 313–321.

Fraser, G., & Pearce, N. (1993) Occupational physical activity and risk of cancer of the colon and rectum in New Zealand males. *Cancer Causes Control, 4,* 45–50.

Frisch, R.E., Wyshak, G., Albright, N.L., Albright, T.E., Schiff, I., Jones, K.P., Witschi, J., Shiang, E., Koff, E., & Marguglio, M. (1985). Lower prevalence of breast cancer and cancers of the reproductive system among former college athletes compared to non-athletes. *British Journal of Cancer, 52,* 885–891.

Garabrant, D.H., Peter, J.M., Mack, T.M., & Bernstein, L. (1984). Job activity and colon cancer risk. *American Journal of Epidemiology, 11,* 1005–1014.

Gittes, R.F. (1991). Carcinoma of the prostate. *New England Journal of Medicine, 324,* 236–245.

Hagberg, J.M. (1990). Exercise, fitness, and hypertension. In Bouchard, C., Shephard, R.J., Stephens, T., Sutton, J.R., & McPherson, B.D. (Eds.). *Exercise, fitness, and health: A consensus of current knowledge (pp. 455–466).* Champaign, IL: Human Kinetics Publishers.

Helmrich, S.P., Ragland, D.R., Loung, R.W., & Paffenbarger, R.S., Jr. (1991). Physical activity and reduced occurrence of non-insulin-dependent diabetes mellitus. *New England Journal of Medicine, 324,* 147–152.

Henderson, B.E., Ross, A.K., & Pike, M.C. (1993). Hormonal chemoprevention of cancer in women. *Science, 259,* 633–638.

Holdstock, D.J., Misiewicz, J.J., Smith, T., & Rowlands, E.N. (1970). Propulsion (mass movements) in the human colon and its relationship to meals and somatic activity. *Gut, 11,* 91–99.

Kelsey, J.L., & Gammon, M.D. (1991). The epidemiology of breast cancer. *Cancer, 41,* 146–165.

Lampe, J.W., Slavin, J.L., & Apple, F.S. (1991). Iron status of active women and the effect of running a marathon on bowel function and gastrointestinal blood loss. *International Journal of Sports Medicine, 12,* 173–179.

Larrabee, R.C. (1902). Leukocytosis after violent exercise. *Journal of Medical Research, 7,* 76–82.

Lee, I-M. (1994). Physical activity, fitness and cancer. In Bouchard, C., Shephard, R.J., & Stephens, T. (Eds.). Physical activity, fitness, and health: International proceedings and consensus statement (pp. 814–831). Champaign, IL: Human Kinetics Publishers.

Lee, I-M., Paffenbarger, R.S., Jr., & Hsieh, C-c. (1991). Physical activity and risk of developing colorectal cancer among college alumni. *Journal of the National Cancer Institute, 83,* 1324–1329.

Lee, I-M., Paffenbarger, R.S., Jr., & Hsieh, C-c. (1992). Physical activity and risk of prostatic cancer among college alumni. *American Journal of Epidemiology, 135,* 169–179.

Le Marchand, L., Kolonel, L.N., & Yoshizawa, C.N. (1991). Lifetime occupational physical activity and prostate cancer risk. *American Journal of Epidemiology, 133,* 103–111.

Levi, F., La Vecchia, C., Negri, E., & Franceschi, S. (1993). Selected physical activities and risk of endometrial cancer. *British Journal of Cancer, 67,* 846–851.

Lew, E.A., & Garfinkel, L. (1979). Variations in mortality by weight among 750,000 men and women. *Journal of Chronic Diseases, 32,* 563–576.

Lupton, J.R., & Meacher, M.M. (1988). Radiographic analysis of the affect of dietary fibers on rat colonic transit time. *American Journal of Physiology, 255,* G633–G639.

Mackinnon, L.T. (1989). Exercise and natural killer cells: What is the relationship? *Sports Medicine, 7,* 141–149.

Markowitz, S., Morabia, A., Garibaldi, K., & Wynder, E. (1992). Effect of occupational and recreational activity on the risk of colorectal cancer among males: A case-control study. *International Journal of Epidemiology, 21,* 1057–1062.

Nieman, D.C. (1994). Exercise, upper respiratory infection, and the immune system. *Medicine and Science in Sports and Exercise, 26,* 128–139.

Oettlé, W. (1991). Effect of moderate exercise on bowel habit. *Gut, 32,* 941–944.

Paffenbarger, R.S., Jr., Hyde, R.T., Wing, A.L., Lee, I-M., Jung, O.L., & Kampert, J.B. (1993). The association of changes in physical-activity level and other lifestyle characteristics with mortality among men. *New England Journal of Medicine, 326,* 538–545.

Pedersen, B.K., & Ullum, H. (1994). NK cell response to physical activity: Possible mechanisms of action. *Medicine and Science in Sports and Exercise, 26,* 140–146.

Peters, C., Litzerich, H., Niemeier, B., Schåle, K., & Uhlenbruck, G. (1994). Influence of moderate exercise training on natural killer cytotoxicity and personality traits in cancer patients. *Anticancer Research, 14,* 1033–1036.

Pukkala, E., Floskiparta, M., Apter, D., & Vihko, V. (1993). Life-long physical activity and cancer risk among Finnish female teachers. *European Journal of Cancer Prevention, 2,* 369–376.

Roitt, I.M., Brostoff, J., & Male, D.K. (1989). *Immunology* (2nd ed.) (pp. 18.1–18.17). London: Gower Medical Publishers.

Shangold, M.M. (1984). Exercise and the adult female: Hormonal and endocrine effects. *Exercise and Sport Sciences Review, 12,* 53–79.

Shephard, R.J. (1991). Physical activity and the immune system. *Canadian Journal of Sport Science, 16,* 169–185.

Slattery, M.L., Schumacher, M.C., Smith, K.R., West, D.W., & Abd-Elghany, N. (1988). Physical activity, diet and risk of colon cancer in Utah. *American Journal of Epidemiology, 128,* 989–999.

United Kingdom Testicular Cancer Study Group. (1994). Aetiology of testicular cancer: Association with congenital abnormalities, age at puberty, infertility, and exercise. *British Medical Journal, 308,* 1393–1399.

Vetter, R., Dosemeci, M., Blair, A., Wacholder, S., Unsal, M., Engin, K., & Fraumeni, J.F., Jr. (1992). Occupational physical activity and colon cancer risk in Turkey. *European Journal of Epidemiology, 8,* 845–850.

Vineis, P., Ciccone, G., & Magnino, A. (1993). Asbestos exposure, physical activity and colon cancer: A case-control study. *Tumori, 79,* 301–303.

Warren, M.P. (1980). The effects of exercise on pubertal progression and reproductive function in girls. *Journal of Clinical Endocrinology Metabolism, 51,* 1150–1157.

Willett, W.C., Stampfer, M.J., Colditz, G.A., Rosner, B.A., & Speizer, F.E. (1990). Relation of meat, fat, and fiber intake to the risk of colon cancer in a prospective study among women. *New England Journal of Medicine, 323,* 1664–1672.

Woods, J.A., & Davis, J.M. (1994). Exercise, monocyte/macrophage function, and cancer. *Medicine and Science in Sports and Exercise, 26,* 147–156.

Zheng, W., Shu, X.O., McLaughlin, J.K., Ghow, W.H., Gao, Y.T., & Blot, W.J. (1993). Occupational physical activity and the incidence of cancer of the breast, corpus uteri and ovary in Shanghai. *Cancer, 71,* 3620–3624.

Physical Activity and the Prevention of Type II (Non–Insulin-Dependent) Diabetes

Andrea Kriska
UNIVERSITY OF PITTSBURGH

A NOTE FROM THE EDITORS

According to the Surgeon General's report, as many as 8 million Americans know they have diabetes and at least 8 million more have diabetes but do not know it. More than 150,000 deaths each year are attributed to this condition. We asked Dr. Andrea Kriska, a researcher who studies diabetes, to write about this physical activity association.

There are two general classes of diabetes. As noted in the Surgeon General's Report, diabetes is a group of disorders that are associated with high blood sugar levels. "Insulin-dependent diabetes mellitus (IDDM or type I) is characterized by an absolute deficiency of circulating insulin . . . (page 125)." Non–insulin-dependent diabetes mellitus (NIDDM, or type II) is characterized by "elevated insulin levels that are ineffective in normalizing . . . blood sugar levels . . . or by impaired insulin secretion (page 125)." Because most cases of diabetes are of the second type (type II) and because physical activity has been shown to be more related to this type of disease, we have asked Dr. Kriska to focus on type II diabetes. In this paper, many questions about diabetes are answered and tables summarize key points. A list of basic definitions of key terms used in the paper is presented in Figure 11.1.

FIGURE 11.1
Basic definitions of key terms.

Insulin. A hormone secreted by the pancreas that regulates levels of sugar in the blood.

Insulin Resistance. A condition that occurs when insulin becomes ineffective or less effective than is necessary to regulate sugar levels in the blood.

Insulin Sensitivity. A person with insulin resistance (see above) is said to have decreased insulin sensitivity. The body's cells are not sensitive to insulin so they resist it and sugar levels are not regulated effectively.

Diabetes. A group of disorders that results in too much sugar in the blood, either because the body does not make enough insulin or makes insulin but cannot properly use it.

Oral Glucose Tolerance Test. A test to determine if a person is diabetic. The test measures the body's ability to clear sugar from the blood in a reasonable time after having taken a standardized oral dose of glucose (sugar).

Blood Glucose. Sugar levels in the blood.

ORIGINALLY PUBLISHED AS SERIES 2, NUMBER 10, OF THE PCPFS *RESEARCH DIGEST*.

"There is a strong link between type II diabetes and sedentary living. The biggest benefits appear to be found among those who incorporate some level of regular physical activity into their daily lives. Physical activity, as recommended by the Surgeon General, would seem to be a prudent strategy for all people, especially those who are at risk for type II diabetes."

WHAT IS TYPE II DIABETES?

Diabetes can be defined simply and succinctly as "too much glucose in the blood" (West, 1978). It is a devastating disease that can often lead to complications such as blindness, kidney failure, coronary heart disease, circulatory problems that may result in amputation, nerve problems, and premature death.

Among those with diabetes, type II is the most common type, accounting for 90–95% of all diabetic cases and affecting about 7% of the US population (DIA; Harris, 1987). Among those with type II diabetes, most (60–90%) but not all are obese when the disease is diagnosed (National Diabetes Data Group, 1979). Symptoms that are usually associated with the onset of type II diabetes are the direct result of the high blood glucose, although in many milder cases of diabetes, there may not be any symptoms (West, 1978). In fact, it has been estimated that the number of individuals in the general population who are not aware that they have type II diabetes is equal to the number of individuals who have been diagnosed with the disease (Harris, 1995).

Just as hypertension is diagnosed at the upper end of a blood pressure distribution, the diagnosis of diabetes is usually made at the upper end of a continuum of blood glucose values. Typically, the diagnosis of type II diabetes is determined based upon a specific test administered in a fasting state (an oral glucose tolerance test) in which the blood glucose values are measured two hours after drinking a specific glucose solution (WHO, 1980). An individual is considered to have diabetes if the blood glucose values two hours after drinking the mixture are 11.1 mmol/l or greater. Just as someone with borderline blood pressure values are at high risk for hypertension, an individual is considered to be at risk for diabetes if his/her blood glucose values two hours after drinking the solution are 7.8–11.0 mmol/l, which is called impaired glucose tolerance (WHO, 1980).

Despite the fact that type II diabetes is a complex condition caused by both genetic and behavioral factors, the basic metabolic abnormalities responsible for the high blood glucose values are resistance of the body's cells to the action of insulin (termed insulin resistance or decreased insulin sensitivity) and the inability of the pancreas to secrete enough insulin to meet the glucose demand (termed insulin deficiency). During the early stages of the disease development in a genetically prone individual, insulin resistance of the insulin-sensitive tissues of the body (muscles and liver) can usually be found (DeFronzo, 1992). Being insulin resistant means that the glucose cannot readily enter the cells, resulting in a rise of blood glucose concentrations. This increase in blood glucose causes the pancreas to secrete more insulin in an attempt to normalize the blood glucose levels. If allowed to continue, this cycle of resistance and secretion proceeds until the amount of insulin that is secreted is no longer sufficient to compensate for an extreme amount of tissue insulin resistance, resulting in elevated blood glucose values and eventually diabetes (Saad, 1988; Knowler, 1995).

WHAT IS THE PHYSIOLOGICAL BASIS BEHIND A POTENTIAL RELATIONSHIP BETWEEN PHYSICAL ACTIVITY AND THE PREVENTION OF TYPE II DIABETES?

Various reviews of the effects of physical activity on insulin resistance and glucose tolerance have identified the physiological reasons why a relationship between physical activity and type II diabetes is possible (Vranic, 1979; Björntorp, 1985; Koivisto, 1986; Lampman, 1991; Horton, 1991; Wallberg-Henriksson, 1992; Zierath, 1992). In general, active individuals have better insulin and glucose profiles than their inactive counterparts (Stevenson, 1995; Lohmann, 1978) with detraining and bed rest shown to deteriorate these metabolic parameters (Lipmann, 1972; Heath, 1983). Equally as convincing, exercise training studies have found physical activity to im-

FIGURE 11.2

Possible mechanisms through which physical activity may prevent or delay the development of type II diabetes.

- Decrease insulin resistance/improve insulin sensitivity
- Improve blood glucose levels (glucose tolerance)
- Decrease overall adiposity
- Reduce central adiposity
- Desirable changes in muscle tissue

prove insulin action or, in other words, decrease insulin resistance (Saltin, 1979; Lindgärde, 1983; Krotkiewski, 1983; Trovati, 1984; Schneider, 1984; Seals, 1984; Rönnemaa, 1986). Less consistently, some exercise training studies have also found activity to improve glucose metabolism in both normal individuals and those with mild type II diabetes (Minuk, 1981; Holloszy, 1986). Based upon the findings of these training studies, it appears that physical activity would most likely impact on insulin action in individuals at high risk for diabetes (with hyperinsulinemia), that is, those individuals whose capacity to secrete insulin is still intact and insulin resistance is the major cause of the abnormal glucose tolerance (Holloszy, 1986).

Obesity and fat distribution (specifically, the distribution of body fat in the central as compared to the peripheral regions) are major contributors to insulin resistance and are therefore, strongly involved in the pathogenesis of type II diabetes (Björntorp, 1988; Björntorp, 1991; Dowse, 1991; Haffner, 1986; Hartz, 1983; Kissebah, 1989; Knowler, 1991; Modan, 1986; Ohlson, 1985; Stern, 1991). Physical activity has also been shown to be inversely associated with obesity and central fat distribution, with studies demonstrating that physical training can reduce both of these parameters (Björntorp, 1979; Brownell, 1980; Despres, 1988; Krotkiewski, 1988). In other words, it is feasible that physical activity may also prevent or delay type II diabetes through decreasing overall fat and/or intra-abdominal fat.

In summary, it appears that physical activity may not only be related to type II diabetes directly but also indirectly through obesity. Since most individuals with type II diabetes are obese, and change in activity is often associated with small but important changes in fat and body composition, complete separation of the effects of activity from the effects of body composition on type II diabetes

is often difficult (Schwartz, 1997). However, clinical studies examining the effects of physical training on patients with type II diabetes have suggested a direct relationship between the two, independent of obesity.

DO EPIDEMIOLOGY STUDIES SUPPORT A RELATIONSHIP BETWEEN PHYSICAL ACTIVITY AND TYPE II DIABETES?

Through the years, from early observations to current epidemiological studies, support for the existence of a relationship between physical activity and type II diabetes has been increasing. Suggestions of a relationship between physical activity and type II diabetes were supported early on by the fact that societies that had abandoned traditional lifestyles (which typically had included large amounts of habitual physical activity) had experienced major increases in type II diabetes (West, 1978). Indirect evidence of this phenomenon was also provided by the observation that groups of subjects who migrated to a more modern environment had more diabetes than their ethnic counterparts who remained in their native land (Hara, 1983; Kawate, 1979; Ravussin, 1994) or that rural dwellers had a lower prevalence of diabetes than their urban counterparts (Cruz-vidal, 1979; Zimmet, 1981; Zimmet, 1983; King, 1984). In these studies, differences in physical activity were suggested as partial explanations for the differences in diabetes prevalence. Results of epidemiology studies are described in the following sections and summarized in Figure 11.3.

Cross-sectional studies collect information about the health outcome (glucose intolerance or type II diabetes) and the potential risk factor (physical inactivity) at the same time within the same group. This type of epidemiological design is limited because it is not possible to establish causality; i.e., did inactivity cause the glucose intolerance or did the condition cause the inactivity.

Cross-sectional epidemiological studies have shown that physical inactivity was associated with type II diabetes and glucose intolerance within populations. Groups of subjects with type II diabetes were found to be less active currently (Taylor, 1983; Taylor, 1984; King, 1984; Dowse, 1990; Ramaiya, 1991; Kriska, 1993) than nondiabetic persons. In addition,

FIGURE 11.3

Epidemiological studies supporting the relationship between physical activity and type II diabetes.

Cross-sectional Study: Both diabetes status (and glucose/insulin levels) and physical activity levels are determined at the same point in time in the same individuals.

- Individuals with type II diabetes are less active than those without diabetes.
- Among those without type II diabetes, more active individuals have lower glucose and insulin values than their inactive counterparts.

Case-Control (or Retrospective) Study: Individuals with and without type II diabetes are asked questions about their past, in this case, their physical activity levels.

- Individuals with type II diabetes reported less physical activity over their lifetime than individuals without diabetes.

Prospective or Longitudinal Study: Inactive and active individuals without type II diabetes are followed over time to determine if physical activity levels play a role in determining who will and will not develop the disease.

- Women alumnae who were former college athletes had a lower prevalence of diabetes than those who were nonathletes.
- For men and women alike, individuals who are relatively more physically active are less likely to develop type II diabetes in the future than those who are sedentary.

Experimental Study or Clinical Trial: Individuals free of type II diabetes are randomly assigned to a group that includes a physical activity program or does not include it. Follow-up of these groups over time will examine which group develops more diabetes in the future.

- Individuals assigned to the group that includes a physical activity program developed less diabetes over time than those who were not assigned to the activity group.

---

cross-sectional studies that have examined the relationship between physical activity and glucose intolerance in individuals without type II diabetes generally showed that blood glucose values after an oral glucose tolerance test (Lindgärde, 1981; Cederholm, 1985; Wang, 1989; Schranz, 1991; Dowse, 1991; Kriska, 1993; Periera, 1995) as well as insulin values (Lindgärde, 1981; Wang, 1989; Dowse, 1991; McKeigue, 1992; Feskens, 1994; Regensteiner, 1995) were significantly higher in the less active compared to the more active individuals.

In case-control (or retrospective) study designs, individuals with and without diabetes are asked questions about their past, particularly their exposure to the specific risk factor in question (i.e., physical activity level). Although this type of study

design is valuable in cases where the disease outcome is rare, it does suffer from potential recall bias, in which the diseased or high-risk individual may remember or recall past events differently. An example of this type of study design was demonstrated in the Pima Indian Study in which those individuals from the Gila River Indian Community with diabetes reported less physical activity over their lifetime than individuals without diabetes (Kriska, 1993).

The most powerful observational study design is the **prospective or longitudinal study design.** This particular design identifies and follows individuals initially free of the health outcome of interest (diabetes) and seeks to establish if initial or subsequent physical activity levels differentiate those who do and do not develop the disease.

The fact that a sedentary lifestyle may play a role in the development of type II diabetes has been demonstrated in prospective studies of college alumni, registered nurses, physicians, and middle-aged British men (Helmrich, 1991; Manson, 1991, 1992; Perry, 1995). Women alumnae who were former college athletes had a lower prevalence of diabetes than those who were nonathletes (Frisch, 1986). A study of male alumni from the University of Pennsylvania (Helmrich, 1991) demonstrated that physical activity was inversely related to the incidence of type II diabetes, a relationship that was particularly evident in men at high risk for developing diabetes (defined as those with a high body mass index, a history of hypertension, or a parental history of diabetes). In a study of female registered nurses aged 34–59 years, women who reported engaging in vigorous exercise at least once a week had a lower incidence of self-reported type II diabetes during the eight years of follow-up than women who did not exercise weekly (Manson, 1991). Similar findings were observed between exercise and incidence of type II diabetes in a five-year prospective study of 40–84-year-old male physicians (Manson, 1992). Finally, the risk of developing diabetes over a 13-year period was reduced by 50% in men engaged in moderate to vigorous levels of physical activity compared to the less active men (Perry, 1995). Although the results of all of these prospective epidemiological studies suggest a causal relationship between physical inactivity and type II diabetes, the strength of their findings is weakened due to the determination of diabetes based upon self-report rather than an oral glucose tolerance test (since an estimated 50% of the general population are not aware that they have type II diabetes).

Similar to measures of physical activity, physical fitness as determined by maximal oxygen uptake or as estimated by vital capacity also appears to play a role in the development of type II diabetes (Eriksson, 1996, 1991). In addition, support that physical fitness may provide some protection against mortality in men at all levels of glucose intolerance (from those with normal blood glucose to those with type II diabetes) was demonstrated in middle-aged men (Kohl, 1992).

Physical activity was a major part of the intervention strategy of a feasibility trial of diabetes prevention in 47–49-year-old men from Malmo, Sweden. Of those with impaired glucose intolerance at baseline, at least twice as many of those who did not take part in the treatment program had developed diabetes at the five-year follow-up compared with those who participated (Eriksson, 1991). However, since the participants were **not** randomly assigned to the intervention treatment groups, and since the treatment groups differed by medical condition at baseline, the results of this study are not conclusive. In other words, the hypothesis that physical activity intervention may prevent type II diabetes was not adequately tested.

The most powerful and by far the most labor-intensive epidemiological study design is the **experimental design or clinical trial** in which efforts are made to prevent or delay the onset of the type II diabetes by manipulating the risk factor of interest, in this case, physical activity levels. In this design, individuals free of type II diabetes would be randomly assigned to receive either the intervention (the physical activity intervention group) or no intervention (the control group). Subsequent follow-up of the two groups over time would determine if the groups differ by the percent who eventually develop the disease outcome.

Results of a more recent clinical trial demonstrated that physical activity intervention led to a decrease in the incidence of diabetes over a six-year period among Chinese individuals initially identified with impaired glucose tolerance (Pan, 1997). At the beginning of the study, 577 individuals with impaired glucose tolerance were identified from a citywide health screening in DaQing and randomized by clinic into one of four groups: exercise only, diet only, diet plus exercise and a control group. In-

dividuals assigned to the exercise group were encouraged to increase their daily leisure physical activity to that comparable to a 30-minute walk. The percent that developed diabetes was significantly lower in each of the three intervention groups compared to the control group (exercise = 44%, diet = 47%, exercise plus diet = 44%, control = 66%).

An example of a randomized, multi-center clinical trial of type II diabetes prevention that incorporates physical activity as one of the possible treatments is currently underway in the United States (Diabetes Prevention Program, sponsored by the National Institutes of Health; NIH, 1993). In this trial, physical activity is combined with dietary modification to comprise the lifestyle intervention arm of the study. Anyone interested in participating in the Diabetes Prevention Program and/or wants to obtain more information about the program should call the following toll-free number (1-888-DDP-JOIN).

PHYSICAL ACTIVITY RECOMMENDATIONS: HOW MUCH IS ENOUGH?

Recent national physical activity recommendations and summary statements suggest that the majority of overall health benefits from physical activity are gained by performing activities that are not necessarily of high intensity (Pate, 1995). In fact, it has been suggested that the sedentary individual who begins to incorporate adequate amounts of **moderate levels** of physical activity into his/her lifestyle such as walking and gardening may attain substantial health benefits and reduce cardiovascular disease risk (Pate, 1995). How can we best incorporate physical activity into our lifestyle to maximize the health benefits specific to type II diabetes?

Type of Physical Activity Recommended

Most of the exercise training and epidemiology studies done to date have focused on aerobic types of activity that require the use of large muscle mass such as walking, running, and biking. Aerobic activities are recommended for the overall public as the primary type of activity because of their potential benefits in regards to improving the type II diabetes and cardiovascular risk profile (Surgeon General's Report, 1996).

Recently, the benefits of incorporating strength training into an overall activity regimen (that includes aerobic activity) for the prevention and treatment of type II diabetes are being recognized. Strength training has been shown to acutely improve glucose tolerance and insulin sensitivity in individuals with both normal and abnormal glucose tolerance (Smutok, 1994; Miller, 1994).

Frequency/Duration of Physical Activity Recommended

A substantial part of the improvements in glucose tolerance and insulin resistance due to exercise are believed to be the result of the cumulative effect of a frequent lowering of the blood glucose levels and decreasing insulin resistance with each specific bout of exercise (Schneider, 1984). In fact, it appears that a large portion of the effect of exercise in decreasing insulin resistance is short-lived, lasting for a few days, whereas the blood glucose lowering effect of activity may not even last that long (Heath, 1983; Koivisto, 1986). Possible additional improvements in glucose tolerance and insulin resistance due to a training effect of regular exercise on these parameters have been suggested as well (Young, 1989).

In addition, the adaptation caused by increased levels of physical activity that can have an impact on insulin resistance over the long term (especially in the older adult) is the change in body composition. This is in light of the fact that a very critical individual goal in regards to glucose intolerance is to attain and maintain an appropriate weight. Physical activity, in conjunction with diet, appears to be the best combination for decreasing weight (preferentially decreasing centrally distributed fat) and to improving glucose tolerance and insulin sensitivity (Yamanouchi, 1995). Furthermore, physical activity has been shown to play an important role in long-term weight maintenance (Wing, 1988; Pavlou, 1989).

Based upon the information provided above, at what frequency should one attempt exercise throughout the week? Since one of the goals for incorporating physical activity into one's lifestyle is to "burn more calories," and since a substantial portion of the improvement in insulin and glucose appears to be short-lived, it seems reasonable to recommend a frequency of exercise of several times per week. In other words, the weekend exerciser should strongly consider adding a few extra bouts of physical activity throughout the week to maximize his/her benefits in regards to glucose tolerance and insulin sensitivity (not to mention the fact that it is safer from a cardiovascular risk point of view).

Intensity of Physical Activity Recommended

In regards to insulin sensitivity and glucose tolerance, physical training studies suggest that higher intensity exercises are more likely to bring about the desired metabolic changes than lower intensity activities (Holloszy, 1986; Seals, 1984). Lower intensity activities appear to follow in the same general direction, although the onset of the effects are much slower and less dramatic (Björntorp, 1995).

In regards to caloric expenditure, intensity of activity is not an issue. The important thing is that activity is being done! In general, lower intensity activities are usually easier to adopt in one's lifestyle and are relatively less likely to result in injury (Pollock, 1991). It is recommended that beginners start any physical activity slowly and gradually speed up the pace and build up the duration over time.

Finally, it appears that the largest and most consistent difference in risk of type II diabetes occurs between those individuals who report relatively no activity and those who report doing something (see the review by Kriska, 1994). This would suggest that the individuals who would benefit the most from any public health effort to prevent type II diabetes would be the sedentary individuals. If you are currently sedentary, or know people who do not incorporate activity into their lifestyle with any regularity, now is the time, and here is the reason, to begin to incorporate moderate levels of physical activity such as walking and gardening. If you have diabetes or coronary heart disease, it is suggested that you talk with your physician before increasing your activity level (ADA Council on Exercise, 1990; Schwartz, 1997). If you are already active, keep up the good work.

REFERENCES

Björntorp, P., Sjostrom, L., & Sullivan, L. (1979). The role of physical exercise in the management of obesity. In J.F. Munro (Ed.), *The treatment of obesity*, Lancaster, England: MTP Press.

Björntorp, P., & Krotkiewski, M. (1985). Exercise treatment in diabetes mellitus. *Acta Med Scan, 21*, 17–37.

Björntorp, P. (1988). Abdominal obesity and the development of non–insulin-dependent diabetes mellitus. *Diab Metab Rev, 4*, 615–622.

Björntorp, P. (1991). Metabolic implications of body fat distribution. *Diabetes Care, 14*, 1132–1143.

Björntorp, P. (1995). Evolution of the understanding of the role of exercise in obesity and its complications. *International Journal of Obesity, 19*, S1–S4.

Brownell, K.D., & Stunkard, A.J. (1980). Physical activity in the development and control of obesity. In A.J. Stunkard (Ed.), *Obesity*, (pp. 300–324). Philadelphia: W.B. Saunders.

Cederholm, J., & Wibell, L. (1985). Glucose tolerance and physical activity in a health survey of middle-aged subjects. *Acta Med Scand, 217*, 373–378.

Cruz-vidal, M., Costas, R., Garcia-Palmieri, M., Sorlie, P., & Hertzmark, E. (1979). Factors related to diabetes mellitus in Puerto Rican men. *Diabetes, 28*, 300–307.

Despres, J.P., Tremblay, A., Nadeau, A., & Bouchard, C. (1988). Physical training and changes in regional adipose tissue distribution. *Acta Med Scand (Suppl), 723*, 205–212.

Dowse, G.K., Gareeboo, H., Zimmet, P.Z., Alberti, K.G.M.M., Tuomilehto, J., Fareed, D., Brissonnette, L.G., & Finch, C.F. (1990). High prevalence of NIDDM and impaired glucose tolerance in Indian, Creole and Chinese Mauritians. *Diabetes, 39*, 390–396.

Dowse, G.K., Zimmet, P.Z., Gareeboo, H., Alberti, K.G.M.M., Tuomilehto, J., Finch, C.F., Chitson, P., & Tulsidas, H. (1991). Abdominal obesity and physical inactivity are risk factors for NIDDM and impaired glucose tolerance in Indian, Creole, and Chinese Mauritians. *Diabetes Care, 14*, 271–282.

Eriksson, K.F., & Lindgarde, F. (1991). Prevention of type II (non–insulin-dependent) diabetes mellitus by diet and physical exercise. *Diabetologia, 34*, 891–898.

Eriksson, K., & Lindgarde, F. (1996). Poor physical fitness, and impaired early insulin response but late hyperinsulinaemia, as predictors of NIDDM in middle-aged Swedish men. *Diabetologia, 39*, 573–579.

Feskens, E.J., Loeber, J.G., & Kromhout, D. (1994). Diet and physical activity as determinants of hyperinsulinemia: the Zutphen elderly study. *American Journal of Epidemiology, 140*, 350–360.

Frisch, R.E., Wyshak, G., Albright, T.E., Albright, N.L., & Schiff, I. (1986). Lower prevalence of diabetes in female former college athletes compared with nonathletes. *Diabetes, 35*, 1101–1105.

Haffner, S.M., Stern, M.P., Hazuda, H.P., Rosenthal, M., Knapp, J.A., & Malina, R.M. (1986). Role of obesity and fat distribution in non–insulin-dependent diabetes mellitus in Mexican Americans and non-Hispanic whites. *Diabetes Care, 9*, 153–161.

Hara, H., Kawate, T., Yamakido, M., & Nishimoto, Y. (1983). Comparative observation of micro- and macroangiopathies in Japanese diabetics in Japan and U.S.A. In H. Abe & M. Hoshi (Eds.), *Diabetic Microangiopathy*. University of Tokyo Press.

Harris, M.I., Hadden, W.C., Knowler, W.C., & Bennett, P.H. (1987). Prevalence of diabetes and impaired glucose tolerance and plasma glucose levels in U.S. population aged 20–74. *Diabetes, 36*, 523–534.

Hartz, A.J., Rupley, D.C., Kalkhoff, R.D., & Rimm, A.A. (1983). Relationship of obesity to diabetes. Influence of obesity and body fat distribution. *Preventive Medicine, 12*, 351–357.

Heath, G., Gavin, J., Hinderlites, J., Hagberg, J., Bloomfield, S., & Holloszy, J. (1983). Effects of exercise and lack of exercise on glucose tolerance and insulin sensitivity. *Journal of Applied Physiology, 55*, 512–517.

Helmrich, S.P., Ragland, D.R., Leung, R.W., & Paffenbarger, R.S. (1991). Physical activity and reduced occurrence of non–insulin-dependent diabetes mellitus. *New England Journal of Medicine, 325*, 147–152.

Holloszy, J.O., Schultz, J., Kusnierkiewicz, J., Hagberg, J.M., & Ehsani, A.A. (1986). Effects of exercise on glucose tolerance and insulin resistance. *Acta Med Scand (Suppl.), 711*, 55–65.

Horton, E.S. (1991). Exercise and decreased risk of NIDDM. *New England Journal of Medicine, 325*, 196–198.

Kawate, R., Yamakido, M., Nishimoto, Y., Bennett, P.H., Hamman, R.F., & Knowler, W.C. (1979). Diabetes mellitus and its vascular complications in Japanese migrants on the island of Hawaii. *Diabetes Care, 2*, 161–170.

King, H., Zimmet, P., Raper, L., & Balkau, B. (1984). Risk factors for diabetes in three Pacific populations. *American Journal of Epidemiology, 119*, 396–409.

Kissebah, A.H., & Peiris, A.N. (1989). Biology of regional body fat distribution: Relationship to non–insulin-dependent diabetes mellitus. *Diab Metab Rev, 5*, 83–109.

Knowler, W.C., Pettitt, D.J., Saad, M.F., Charles, M.A., Nelson, R.G., Howard, B.V., Bogardus, C., & Bennett, P.H. (1991). Obesity in the Pima Indians: Its magnitude and relationship with diabetes. *American Journal of Clinical Nutrition, 53*, S1543–S1551.

Knowler, W., Narayan, V., Hanson, R. et al. (1995). Perspectives in diabetes: Preventing non–insulin-dependent diabetes. *Diabetes, 44*, 483–488.

Kohl, H.W., Gordon, N.F., Villegas, J.A., & Blair, S.N. (1992). Cardiorespiratory fitness, glycemic status, and mortality risk in men. *Diabetes Care, 15*, 184–192.

Koivisto, V.A., Yki-Jarvinen, H., & DeFronzo, R.A. (1986). Physical training and insulin sensitivity. *Diab Metab Rev, 1*, 445–481.

Kriska, A., LaPorte, R., Pettitt, D., Charles, M., Nelson, R., Kuller, L., Bennett, P., & Knowler, W. (1993). The association of physical activity with obesity, fat distribution and glucose intolerance in Pima Indians. *Diabetologia 36*, 863–869.

Kriska, A.M., Blair, S.N., & Pereira, M.A. (1994). The potential role of physical activity in the prevention of non–insulin-dependent diabetes mellitus: The epidemiological evidence. *Exercise and Sports Science Reviews, 22*, 121–143.

Krotkiewski, M. (1983). Physical training in the prophylaxis and treatment of obesity, hypertension and diabetes. *Scandinavian Journal of Rehabilitation and Medicine Suppl*, 55–70.

Krotkiewski, M. (1988). Can body fat patterning be changed? *Acta Med Scand Suppl, 723*, 213–223.

Lampman, R.M., & Schteingart, D.E. (1991). Effects of exercise training on glucose control, lipid metabolism, and insulin sensitivity in hypertriglyceridemia and non–insulin-dependent diabetes mellitus. *Medicine and Science in Sports and Exercise, 23*, 703–712.

Lindgärde, F., & Saltin, B. (1981). Daily physical activity, work capacity and glucose tolerance in lean and obese normoglycaemic middle-aged men. *Diabetologia, 20* 134–138.

Lindgarde, F., Malmquist, J., & Balke, B. (1983). Physical fitness, insulin secretion, and glucose tolerance in healthy males and mild type II diabetes. *Acta Diabet Lat, 20*, 33–40.

Lipman, R.L., Raskin, P., Love, T., Triebwasser, J., Lecocq, F.R., & Schnure, J.J. (1972). Glucose intolerance during decreased physical activity in man. *Diabetes, 21*, 101–107.

Lohmann, D., Liebold, F., Heilmann, W., Senger, H., & Pohl, A. (1978). Diminished insulin response in highly trained athletes. *Metabolism, 27*, 521–524.

Manson, J.E., Rimm, E.B., Stampfer, M.J., Colditz, G.A., Willett, W.C., Krolewski, A.S., Rosner, B., Hennekens, C.H., & Speizer, F.E. (1991). Physical activity and incidence of non–insulin-dependent diabetes mellitus in women. *Lancet, 338*, 774–778.

Manson, J.E., Nathan, D.M., Krolewski, A.S., Stampfer, M.J., Willett, W.C., & Hennekens, C.H. (1992). A prospective study of exercise and incidence of diabetes among U.S. male physicians. *Journal of the American Medical Association, 268*, 63–67.

McKeigue, P.M., Pierpoint, T., Ferrie, J.E., & Marmot, M.G. (1992). Relationship of glucose intolerance and hyperinsulinaemia to body fat pattern in South Asians and Europeans. *Diabetologia, 35*, 785–791.

Modan, M., Karasik, A., Halkin, H., Fuchs, Z., Lusky, A., Shitrit, A., & Modan, B. (1986). Effect of past and concurrent body mass index on prevalence of glucose intol-erance and type II diabetes and non–insulin response. *Diabetologia, 29*, 82–89.

National Diabetes Data Group. (1979). Classification and diagnosis of diabetes and other categories of glucose intolerance. *Diabetes, 28*, 1039–1057.

Ohlson, L.O., Larsson, B., Svardsudd, K., Welin, L., Eriksson, H., Wilhelmsen, L., Bjorntorp, P., & Tibblin, G. (1985). The influence of body fat distribution on the incidence of diabetes mellitus: Thirteen and one-half years of follow-up of the participants in the study of men in 1913. *Diabetes, 34*, 1055–1058.

Pan, X., Li, G., Hu, Y. et al. (1997). Effects of diet and exercise in preventing NIDDM in people with impaired glucose tolerance: The Da Qing IGT and diabetes study. *Diabetes Care, 20*, 537–544.

Pate, R.R., Pratt, M., Blair, S.N., Haskell, W.L., Macera, C.A., Bouchard, C., Buckner, D., Caspersen, C.J., Ettinger, W., Heath, G.W., King, A., Kriska, A.M., Leon, A.S., Marcus, B.H., Morris, J., Paffenbarger, R., Patrick, K., Pollock, M., Rippe, J.M., Sallis, J., & Wilmore, J.H. (1995). Physical activity and health: A recommendation from the Centers for Disease Control and Prevention and the American College of Sports Medicine. *Journal of the American Medical Association, 273*, 402–407.

Pavlou, K.N., Krey, S., & Steffe, W.P. (1989). Exercise as an adjunct to weight loss and maintenance in moderately obese subjects. *American Journal of Clinical Nutrition, 49*, 1115–1123.

Pereira, M., Kriska, A., Joswiak, M., Dowse, G., Collins, V., Zimmet, P., Gareeboo, H., Chitson, P., Hemraj, F., Purran, A., & Fareed, D. (1995). Physical inactivity and glucose intolerance in the multi-ethnic island of Mauritius. *Medicine and Science in Sports and Exercise, 27*, 1626–1634.

Perry, I., Wannamethee, S., Walker, M. et al. (1995). Prospective study of risk factors for development of non–insulin-dependent diabetes in middle-aged British men. *British Medical Journal, 310*, 560–564.

Physical Activity and Health: A Report of the Surgeon General. Invited author. U.S. Department of Health and Human Services. Centers for Disease Control and Prevention. National Center for Chronic Disease Prevention and Health Promotion. President's Council on Physical Fitness and Sports. 1996.

Pollock, M.L., Carroll, J.F., Graves, J.E., Leggett, S.H., Braith, R.W., Limacher, M., & Hagberg, J.M. (1991). Injuries and adherence to walking to walk/jog and resistance training programs in the elderly. *Medicine and Science in Sports and Exercise, 23*, 1194–1200.

Ravussin, E., Bennett, P.H., Valencia, M.E., Schulz, L.O., & Esparza, J. (1994). Effects of traditional lifestyle on obesity in Pima Indians. *Diabetes Care, 17*, 1067–1074.

Regensteiner, J.G., Shetterly, S.M., Mayer, E.J., Eckel, R.H., Haskell, W.L., Baxter, J., & Hamman, R.F. (1995). Relationship between habitual physical activity and insulin area among individuals with impaired glucose tolerance. *Diabetes Care, 18*, 490–497.

Rönnemaa, T., Mattila, K., Lehtonen, A., & Kallio, V. (1986). A controlled randomized study on the effect of long-term physical exercise on the metabolic control in type II diabetic patients. *Acta Med Scand, 220,* 219–224.

Saad, M.F., Knowler, W.C., Pettitt, D.J., Nelson, R.G., Mott, D.M., & Bennett, P.H. (1988). The natural history of impaired glucose tolerance in the Pima Indians. *New England Journal of Medicine, 319,* 1500–1506.

Saltin, B., Lindgärde, F., Houston, M., Horlin, R., Nygaard, E., & Gad, P. (1979). Physical training and glucose tolerance in middle-aged men with chemical diabetes. *Diabetes, 28,* 30–32.

Schneider, S.H., Amorosa, L.F., Khachadurian, A.K., & Ruderman, N.B. (1984). Studies on the mechanism of improved glucose control during regular exercise in type II diabetes. *Diabetologia, 26,* 355–360.

Schranz, A., Tuomilehto, J., Marti, B., Jarrett, R.J., Grabauskas, V., & Vassallo, A. (1991). Low physical activity and worsening of glucose tolerance: results from a 2-year follow-up of a population sample in Malta. *Diabetes Res Clin Prac, 11,* 127–136.

Schwartz, R. (1997). Physical activity, insulin resistance, and diabetes. In A. Leon (Ed.), *Physical Activity and Cardiovascular Health: A National Consensus* (pp. 218–227). Champaign, IL: Human Kinetics Publishers.

Seals, D., Hagberg, J., Hurley, B., Ehsani, A., & Holloszy, J. (1984). Effects of endurance training on glucose tolerance and plasma lipid levels in older men and women. *Journal of the American Medical Association, 252,* 645–649.

Smutok, M., Reece, C., Kokkinos, P. et al. (1994). Effects of exercise training modality on glucose tolerance in men with abnormal glucose regulation. *International Journal of Sports Medicine, 15,* 283–289.

Stern, M.P. (1991). Kelly West lecture; Primary prevention of type II diabetes mellitus. *Diabetes Care, 14,* 399–410.

Taylor, R.J., Bennett, P.H., LeGonidec, G., Lacoste, J., Combe, D., Joffres, M., Uili, R., Charpin, M., & Zimmet, P.Z. (1983). The prevalence of diabetes mellitus in a traditional-living Polynesian population: The Wallis Island survey. *Diabetes Care, 6,* 334–340.

Taylor, R.J., Ram, P., Zimmet, P., Raper, L., & Ringrose, H. (1984). Physical activity and prevalence of diabetes in Melanesian and Indian men in Fiji. *Diabetologia, 27,* 578–582.

Trovati, M., Carta, Q., Cavalot, F., Vitali, S., Banaudi, C., Lucchina, P.G., Fiocchi, F., Emanuelli, G., & Lenti, G. (1984). Influence of physical training on blood glucose control, glucose tolerance, insulin secretion, and insulin action in non–insulin-dependent diabetes patients. *Diabetes Care, 7,* 416–420.

Wallberg-Henriksson, H. (1992). Exercise and diabetes mellitus. In J.O. Holloszy (Ed.), *Exercise and Sport Sciences Reviews* (pp. 339–368). Williams and Wilkins.

Wang, J.T., Ho, L.T., Tang, K.T., Wang, L.M., Chen, Y.D.I., & Reaven, G.M. (1989). Effect of habitual physical activity on age-related glucose intolerance. *Journal of the American Geriatric Society, 37,* 203–209.

West, K.M. *Epidemiology of diabetes and its vascular lesions.* New York: Elsevier, 1978.

Wing, R.R., Epstein, L.H., Bayles, M.P., Kriska, A.M., Nowalk, M.P., & Gooding, W. (1988). Exercise in a behavioural weight control programme for obese patients with type II (non–insulin-dependent) diabetes. *Diabetologia, 31,* 902–909.

World Health Organization Expert Committee. *Second report on diabetes mellitus.* Technical Report Series No. 646, Geneva, Switzerland, 1980.

Yamanouchi, K., Shinozaki, T., Chikada, K. et al. (1995). Daily walking combined with diet therapy is a useful means for obese NIDDM patients not only to reduce body weight but also to improve insulin sensitivity. *Diabetes Care, 18,* 775–778.

Young, J., Enslin, J., & Kuca, B. (1989). Exercise intensity and glucose tolerance in trained and nontrained subjects. *Journal of Applied Physiology, 67,* 39–43.

Zimmet, P.Z., Faauiso, S., Ainuu, S., Whitehouse, S., Milne, B., & DeBoer, W. (1981). The prevalence of diabetes in the rural and urban Polynesian population of Western Samoa. *Diabetes, 30,* 45–51.

Zimmet, P.Z., Taylor, R., Ram, P., King, H., Sloman, G., Raper, L., & Hunt, D. (1983). Prevalence of diabetes and impaired glucose tolerance in the biracial population of Fiji: A rural-urban comparison. *American Journal of Epidemiology, 118,* 673–688.

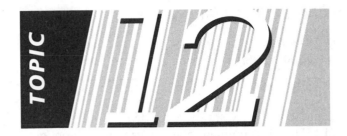

Osteoporosis and Physical Activity

Janet M. Shaw
UNIVERSITY OF UTAH

Christine Snow
OREGON STATE UNIVERSITY

INTRODUCTION

The National Osteoporosis Foundation (NOF) has defined osteoporosis as a disease characterized by low bone mass and microarchitectural deterioration of bone tissue leading to enhanced bone fragility and a consequent increase in fracture risk. In other words, osteoporosis is the loss of bone tissue that makes bones weaker. It has been projected that over 5 million fractures of the hip, spine, and wrist will occur in women over the age of 45, which will account for more than $45 billion in direct health care costs over the next ten years (Chrischilles, Shireman, & Wallace, 1994). This is a conservative estimate of the future public health impact of osteoporosis, since the projections are based on only three fracture sites and limited to females. No doubt the estimate would be greater if it included men, who also are at risk of osteoporosis as they grow older.

In addition to the financial burden attributed to this disease, osteoporosis has a profound effect on the quality of life of older individuals. Those afflicted typically experience reduced mobility, pain, loss of independence, and psychological distress associated with postural disfigurement and the fear of additional fractures. Hip fractures are the most severe fractures since they carry the highest incidence of morbidity and mortality. The postural abnormality associated with vertebral fractures results in reduced cardiovascular capacity and affects other internal organs due to compression of the chest and abdominal regions. In order to define effective preventive strategies, it is important to determine the lifestyle factors that influence fracture risk. The two primary determinants of fracture risk are low bone mass and falls.

Physical activity has been proposed as one strategy to reduce fractures by increasing bone mass and by preventing falls through improved functional ability. Although the mechanism by which exercise increases bone mass is not clear, it likely influences bone directly through mechanical forces (loading) transferred to bone. Bone responds to changes in mechanical loading and the regulation of bone strength is a function of the loads to which the skeleton is exposed. The most striking examples of this adaptation are the reports that demonstrate marked bone loss in the absence of weight-bearing activity, such as occurs in space travel and prolonged bed rest

ORIGINALLY PUBLISHED AS SERIES 2, NUMBER 3, OF THE PCPFS RESEARCH DIGEST.

"Bone health is promoted through regular weight-bearing physical activities that use muscular strength and power, and exert force on the skeleton above normal amounts."

(Mack et al., 1967; Nishimura et al., 1994). Conversely, many reports have shown that bone mass among physically active individuals and athletes is significantly higher compared to their nonactive and nonathletic counterparts. Some studies that have imposed significant mechanical forces via exercise intervention report positive effects on bone mass, although the magnitude of effect is much less impressive than would be predicted from studies on athletes and active individuals. Therefore, the ideal exercise program that maximizes bone response remains elusive. Evidence is accumulating to suggest, however, that exercise that increases muscle strength, mass, and power, may provide the best osteogenic stimulus. Activities of this type provide additional skeletal protection in the older adult by preventing falls, which are highly related to the incidence of fractures, particularly at the hip.

This review presents the recent literature in the field and provides recommendations for exercise design that may aid in fracture prevention. In this review, the terms "bone mass" and "bone mineral density (BMD)" will be used as synonyms.

PHYSICAL ACTIVITY AND BONE MASS

Physical activity transmits loads to the skeleton in two ways: by muscle pull and by gravitational forces from weight-bearing activity. It is generally assumed that a high level of activity corresponds to a high level of mechanical loading. However, despite the intensity of muscular activity associated with competitive swimming, studies comparing athletic groups have demonstrated that swimmers generally have BMD values lower than those of nonathletic controls (Taaffe et al., 1995). Therefore, activities that require full support of body weight (i.e., those that are performed on the feet) are recommended if skeletal response is a desired outcome of exercise participation. Sports with unilateral activity, such as tennis, continue to provide the best representation of the positive effects of exercise on bone in humans (Huddleston et al., 1980; Kannus et

al., 1994). These studies have demonstrated greater BMD in the dominant playing arm vs. the nondominant arm across different age groups. However, most forms of activity are not as easily characterized by such specific, localized loading patterns.

Other indicators that physical activity exerts a positive influence on the skeleton is the finding that certain measures of physical fitness are correlated with BMD. Specifically, body composition and muscular strength exhibit positive associations with bone mass. Investigations of BMD and body composition have arisen out of the common finding that body weight is associated with bone density. Research has attempted to specify which aspect of body composition, lean (muscle) or fat mass, is the best predictor of bone mass. Muscle directly attaches to bone and may influence the skeletal system via this mechanism, while fat mass contributes to body weight in a nonspecific manner. It has been proposed that fat mass has the potential to increase circulating levels of estrogen, although this explanation for its beneficial influence on bone has yet to be established. Associations between both fat and lean mass and BMD have been demonstrated (Reid, Plank, & Evans, 1992; Sowers et al., 1992). Although fat mass has been associated with bone and can provide cushioning in the fall-prone elderly, there are known health problems associated with excess body fat (e.g., cardiovascular disease, type II diabetes). On the other hand, adequate muscle mass is necessary for optimal function throughout the life span and muscular atrophy that accompanies the aging process is associated with falling and fracture. Therefore it is prudent to recommend that a fracture prevention program include activities that encourage muscle mass development.

Mechanical forces are directly applied to bone by muscular attachments and individuals with high muscle strength are able to generate large forces during contraction. Thus, muscle strength is a measure of physical fitness that has been studied with respect to skeletal health. Research has shown that the relationship between muscle strength and bone demonstrates site-specificity. Strength of the hip muscles has been related to hip BMD, and grip strength has been associated with forearm BMD (Snow-Harter et al., 1993; Snow-Harter et al., 1990). The contribution of muscle strength to BMD in various cross-sectional studies has ranged from 9 to 38% in nonathletic adults. Since approximately 60–80% of bone mass is estimated to be genetically determined, the relationship between muscle strength and bone is not trivial and again points to the importance of the muscular system with respect to bone health.

Research has demonstrated that male and female athletes who participate in sports that require muscular strength and power (e.g., weight lifting, gymnastics, wrestling) exhibit higher bone mass than those whose sports involve primarily muscular endurance (e.g., distance running, triathlon) (Robinson et al., 1995). Information on the loading characteristics of various activities suggests that walking and slow running provide loads equal to or slightly higher than body weight alone at the spine. In comparison, forces at the spine have been estimated to be five to six times body weight while weight lifting (Granhad, Jonson, & Hansson, 1987). Jumping associated with gymnastics training may elicit forces as high as 10 to 12 times body weight.

The research on athletes and the size of the load for a specific sport suggests that the skeleton's response to mechanical loading depends on the *magnitude* of the force. In practical terms, the skeleton must encounter forces that are *greater* than those it experiences on a day-to-day basis. Even though walking is a weight-bearing activity, its ability to evoke a skeletal response is limited to the older adult who was previously bedridden and unable to ambulate for a period of time. On the other hand, one who performs activities of daily living without assistance will be in a weight-bearing posture much of the day. For this person, walking as an exercise will not exceed the loading threshold of daily activities and therefore will not improve bone mass.

Exercise intervention studies have attempted to introduce various exercise programs in humans to determine the best exercise prescription for bone health. The results of these studies are equivocal. While some reports indicate that BMD increases slightly with exercise, some report no change or slight decreases. In order to detect changes in bone mass, an intervention must be several months in du-

ration, depending on the age group and type of program (six months minimum). Relative to other exercise interventions, these are long time intervals (e.g., muscular strength increases can be observed in eight weeks). Over the life span, however, these time intervals are relatively short. This may be one reason why remarkable changes have not been observed within the time frame of training studies. In addition, the expected magnitude of skeletal response is much less than that observed in the muscular system. To illustrate, muscular strength improvements on the order of 50–100% during the course of a resistance training program are not unusual, especially if initial values were low. A 1.5% increase in bone mass over a period of nine months is meaningful, since average rates of loss are approximately 0.5–1% per year. To date, most exercise studies have not designed their exercise training programs according to the principles of training. This may be the main reason why many studies have observed minimal or no training effects on the skeleton (Drinkwater, 1994). The application of these principles to bone loading is outlined in Table 12.1.

PREVENTION STRATEGIES THROUGHOUT THE LIFE SPAN

Bone is a dynamic tissue that is constantly undergoing remodeling activity, a function of bone cells, during which old bone is removed and new bone is formed. The factors that determine the level of

TABLE 12.1

Principles of training.

Specificity	The impact of the training should be at the bone site of interest since loading seems to have a localized effect.
Overload	The training stimulus must include forces much greater than that afforded by habitual activity.
Reversibility	In the absence of the training stimulus, the positive effect on bone will be lost.
Initial values	Individuals with low BMD will have the greatest potential to gain from increased mechanical loading.
Diminishing returns	Each individual's biological ceiling determines the extent of adaptation to the training.

bone cell activity are mechanical loading, calcium intake, and reproductive hormones. Strategies to decrease risk for osteoporotic fracture should take these factors into consideration throughout the life span since bone mass in the older adult is a product of the amount of bone acquired during growth and subsequent rates of loss during adulthood.

Physical activity has been shown to be an important contributor to bone mass in children prior to adolescence (Slemenda et al., 1991). In addition, this group should have adequate calcium intake so that the necessary blocks for building bone mineral are present during growth. It has been proposed that young bone may be more responsive to mechanical loading than old bone (Forwood & Burr, 1993). Given that approximately 60% of the final skeleton is acquired during adolescence, one preventive strategy is to maximize skeletal loading during this rapid phase of growth. It is also important to consider reproductive endocrine status at this time of life. The negative effects of abnormally low estrogen on BMD in amenorrheic women with a high volume of physical training and very low body weight (primarily distance running and ballet dancing) are well documented (Drinkwater et al., 1984). These effects are even more dramatic in amenorrheic women with anorexia nervosa. Although there is little if any documentation in men, abnormally low testosterone levels are theoretically detrimental for bone.

Preventive strategies in adults are generally aimed at maintaining bone mass or reducing the rate of loss. However, recent studies on young adult women indicate that physical activity may play an important role with respect to the capacity to increase bone mass after growth has stopped (Recker et al., 1992; Bassey & Ramsdale, 1994). Recker and colleagues observed increases in spine BMD over a period of five years in a large group of women in their twenties. The increases were related to self-selected physical activity patterns. Bassey and Ramsdale (1994) administered high- and low-impact exercise programs to young women for six months and observed BMD increases at the hip in the high-impact group only. The authors note that small improvements in bone mass in young to middle adulthood may result in quite significant reductions in risk for osteoporotic fracture in later years. It is important to note that BMD increases with physical activity are likely to be most dramatic in

young adulthood when bone appears to be more responsive to mechanical loading. In addition, loading characteristics must be substantial, as demonstrated by the high-impact activity administered by Bassey and Ramsdale (1994), which included jumping. Adequate calcium intake and maintenance of normal circulating levels of reproductive hormones are still important factors for optimal bone health in adulthood. However, since growth has ceased, recommendations for calcium intake are slightly lower than in adolescence.

Older adults face multiple challenges with advancing age. Age-related reductions in bone mass, muscle strength and power, and postural stability make this group at highest risk for fracture. Impaired musculoskeletal function and dynamic balance associated with aging and disuse ultimately result in decreased mobility. In addition, these declines in musculoskeletal function have been associated with an increase in falls and incidence of hip fracture. Vandervoort et al. (1990) report that once function has declined to the point where mobility is significantly reduced, older individuals may refuse to ambulate due to a fear of falling, which is the beginning of a downward spiral that ultimately results in loss of independence. This situation, in which very few physical attempts are made, leads to marked reductions in strength and power of the lower extremities, which have been specifically linked to fall risk. Although bone mass is a major risk factor for osteoporosis, falls and their severity are highly related to fractures in the elderly. In fact, 90% of all hip fractures occur as a result of a fall (Melton, 1993).

Falls are caused by many different factors. Epidemiological research has consistently found that lower limb strength, reaction time, sensory impairment, and postural instability are important risk factors for falls. Greenspan et al. (1994) have proposed that not all falls are potentially injurious and that fall *severity* in combination with bone mass at the hip are the two primary determinants of hip fracture in ambulatory elderly. Specifically, those who fall to the side and have no ability to alter fall direction or speed of impact and land directly on the hip, are more likely to fracture, particularly if BMD at that site is low (Hayes et al., 1993). The link of muscular strength and power to fall risk is most logically in the stabilization and control required for voluntary movements as well as for the ability to recover from a stumble. One study determined that leg extensor (quadriceps) power in older men and women was the best predictor of functional performance (Bassey et al., 1992).

Strategies to prevent fracture in older adults must target bone mass as well as factors associated with falls. Several studies have observed beneficial effects of weight training in older populations including increased bone mass, muscular strength, power, dynamic balance, and functional independence. Thus, this may be the best choice of exercise training at this stage in the life span. Most research has focused on machine-based training (e.g., Universal Gym, Nautilus), which requires a seated posture for lower body exercises. While this isolates muscle groups in the legs, it effectively reduces loads at the hip and does not require postural control and balance. To encourage optimal function in a standing posture, older adults should be encouraged to perform exercises such as stepping and rising from a chair. These exercises target muscle groups and actions important for everyday function. While it may seem dangerous for older adults to engage in this type of training, resistance training has proven successful among nursing-home residents, even among quite old adults. The benefits of participation clearly outweigh the risks of immobility, decreased function, and increased likelihood of falls and fracture.

Assessing Your Risk for Osteoporosis

For each of the following questions, check either yes or no.

	Yes	No
1. Do you have a family history of osteoporosis? (Have any of your relatives broken a wrist or hip or had a dowager's hump?)	___	___
2. Did you go through menopause or have your ovaries removed by surgery before age 50?	___	___
3. Did your menstrual periods ever stop for more than a year for reasons other than pregnancy or nursing?	___	___
4. Did your ancestors come from England, Ireland, Scotland, Northern Europe, or Asia, or do you have a small, thin body frame?	___	___
5. Have you had surgery in which a part of your stomach or intestines was removed?	___	___
6. Are you taking or have you taken drugs like cortisone, steroids, or anticonvulsants over a prolonged period?	___	___
7. Do you have a thyroid or parathyroid disorder (hyperthyroidism or hyperparathyroidism)?	___	___
8. Are you allergic to milk products or are you lactose intolerant?	___	___
9. Do you smoke cigarettes?	___	___
10. Do you drink wine, beer, or other alcoholic beverages daily?	___	___
11. Do you do less than one hour of exercising such as aerobics, walking, or jogging per week?	___	___
12. Have you ever exercised so strenuously that you had irregular periods or no periods at all?	___	___
13. Have you ever had an eating disorder (bulimia or anorexia nervosa)?	___	___

If you answered "yes" to many of these questions, you may be at an increased risk for osteoporosis.

Source: From *Wellness: Choices for Health and Fitness,* by R. Donatelle, C. Snow-Harter, and A. Wilcox. Copyright © 1995 Benjamin/Cummings Publishing Company. By permission of Brooks/Cole Publishing Company, Pacific Grove, CA 93950, a division of International Thompson Publishing Inc.

CONCLUSIONS

Exercise may benefit the skeleton and reduce osteoporosis and fracture risk in the following ways: (1) increase bone mass up to and through adolescence, which will result in higher BMD levels across the life span; (2) improve and maintain bone density during early adulthood; and (3) reduce or slow the rate of age-related loss during middle and older age. In order to have an effect on bone, exercise must be different from daily activities, that is, an *overload* must be applied to the skeleton. It is important to remember that physical activity has not been shown to offset the transient increase in bone loss resulting from estrogen deficiency that is observed in the first five to seven years past menopause. Although still uncertain, the gap is beginning to narrow with respect to the types and amount of activities that confer the best osteogenic stimulus. Participation in activities of high load and low repetitions, which increase muscle strength and power, may ultimately prove to be the most beneficial to bone mass. Research to quantify forces from activities that promote strength and power will substantiate these predictions and the models should be evaluated in populations at different stages of skeletal development.

The importance of building lower extremity strength and cardiovascular health cannot be over-emphasized with respect to fall prevention and general health. Low bone mass is a primary risk factor for fractures, with 90% of hip fractures occurring as the result of a fall. Perhaps the most significant benefit of participation in exercise relates to improvements in neuromuscular function. Sound neuromuscular function is essential for both static and dynamic postural stability. The ability to avoid an obstacle, recover from a stumble, or alter the direction of a fall may significantly reduce fall severity (Greenspan et al., 1994). Muscle mass, strength, and power decline with age, particularly in the lower extremities (Annianson et al., 1984) and this has been attributed, in part, to a decrease in physical activity. As a result, it is more difficult for the elderly to perform activities of daily living, particularly ambulation. Resistance training programs have demonstrated significant improvement in neuromuscular function in the elderly through the tenth decade, which translates to reduced risk of fall-related fractures.

"The foundation for bone health begins early in life. Physical activity that places a load on the bones is essential throughout childhood and the adolescent years."

Editors

REFERENCES

Annianson, A.C., Zitterberg, C., Hedberg, C., et al. (1984). Impaired muscle function with aging. *Clinical Orthopaedics and Related Research, 191,* 193–210.

Bassey, E.J., & Ramsdale, S.J. (1994). Increase in femoral bone density in young women following high-impact exercise. *Osteoporosis International, 4,* 72–75.

Bassey, E.J., Fiatarone, M.J., O'Neill, E.F., et al. (1992). Leg extensor power and functional performance in very old men and women. *Clinical Science, 82,* 321–327.

Cavanaugh, D.J., & Cann, C.E. (1988). Brisk walking does not stop bone loss in postmenopausal women. *Bone, 9,* 201–204.

Chrischilles, E., Sherman, T., & Wallace, R. (1994). Cost and health effects of osteoporotic fractures. *Bone, 15,* 377–386.

Donatelle, Snow-Harter, C., & Wilcox (1995). *Wellness: Choices for health and fitness.* Pacific Grove, CA: Brooks/Cole.

Drinkwater, B.L. (1994). C.H. McCloy Research Lecture: Does physical activity play a role in preventing osteoporosis? *Research Quarterly for Exercise and Sport, 65,* 197–206.

Drinkwater, B.L., Nilson, K., Chestnut, C.H., Bremner, W.J., Shainholtz, S., et al. (1984). Bone mineral content of amenorrheic and eumenorrheic athletes. *New England Journal of Medicine, 311,* 277–281.

Forwood, M.R. & Burr, D.B. (1993). Physical activity and bone mass: Exercises in futility? *Bone Mineral, 21,* 89–112.

Granhad, H., Jonson, R., & Hansson, T. (1987). The loads on the lumbar spine during extreme weight lifting. *Spine, 12,* 146–149.

Greenspan, S.L., Meyers, E.R., Maitland, L.A., et al. (1994). Fall severity and bone mineral density as risk factors for hip fracture in ambulatory elderly. *Journal of the American Medical Association, 271,* 128–133.

Hayes, W.C., Meyers, E.R., Morris, J.N., et al. (1993). Impact near the hip dominates fracture risk in elderly nursing home residents who fall. *Calcified Tissue International, 52,* 192–198.

Huddleston, A.L., Rockwell, D., Kulund, D.N., et al. (1980). Bone mass in lifetime tennis players. *Journal of the American Medical Association, 244,* 1107–1109.

Kannus, P., Haapasalo, H., Sievanen, H., et al. (1994). The site-specific effects of long-term unilateral activity on bone mineral density and content. *Bone, 15,* 279–284.

Mack, P.B., LaChance, P.A., Vose, G.P., et al. (1967). Bone demineralization of foot and hand of Gemini Titan IV, V and VII astronauts during orbital flight. *American Journal of Roentgenology: Radium Therapy and Nuclear Medicine, 100,* 503–511.

Melton, L. J. (1993). Hip fractures: A worldwide problem today and tomorrow. *Bone, 14,* S1–S8.

Nishimura, H., Fukuoka, H., Kiriyama, M., et al. (1994). Bone turnover and calcium metabolism during 20 days bed rest in young healthy males and females. *Acta Physiol Scand, 150, Suppl 616,* 27–35.

Recker, R.R., Davies, K.M., Hinders, S.M., et al. (1992). Bone gain in young adult women. *Journal of the American Medical Association, 268,* 2403–2408.

Reid, I.R., Plank, L.D., & Evans, M.C. (1992). Fat mass is an important determinant of whole body bone density in premenopausal women but not in men. *Journal of Clinical Edocrinal Metabolism, 75,* 779–782.

Robinson, T.L., Snow-Harter, C., Taaffe, D.R., et al. (1995). Gymnasts exhibit higher bone mass than runners despite similar prevalence of amenorrhea and oligomenorrhea. *Journal of Bone Mineral Research, 10,* 26–35.

Slemenda, C.W., Miller, J.Z., Hui, S.L., et al. (1991). Role of physical activity in the development of skeletal mass in children. *Journal of Bone Mineral Research, 6,* 1227–1233.

Snow-Harter, C., Bouxsein, M., Lewis, B., et al. (1990). Muscle strength as a predictor of bone mineral density in young women. *Journal of Bone Mineral Research, 5,* 589–595.

Snow-Harter, C., Robinson, T., Shaw, J., et al. (1993). Determinants of femoral neck mineral density in pre- and postmenopausal women. *Medicine and Science in Sports and Exercise, 25, Suppl Sl53.*

Sowers, M.R., Kshirsagar, A., Crutchfield, M.M., & Updike, S. (1992). Joint influence of fat and lean body composition compartments on femoral bone mineral density in premenopausal women. *American Journal of Epidemiology, 136,* 257–265.

Taaffe, D.R., Snow-Harter, C., Connolly, D.A., et al. (1995). Differential effects of swimming versus weight bearing activity on bone mineral status of eumenorrheic athletes. *Journal of Bone Mineral Research, 10,* 586–593.

Vandervoort, A., Hill, K., Sandrin, M., et al. (1990). Mobility impairment and failing in the elderly. *Physical Therapy Canada, 42,* 99–107.

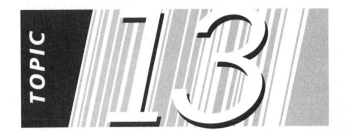

Physical Fitness and Healthy Low Back Function

Sharon Ann Plowman
NORTHERN ILLINOIS UNIVERSITY

Papers 6 and 7 in Section II gave a general overview of the benefits of physical activity and how those benefits related to major lifestyle diseases and the *Healthy People 2000* promotion and disease prevention priorities. This paper focuses on physical activity, physical fitness, healthy back function, and low back pain.

The following key points are discussed in detail in this article:

- At some time in their lives, 60–80% of all individuals experience low back pain. The condition is disabling to 1–5% of this population.

- To have a healthy, well-functioning back, flexible lumbar muscles, hamstrings, and hip flexors, and strong fatigue-resistant abdominal and back extensor muscles are necessary.

- The *Healthy People 2000* goals aim to decrease disability from chronic disabling disease and to increase the proportion of the population who regularly perform activities to enhance muscular strength, endurance, and flexibility. In terms of low back health, the latter goal may be one way of achieving the former goal.

- Exercises to maintain or increase muscular function in the low back region are presented in Table 13.1.

- The anatomical logic (presented in Table 13.2) linking low back health and physical activity is stronger than the research evidence at this time.

Studies (see body of text) support the fact that individuals who have suffered low back pain (LBP) have weaker, more fatigable, and less flexible muscles in the trunk region even after the acute pain episode has subsided than do those who are pain free. Continued weakness, low endurance, and restricted range of movement appear to be contributing factors to recurrent LBP. The ability to predict first-time LBP from muscular strength, endurance, or flexibility values has not been established. Likewise, a direct relationship between LBP and cardiovascular or body composition fitness has not been established. On the other hand, with one exception, which is noted in the following text, the studies reviewed have not shown that high levels of any of these fitness components are in any way linked as causal factors to LBP. Therefore, it appears prudent at this

---

ORIGINALLY PUBLISHED AS SERIES 1, NUMBER 3, OF THE PCPFS *RESEARCH DIGEST*.

HIGHLIGHT ▌█▌ ▌▌▐██▌ █▌ ▐██▌▌ ▐▐ █▐▐ ▐█▐   ▐ ▐ ▐▐█▐ ▐█▐▐▐█▐▐▌ ▐ ▐ ▐▐█▐ ▐█▐ ▐▐ ▐▐ █▐▐▐█ █ ▐▐█▐▐▌ ▐▌

The development and maintenance of healthy low back function requires a balance of flexibility, strength, and endurance. Specifically, the critical components are:

a. low back lumbar flexibility;
b. hamstring flexibility;
c. hip flexor flexibility;
d. strength and endurance of the forward and lateral abdominals; and
e. strength and endurance of the back extensor muscles.

Include appropriate exercises for each group in your workouts, paying particular attention to your personal weaknesses.

TABLE 13.1   ▌█▌ ▌▌▐██▌ █▌ ▐██▌▌ ▐▐ █▐▐ ▐█▐   ▐ ▐ ▐▐█▐ ▐█▐▐▐█▐▐▌ ▐ ▐ ▐▐█▐ ▐█▐ ▐▐ ▐▐ █▐▐▐█ █ ▐▐█▐▐▌ ▐▌

Suggested exercises for various fitness levels.

NEUROMUSCULAR FITNESS COMPONENTS	LOW	MODERATE	HIGH
a. Lumbar mobility*	**Knee to Chest** In supine lying position bring one or both knees to the chest, grasping the leg, under the thigh(s), raise and lower head slowly.	**"Mad Cat"** Kneeling on all fours alternate head up with sway back and head tucked with rounded back.	**Crossed Leg Flexion** Sitting position with knees flexed and ankles crossed. Slowly bend forward until head approaches floor.
b. Hamstring flexibility*	**Modified Hurdler's Stretch** Sit with one leg straight, the other flexed. Move the flexed knee to the side and bend forward.	**PNF Supine Position** Place jump rope around foot or ankle with leg raised as straight as possible. Contract against rope, relax, and pull leg straighter. Repeat.	**Standing Stretch** Stand with one leg placed on a support at about 90° hip flexion. Keeping back straight with shoulders back, flex forward.
c. Hip flexor flexibility*	**Hip Extension** Stand with pelvis in neutral position. Extend leg backward at hip.	**Lying Stretch** Lie on table with knees over the edge and back flat. Pulling one leg to the chest (hands on thigh) stretches the opposite hip.	**Standing Stretch** Stand in forward backward stride position. Bend front knee and thrust back hip forward. Keep front knee over ankle.
d. Abdominal strength/ endurance**	**Pelvic Tilt** In supine lying or standing position—press pelvis to floor or wall.	**Partial Curl (crunch)** Hook lying position, feet not held, tilt pelvis, curl up, sliding hands at side 3–4½ inches.	**Oblique Curl** Lying on side — twist trunk and curl up reaching for top leg with opposite arm.
e. Back extensor strength/endurance**	**Hyperextension—1** Lying in prone position with hands at thighs. Keep neck and chin in neutral position and raise shoulders off floor.	**Hyperextension—2** Lying in prone position with arms and hands extended forward. Keep neck and chin in neutral position and raise shoulders off floor.	**Hyperextension—3** Lying in prone position on a table or bench with body supported and stabilized from top of pelvis down. Flex waist to 90° and extend to several inches above level.

*Move into stretch positions slowly and hold for 10–60 seconds.
**Repeat controlled movements 5–25 times.

point to continue recommending a specific program of truncal muscular fitness as a part of a comprehensive physical fitness activity program. This recommendation is in accordance with the *Healthy People 2000* goal, which states the aim of increasing to at least 40% the proportion of the population six years old and above who regularly perform physical activities that enhance and maintain muscular strength, muscular endurance, and flexibility (Public Health Service, 1990). A comprehensive program would, of course, utilize the entire body and, along with the trunk region, stress upper arm and shoulder girdle areas. While baseline data suggest that the goal is close to being met for high school students, for the total population the 1991 estimate is that only 16% are involved in such programs.

For the trunk and low back region, it is imperative that the neuromuscular program go beyond traditional sit-ups for abdominal strength (actually, partial curls should be substituted for sit-ups) and modified hurdler's stretches for hamstring flexibility. The exercise program should be designed to include all five major anatomical areas and abilities listed in Table 13.1 without overemphasizing lumbar flexibility. Ignoring any element in the whole may lead to imbalances. Table 13.1 presents suggested flexibility and muscular strength/endurance exercises for the five identified areas with a progression from relatively easy to reasonably hard. Individual selections can be made from this chart for each area. Even if these components have not been shown irrevocably to be protective against the development of LBP, truncal muscular strength, endurance, and flexibility are important aspects of a healthy, fully functioning, fit body.

It should be noted that the activities listed in Table 13.1 are limited to those that require no specialized equipment, not even free weights. They may, thus, be less than the optimal exercise. For example, evidence is accumulating that back extensor exercises done on a specialized machine (the MedX™) that stabilizes the pelvis provides the best results. Without pelvic stabilization, back extension strength may not be developed (Foster & Fulton, 1991; Risch et al., 1993).

THE PROBLEM

The incidence of low back pain has been and continues to be consistently high. At some time in their lives, 60–80% of all individuals experience back pain. Both sexes are affected equally. Most cases occur between the ages of 25 and 60 years, but no age is completely immune. Fortunately, most LBP is acute and, with or without treatment of any kind, resolves itself within three days to six weeks. After six weeks to a year, the condition is considered to be chronic. For the 1–5% so afflicted, the condition is disabling. This statistic speaks directly to the *Healthy People 2000* priority of reducing disability from chronic disease, for while LBP is not the most prevalent disabling disease in the U.S., it is one of the many (Public Health Service, 1990). The psychological, social, and physical costs to individuals cannot begin to be calculated. The medical, insurance, and business/industry costs have been estimated into the billions of dollars per year (Cailliet, 1988; Plowman, 1992; Kumar, 1994).

Most cases of acute LBP arise spontaneously from no known cause. Without knowing the exact cause or causes of LBP, it is difficult to determine risk factors that might predispose an individual to LBP. Among the possible risk factors most commonly linked with LBP is a lack of physical fitness. Indeed, LBP has often been labeled as a hypokinetic disease, that is, as a disease caused by and/or associated with a lack of exercise (Kraus and Raab, 1961).

THE THEORETICAL LINK BETWEEN PHYSICAL ACTIVITY, PHYSICAL FITNESS, AND LOW BACK PAIN

The theoretical link between physical activity, physical fitness, and LBP is largely based on functional anatomy Anatomically, back pain is primarily located in the lumbosacral region of the back, which normally forms a lordotic curve. Twenty-four vertebrae comprise the entire spine. Effective functioning of the back requires coordination of all of the vertebra, the pelvis, the hip and thigh joints, and the muscles, fascia, and ligaments which originate and insert on these bones. Such coordination is task-specific, but to be normal it should be completed with minimal and equalized stresses within the spine (Cailliet, 1988; Gracovetsky, 1990).

Table 13.2 presents the theoretical relationships between all of the components of health-related physical fitness and healthy and unhealthy functioning of the low back. It can be seen that there is a

TABLE 13.2

Theoretical relationship between physical fitness components and healthy/unhealthy low back/spinal function.

Physical Fitness Component	Normal Anatomical Function in Low Back—Healthy	Dysfunction	Results of Dysfunction—Unhealthy
Cardiovascular Respiratory Endurance	Discs obtain nutrients and dispose of wastes by absorption from adjacent blood supply.	Poor circulation, low CVR endurance; atherosclerosis	May speed up disc degeneration.
Body Composition	High musculature allows for proper functioning as outlined below and provides mechanical loading on the vertebrae for maintenance of bone mass.	High % body fat content	Increases the weight the spine must support; may lead to increased pressure on discs or other vertebral structures.
Neuromuscular a. Lumbar flexibility	Allows the lumbar curve to be almost reversed in forward flexion.	Inflexible	Disrupts forward and lateral movement; places excessive stretch on hamstrings, leading to low back and hamstring pain.
b. Hamstring flexibility	Allows anterior rotation (tilt) of the pelvis in forward flexion and posterior rotation in sitting position.	Inflexible	Restricts anterior pelvic rotation and exaggerates posterior tilt; both cause increased disc compression; excessive stretching causes strain and pain.
c. Hip flexor flexibility	Allows achievement of neutral pelvic position.	Inflexible	Exaggerates anterior pelvic tilt if not counteracted by strong abdominal muscles, thereby increasing disc compression.
d. Abdominal strength/endurance	Maintains pelvic position; reinforces back extensor fascia and pulls it laterally on forward flexion providing support.	Weak, easily fatigued	Allows abnormal pelvic tilt; increases strain on back extensor muscles.
e. Back extensor strength/endurance	Provides stability for spine; maintains erect posture; controls forward flexion.	Weak, easily fatigued	Increases loading on spine; causes increased disc compression.

strong anatomical rationale for all components of fitness. The actual research-based support is not as strong as the anatomical relationships.

THE RESEARCH LINK BETWEEN PHYSICAL ACTIVITY, PHYSICAL FITNESS, AND LOW BACK PAIN

Types of research studies. Studies that have attempted to determine the relationship between physical activity and/or fitness and low back function or pain/injury are of two primary types. The first are retrospective studies. In a retrospective study, the relationship between the activity or fitness component and LBP is examined, or an attempt is made to distinguish between those who do and do not have low back pain based on the activity or fitness score. Retrospective studies must be interpreted cautiously since there are at least three possible confounding problems. First, activity or fitness measures in individuals already suffering from LBP may represent less than maximal effort due to real or feared pain. Second, physical activity is generally spontaneously decreased in individuals suffering from LBP, with the result that scores may reflect detraining as much as LBP per se. Third, these studies statistically establish just relationships (some of which may be statistically significant but not practically meaningful) and not cause and effect.

The second type of study is prospective. Prospective studies are longitudinal studies that test either normal individuals with no history of LBP, individuals with a history of LBP, or both, and then wait a specified time to see who develops LBP. The initial activity or fitness variables are then statistically analyzed to determine which, if any, had the most predictive value for the development of LBP. Prospective studies are obviously more valuable but they are also harder to conduct.

Throughout this section it has been emphasized that either physical activity or physical fitness can be used to determine the linkage with low back health or pain. In point of fact, very few studies have even attempted to relate physical activity per se in nonathletic populations with LBP. Those that have examined activity are weak in design and contradictory in outcome, precluding any meaningful comments or conclusions. The biggest difficulty is the inconsistent classification of physical activity and a primary reliance on frequency of participation to the exclusion of duration and intensity (Plowman, 1992). Even the most direct study by Porter, Adams, and Hutton (1989), which found a significant positive relation between spinal motion segment compressive strength and physical activity in young men killed in motorcycle accidents, relied only on a sports history obtained from the next of kin.

A more recent 10-year prospective study by Leino (1993) did attempt to classify activity levels into an exercise activity score (EAS = duration $\times$ estimated energy expenditure for light, moderate, or strenuous intensity), a strenuous activity score (SAS = 500 kcal day^{-1} or more), and a total activity score (travel to and from work, housework, and exercise). Back morbidity was assessed by both subject symptoms and clinical examination. At baseline, none of the physical activity scores was statistically related to low back problems. Males exhibited greater stability in EAS and SAS than females. Prospectively, for the males but not the females, the lower EAS and/or SAS scores at baseline and five years, the higher the low back problems after 10 years. When adjusted for other lifestyle factors, the SAS rating was not as consistently predictive as that of the EAS. Part of the difficulty in discerning the relationship between physical activity and low back pain is that it may be U-shaped. That is, both no or too little activity and extremely strenuous activity (either absolute or relative to an individual's capabilities) may predispose an individual to low back problems. Thus, no exercise prescription guidelines specific for low back health can be documented from the literature. This is a fertile area for research.

The rest of this report will concentrate on the linkage between physical fitness and low back health or pain. Some specific studies will be mentioned for illustrative purposes, but the primary emphasis will be on general consensus. For a more in-depth presentation of the research literature, the reader is referred to Plowman (1992). Complete references are also provided there.

CARDIOVASCULAR FITNESS AND LBP

As stated in Table 13.2, a properly functioning cardiovascular system is necessary for disc nourishment and to slow disc degeneration. The exact relationship with total body cardiovascular fitness has received little attention. Only two retrospective studies have measured cardiovascular fitness, and neither established a definitive linkage with low back function (Plowman, 1992).

Likewise, only two prospective studies have designs specific enough to draw conclusions from, but unfortunately the conclusions that must be drawn are in opposition to each other. The first study was completed on fire fighters by Cady, Thomas, and Karwasky (1985). Cardiovascular condition was assessed by physical working capacity (PWC). The 20 fire fighters with the lowest PWC incurred much higher low back injury costs than the 20 with the highest PWC, showing a beneficial effect. The second study is the study with the stronger design. It was conducted by Battié et al. (1989). Maximal oxygen consumption (VO_2max) was predicted from a submaximal treadmill test on over 2,400 Boeing airplane employees. VO_2max was not found to be predictive of the 228 back problems which occurred in these employees over the subsequent four years.

Haliovaara et al. (1995) have presented epidemiological evidence against the theory that atherosclerosis (the narrowing of blood vessels as a result of the build-up of plaque) contributes to the development of LBP by determining death rates from cardiovascular disease in individuals with and without LBP. Comprehensive health examinations were performed on 7,217 individuals representative of the Finnish population. Seventy-six percent had a history of LBP complaints; 17% were diagnosed with chronic LBP. Twelve to 14 years later, 1,487 individuals had died from cardiovascular disease. Neither a history of LBP complaints nor diagnosed chronic LBP predicted cardiovascular mortality.

There is no evidence that a highly fit cardiovascular system is detrimental in any way, but the evidence of benefit is minimal. This is another area which requires further research.

BODY COMPOSITION AND LBP

The skeletal system in general and the spine in particular are the primary supporting structures of the body. As pointed out in Table 13.2, if the weight the spine supports is largely muscular and the muscles are both strong and flexible, healthy functioning should result. However, if a large portion of the body mass is fat, this adds excess weight and pressure on the discs without any positive assistance. The few studies which have utilized body mass index (WT/HT^2) (BMI) and/or skinfolds as an indication of body composition have shown split results. However, an analysis of the NHANES-II national probability sample data set did show a substantial increase in LBP prevalence (1.7 times higher) in the most obese 20% compared with the least obese 20% of the 10,404 adult subjects when obesity was defined by both BMI and skinfold measures. No studies have been done on LBP in which body composition has been directly assessed by a laboratory criterion measure such as underwater weighing (Plowman, 1992).

NEUROMUSCULAR FITNESS AND LBP

The most important components of fitness in relation to healthy functioning of the low back are muscular strength, muscular endurance, and flexibility. It is necessary that each separate muscle group possess both strength/endurance and flexibility, and

that anatomically opposing muscle groups are balanced in strength/endurance and flexibility. The goal in relation to the low back region is that the vertebra will be kept in proper alignment without excessive disc pressure throughout the full range of possible motions. In addition, the pelvis must freely rotate both posteriorly and anteriorly without strain on the muscles or fascia. Table 13.2 presents the specific actions of the back, hip, abdominal, and hamstring muscles and what can theoretically happen if these muscles are allowed to become weak, easily fatigued, and/or inflexible.

The research evidence shows that regardless of the testing mode (that is, whether the test is one of static or dynamic function), individuals with low back pain exhibit lower strength values of both the abdominals and back extensor groups than do individuals without LBP. Only two studies looked at trunk extensor endurance specifically, but both of these found that individuals with LBP severe enough to limit function had scores lower than those without such limitations (Plowman, 1992).

Perhaps the most interesting studies in this area are those utilizing electromyographic (EMG) analysis of back extensor fatigue. In each of the three studies (DeVries, 1968, Roy, DeLuca, & Casavant, 1989; Roy et al., 1990), 80–100% of those with LBP showed increased electrical activity during sustained static muscle contraction. While these were not intended to be prospective studies, in one case an individual who showed high EMG activity but no history of LBP developed LBP the following year. Retrospective studies of low back pain and hamstring flexibility have shown the same trend. That is, there is a significant relationship between tightness in those muscle groups and LBP (Plowman, 1992).

Prospective studies of neuromuscular fitness are neither as numerous nor as definitive as the retrospective ones. Only one strength/endurance study found any variable predictive of first-time low back pain, and this showed the predictive variable to be limited (low) back extensor endurance (Biering-Sorensen, 1984a). Unfortunately, this was the only study using this variable, but since it is consistent with the results of the retrospective studies it would seem that back extensor endurance needs to be given more attention. Recurrent back pain has been successfully predicted in about half of the studies of trunk and back extensor strength/endurance with, as expected, low scores preceding the reoccurrence of back pain (Plowman, 1992).

One prospective study found lumbar flexibility to be predictive of first-time LBP (Biering-Sorensen, 1984b). In it, increased (not decreased as might be expected) lumbar mobility was found to be predictive of first-time back pain in males but not females. It is anatomically possible that extreme lumbosacral flexion stresses the discs at that site (Sharpe, Liehmon, & Snodgrass, 1988). Recurrent back pain has been found to be predictable from both low lumbar extension range of motion and low hamstring flexibility.

No specific level of strength, endurance and/or flexibility has emerged as critical in any of these studies. Hopefully, further research to clarify these issues will be forthcoming.

Part of the difficulty in experimentally being able to provide evidence concerning the relationship of lumbar extension and flexion strength, endurance, and flexibility and low back pain may be in the previously available equipment. Specifically, testing of the lumbar extensor muscles without stabilization of the pelvis may have led to inaccurate results and conclusions. If the pelvis moves during testing, the force measured also includes some unknown contribution from the hip extensors and is not truly a measure of back extension strength (Jones, 1993).

CHILDREN/ADOLESCENTS AND LBP

Historically, LBP in adolescents and especially children was considered indicative of a serious pathological condition, either anatomical or physiological (King, 1986). Statements such as "backache is so rare in the prepubertal and early pubertal patient that such patients should undergo a complete work-up for a serious cause. . . ." (Dymet, 1991, p. 170) were commonplace. Today, however, evidence is mounting that LBP is no longer rare in this age group. Over half a dozen large sample studies of Scandinavian and European children in the past decade (Balague, Dutoit, & Waldburger, 1988; Balague et al., 1993; Burton et al., 1996; Mierau, Cassidy, & Yong-Hing, 1989; Salminen, Pentti, & Terho, 1992; Taimela et al., 1997; Troussier et al., 1994) have shown that the incidence of LBP is relatively low prior to puberty (1–28%) but falls very close (50–80%) to the adult range by the early- to

mid-teen years. Some studies report that young females have more LBP than young males, but the role of back discomfort associated with the menstrual cycle does not appear to have been clarified in these studies.

The relationship between physical activity and LBP in children and adolescents suffers from the same ambiguities as for adults. In most studies, youngsters both with and without LBP have been evenly distributed into low, moderate, and high activity groups (Balague et al., 1993; Kujala et al., 1992; Salminen, 1984; Taimela et al., 1997; Troussier et al., 1994). In one study (Salminen et al., 1995) low participation in activity was associated with increased frequency of LBP. However, in still others, high participation, especially in heavy sports training, has been associated with an increased incidence of LBP (Balague, Dutoit, & Waldburger, 1988; Burton et al., 1996; Kujala et al., 1992; Taimela et al., 1997).

Cardiovascular fitness has not been investigated in relation to LBP in this age range, but several attempts have been made to relate anthropometric variables to LBP. Neither height, weight, nor body mass index (BMI) has been shown to be predictive of future LBP (Salminen et al., 1993; Salminen et al., 1995). However, a tall sitting height and a high degree of asymmetry as measured by the forward bending test may play a modest role in LBP (Fairbank et al., 1984; Nissinen et al., 1994).

Isokinetic trunk flexion and extension strength were found to be no different between 10- and 16-year-olds with and without LBP (Balague et al., 1993); however, both abdominal and back extensor muscular endurance did differ significantly between youngsters with and without LBP (Salminen et al., 1993). These muscular endurance measures, however, were not predictive of LBP in a three-year follow-up study (Salminen et al., 1995).

Flexibility measures have been shown to be positively, negatively, and nonsignificantly related to LBP (Burton et al., 1989; Burton et al., 1996). A positive relationship means that a high degree of mobility is associated with LBP. High lumbar mobility was apparent in children and adolescents with LBP but, unlike the Biering-Sorensen (1984a) results in adults, was not found to be predictive of LBP in youngsters (Salminen et al., 1993; Salminen et al., 1995). Decreased hamstring flexibility (Mierau, Cassidy, & Yong-Hing, 1989; Salminen et al.,

1993; Salminen et al., 1995), decreased femoral and tibial rotation (Fairbank et al., 1984), and decreased lumbar extension and flexion (Salminen et al., 1993; Salminen et al., 1995) have all been associated with increased LBP in children and adolescents, but no evidence exists that any of these can predict future LBP.

Thus, the pattern of the relationship between physical activity and/or physical fitness variables is no clearer in children and adolescents than in adults. It does seem that LBP is more of a problem in children and adolescents than previously thought. However, for individuals of all ages the key may be in the degree of the predisposing factors, not just whether an individual is active, strong, or flexible. Continued investigation into factors predictive of LBP in children and adolescents is important to try to avoid LBP at this age, but it is also important because a better understanding of LBP in children and adolescents may yield clues to the origins of adult LBP and to a means of prevention. In the meantime, moderate levels of activity are to be encouraged for all since, at the very least, this level of activity appears to do no harm to the back.

REFERENCES

Balague, F., Damidot, P., Nordin, M., Parnianpour, M., & Waldburger, M. (1993). Cross-sectional study of the isokinetic muscle trunk strength among school children. *Spine, 18,* 1199–1205.

Balague, F., Dutoit, G., & Waldburger, M. (1988). Low back pain in school children: An epidemiological study. *Scandinavian Journal of Rehabilitative Medicine, 20,* 175–179.

Battié, M.C., Bigos, S.J., Fisher, L.D., Hansson, T.H., Nachemson, A.L., Spengler, D.M., Wortley, M.D., & Zeh, J. (1989). A prospective study of the role of cardiovascular risk factors and fitness in industrial back pain complaints. *Spine, 12,* 141–147.

Biering-Sorensen, F. (1984a). A one-year prospective study of low back trouble in a general population. *Danish Medical Bulletin, 31,* 362–375.

Biering-Sorensen, F. (1984b). Physical measurements as risk indicators for low-back trouble over a one-year period. *Spine, 9,* 106–119.

Burton, A.K., Clarke, R.D., McClune, T.D., & Tillotson, K.M. (1996). The natural history of low back pain in adolescents. *Spine, 21,* 2323–2328.

Burton, A.K., Tillotson, K.M., & Troup, J.D.G. (1989). Variation in lumbar sagittal mobility with low-back trouble. *Spine, 14,* 584–590.

Cady, L.D., Thomas, P.C., & Karwasky, R.J. (1985). Program for increasing health and physical fitness for fire fighters. *Journal of Occupational Medicine, 27,* 110–114.

Cailliet, R. (1988). *Low back pain syndrome,* 4th edition. Philadelphia: F.A. Davis.

DeVries, H.A. (1968). EMG fatigue curves in postural muscles. A possible etiology for idiopathic low back pain. *American Journal of Physical Medicine, 47,* 175–181.

Deyo, R.A., & Bass, J.E. (1989). Lifestyle and low-back pain: The influence of smoking and obesity. *Spine, 14,* 501–506.

Dymet, P.G. (1991). Low back pain in adolescents. *Pediatric Annals, 20,* 170–178.

Fairbank, J.C.T., Pynsent, P.B., van Poortvliet, J.A., & Phillips, H. (1984). Influence of anthropometric factors and joint laxity in the incidence of adolescent pain. *Spine, 9,* 461–464.

Foster, D.N., & Fulton, M.N. (1991). Back pain and the exercise prescription. *Clinics in Sports Medicine, 10,* 197–209.

Gracovetsky, S., Kary, M., Levy, S., Ben Said, R., Pitchen, I., & Helie, J. (1990). Analysis of spinal and muscular activity during flexion/extension and free lifts. *Spine, 15,* 1333–1339.

Heliovaara, M., Makela, M., Aromaa, A., Impivaara, O., Knekt, P., & Reunanen, A. (1995). Low back pain and subsequent cardiovascular mortality. *Spine, 20,* 2109–2111.

Jones, A. (1993). *The lumbar spine, the cervical spine and the knee: Testing and rehabilitation.* Ocala, FL: MedX Corporation.

King, H.A. (1986). Evaluating the child with back pain. *The Pediatric Clinics of North America, 33,* 1489–1493.

Kraus, H., & Raab, W. (1961). *Hypokinetic disease.* Springfield, IL: Charles C. Thomas.

Kujala, U.M., Salminen, J.J., Taimela, S., Oksanen, A., & Jaakkola, L. (1992). Subject characteristics and low back pain in young athletes and nonathletes. *Medicine and Science in Sports and Exercise, 24,* 627–632.

Kumar, S. (1994). The epidemiology and functional evaluation of low-back pain: A literature review. *Physical Medicine and Rehabilitation, 4,* 15–27.

Leino, P.I. (1993). Does leisure time physical activity prevent low back disorders? A prospective study of metal industry employees. *Spine, 18,* 863–871.

Mierau, D., Cassidy, J.D., & Yong-Hing, K. (1989). Low-back pain and straight leg raising in children and adolescents. *Spine, 14,* 526–528.

Nissinen, M., Heliovaara, M., Seitsamo, J., Alaranta, H., & Poussa, M. (1994). Anthropometric measurements and the incidence of low back pain in a cohort of pubertal children. *Spine, 19,* 1367–1370.

Plowman, S.A. (1992). Physical activity, physical fitness, and low back pain. In J.O. Holloszy (Ed.), *Exercise and Sport Sciences Review, 20,* 221–242.

Porter, R.W., Adams, M.A., & Hutton, W.C. (1989). Physical activity and the strength of the lumbar spine. *Spine, 14,* 201–203.

Public Health Service. (1990). *Healthy People 2000.* Washington, D.C.: U.S. Government Printing Office.

Risch, S.V., Norvell, N.K., Pollock, M.L., Risch, E.D., Langer, H., Fulton, M., Graves, J.E., & Leggett, S.H. (1993). Lumbar strengthening in chronic low back pain patients: Physiologic and psychological benefits. *Spine, 18,* 232–238.

Roy, S.H., DeLuca, C.J., & Casavant, D.A. (1989). Lumbar muscle fatigue and chronic lower back pain. *Spine, 14,* 992–1001.

Roy, S.H., DeLuca, C.J., Snyder-Mackler, L., Emley, M.S., Crenshaw, R.L., & Lyons, J.P. (1990). Fatigue, recovery, and low back pain in varsity rowers. *Medicine and Science in Sports and Exercise, 22,* 463–469.

Salminen, J.J. (1984). The adolescent back: A field survey of 370 Finnish schoolchildren. *Acta Paediatrica Scandinavica, Supplement 315,* 8–122.

Salminen, J.J. (1992). Spinal mobility and trunk muscle strength in 15-year-old schoolchildren with and without low-back pain. *Spine, 17,* 405–411.

Salminen, J.J. (1995). Low back pain in the young. *Spine, 19,* 2101–2108.

Salminen, J.J., Oksanen, A., Maki, P., Pentti, J., & Kujala, U.M. (1993). Leisure time physical activity in the young: Correlation with low-back pain, spinal mobility and trunk muscle strength in 15-year-old school children. *International Journal of Sports Medicine, 14,* 406–410.

Salminen, J.J., Pentti, J., & Terho, P. (1992). Low back pain and disability in 14-year-old schoolchildren. *Acta Paediatrica, 81,* 1035–1039.

Sharpe, G.L., Liehman, W.P., & Snodgrass, L.B. (1988). Exercise prescription and the low back-kinesiological factors. *Journal of Health, Physical Education, Recreation and Dance, 59(8),* 74–78.

Taimela, S., Kujala, U.M., Salminen, J.J., & Viljanen, T. (1997). The prevalence of low back pain among children and adolescents: A nationwide, cohort-based questionnaire survey in Finland. *Spine, 22,* 1132–1136.

Troussier, B., Davoine, P., deGaudemaris, R., Fauconnier, J., & Phelip, X. (1994). Back pain in school children: A study among 1178 pupils. *Scandinavian Journal of Rehabilitative Medicine, 26,* 143–146.

IV

Fitness, Economic, and Mental Health Benefits of Physical Activity

The benefits of physical activity are not limited to reduction of risk of chronic diseases discussed in the previous section. Regular activity produces fitness gains that can enhance performance and provide health benefits. Michael Pollock and Kevin Vincent discuss the benefits of resistance training and the impact it has on muscular strength and endurance. Jack Wilmore focuses on body composition changes associated with regular activity. Coverage of the benefits of physical activity would be incomplete without a discussion of its mental health benefits. Daniel Landers discusses the impact of physical activity on mental health. The paper by Larry Gettman completes this section with a discussion of the economic benefits of physical activity.

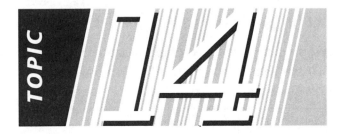

Resistance Training for Health*

Michael L. Pollock, Kevin R. Vincent

UNIVERSITY OF FLORIDA

INTRODUCTION

Increasing physical activity and participation in an aerobic endurance exercise program have been shown to decrease the risk of chronic diseases (e.g., coronary heart disease [CHD], stroke, osteoporosis, diabetes, obesity/weight control), which have become the leading causes of morbidity and mortality in the United States. The American Heart Association (AHA) has identified physical inactivity as a primary risk factor for the development of CHD along with cigarette smoking, high blood pressure, and elevated levels of cholesterol. As an intervention, the American College of Sports Medicine (ACSM), the AHA, and the Surgeon General's Report on Physical Activity and Health all have established guidelines for aerobic exercise programs designed to positively affect health status. These recommendations are based on a pre-ponderance of evidence establishing the effect of exercise on disease prevention (see Figure 14.1).

The effects of resistive type exercise (strength training) on health status have been largely overlooked. Traditionally, strength training has been seen as a means of improving muscular strength and endurance (muscle mass) and power, but not as a means for improving health. There is increasing evidence that strength training plays a significant role in many health factors (see Figure 14.1). The ACSM (1990, 1995), AHA (1995), and the Surgeon General's Report on Physical Activity and Health (1996) all have recognized the importance of strength training as an important component of health. These organizations have recommended performing 1 set of 8–12 repetitions of 8–10 exercises 2–3 times per week for persons under 50 years of age and the same regimen using 10–15 repetitions for persons over 50 years of age. The

ORIGINALLY PUBLISHED AS SERIES 2, NUMBER 8, OF THE PCPFS *RESEARCH DIGEST*.

*Since publication of this issue of the *Research Digest* on "Resistant Training for Health," the American College of Sports Medicine has accepted for publication in their journal *Medicine and Science in Sports and Exercise* the publication of a symposium issue on Resistance Training for Health and Disease edited by Michael Pollock, Ph.D., and William Evans, Ph.D. This issue will highlight the effect of resistance on bone density, body composition, and function of the elderly, low-back pain and disability, acute responses to resistance training and safety, and finally, a prescription of resistance training for health and disease. These timely papers will supplement this *Research Digest* topic.

HIGHLIGHT

"Adding strength training to a program of regular physical activity will help to decrease the risk of 'chronic diseases' while improving quality of life and functionality, allowing people of all ages to improve and maintain their health and independent lifestyle."

research and rationale for this exercise prescription have been reviewed (ACSM, 1990; Pollock et al., 1994; Feigenbaum & Pollock, 1997). Although greater intensity (fewer repetitions and greater weight) with multiple sets can elicit greater improvements in strength and power, it may not be appropriate for older nonathletic participants. A regimen of 8–12 or 10–15 repetitions appears to be an adequate balance for developing both muscular strength and endurance. The research suggests that 80–90% of the strength gains can be elicited using this regimen compared to the high volume types of programs. Thus, because time is an important factor for program compliance, the above recommended guidelines seem appropriate. Although more research is necessary to confirm the best combination of intensity (repetitions, weight, sets) for older or more fragile participants, it appears that the 10–15 repetition guideline may create less joint stress and injury than the 8–12 repetition program.

Improving muscular strength has been traditionally viewed as important for athletes, competitive weightlifters, and bodybuilders, but not for improving health status. Recent evidence indicates that this conception is no longer true. In this paper we will provide information concerning how strength training can influence health and disease prevention.

IMPROVEMENTS IN STRENGTH AND FUNCTION

Aging has been associated with a decrease in muscle mass and strength (Larsson et al., 1979). This decrease in strength is linked to decreased mobility, decreased functionality, and increased risk of falling in older people (Bendall et al., 1989; Fiatarone & Evans, 1990). Falls have been identified as the most frequent cause of injury-related mortality in the elderly (Fife et al., 1984). According to Greenspan et al. (1994), 90% of all hip fractures in

the elderly occur as a result of a fall. The authors also suggested that to help prevent the risk of falling, interventions should include exercise designed to improve quadriceps strength, neuromuscular function, and gait. Nevitt et al. (1991) conducted a prospective study to determine the risk factors that lead to injurious falls in the elderly. They reported that the fallers' ability to protect him- or herself during the fall affected the risk of injury. Upper and lower extremity strength, reaction time, and time to complete a cognitive test were associated with risk of falling and injury. The authors recommended that interventions intended to reduce the risk of falling and injury should include strength training and exercise. Fiatarone et al. (1994) examined the effect of 10 weeks of resistance exercise for the legs only on muscle strength and function in elderly adults (mean age, 87± 0.6 yr). Resistance exercise increased muscle strength (113%), gait velocity (12%), stair climbing power (28%). Fiatarone et al. (1990) reported that eight weeks of resistance exercise for the legs improved strength and function in nonagenarians (mean age 90±1 yr). Quadriceps strength improved 174% and tandem gait speed increased 48% following resistance training.

The Surgeon General's Report on Physical Activity and Health stated that developing muscular strength can improve one's ability to perform tasks and reduce the risk of injury. The report goes on to say that "resistance training may contribute to better balance, coordination, and agility that may help prevent falls in the elderly."

LOW BACK PAIN AND STRENGTH

Low back pain and spinal disorders are the predominant reason for disability in the workforce. It is estimated that chronic low back pain accounts for nearly 80% of the annual cost of low back disorders even though this classification represents only 10% of all spinal disorders (Spengler et al., 1986). Lack of lumbar strength has been associated with the development of low back pain and dysfunction.

Russell et al. (1990) reported increased lumbar strength and decreased low back pain following eight weeks of isolated lumbar extension exercise in subjects with chronic low back pain. Risch et al. (1993) examined the effect of 10 weeks of lumbar extension exercise on patients with chronic low back and reported decreased low back pain, physical and psychosocial dysfunction. The results also showed a significant improvement in lumbar extension strength. Nelson et al. (1995) examined the effect of isolated lumbar extension exercise on 895 chronic low back pain patients who had failed an average of six other treatment modalities prior to enrolling in the study. The patients performed lumbar extension and torso rotation exercise for 10 weeks. The results showed that most of the patients increased low back strength, decreased low back and leg pain, and improved their ability to perform daily activities. Seventy-two percent were able to return to work.

Some evidence is also available suggesting that improving low back strength is effective in reducing the incidence of low back dysfunction in the work place. Mooney et al. (1995) reported that the prevalence of low back injuries was reduced at a coal mine following a program of 20 weeks of lumbar extension exercise.

BONE MINERAL DENSITY

Osteoporosis is a degenerative disease that is characterized by a decrease in bone mineral density (BMD). This loss makes the bones more susceptible to fractures. These fractures can lead to decreased physical activity and possibly increased susceptibility to further health problems and mortality. Research has indicated that bone formation can be stimulated by placing a strain on the bone as is seen during resistive and aerobic exercise (Rubin & Lanyon, 1984). Although both forms of exercise can increase BMD, the increase is site-specific to the joints exercised. Hamdy et al. (1994) reported higher BMD in the upper arm in persons who weight trained compared to runners, but that there was no difference for lower body BMD between the two groups. Karlsson et al. (1993) reported that active and retired weightlifters had higher BMD for the spine, hip, tibia, and forearm when compared to controls. In a comparison of BMD between female weightlifters, cyclists, cross-country skiers, and orienteers, Heinonen et al. (1993) reported that the weightlifters had the highest weight adjusted BMD in the distal radius, lumbar spine, distal femur, and patella. Snow-Harter et al. (1992) showed that eight months of either resistance exercise or jogging improved lumbar BMD when compared to controls, but no difference was seen between the exercise groups. Braith et al. (1996) examined the effects of six months of resistance exercise on BMD following heart transplant surgery. Typically, BMD decreases during the post-operative period as a consequence of glucocorticoid therapy. The group that performed strength training for six months was able to return their lumbar, total body, and femoral neck BMD to near baseline levels while the non-strength-training groups' BMD remained depressed. Pollock et al. (1992) showed that six months of isolated lumbar training improved lumbar BMD compared to controls in men and women 60 to 79 years of age. Menkes et al. (1993) reported a significant increase in femoral neck BMD in middle-aged to older men following 16 weeks of strength training. These data indicate that resistance and aerobic exercise can both positively affect BMD, but that this influence is site-specific to the mode of exercise.

AEROBIC CAPACITY

Exercise programs that emphasize endurance exercise usually elicit a 15–30% increase in maximum oxygen uptake (VO_2max). Available evidence indicates that traditional weight training (greater than 1–2 minutes rest between exercises) does not increase VO_2max (Pollock & Wilmore, 1990). However, it has been shown that performing circuit training regimens can increase VO_2max 5–8%. These regimens consist of a circuit of approximately 10 exercises. A weight is chosen that can be lifted for 15 repetitions for each exercise with a short (15–30 second) rest period between exercises. Thus, circuit weight training has only a modest effect on VO_2max and should not be used for that sole purpose. Although weight training has only a modest effect on VO_2max, it has a dramatic effect on strength, endurance, and physical function. For example, Hickson et al. (1980) found that strength training the legs for 10 weeks improved performance time on both a treadmill (12%) and a stationary cycle (47%), while

VO$_2$max only increased 4%. Ades et al. (1996) reported that 12 weeks of strength training improved submaximal treadmill walking time by 38% while no change was reported for controls.

BODY COMPOSITION

Obesity is a risk factor for several health problems including diabetes mellitus, arthritis, cardiovascular disease (CVD), and kidney dysfunction (Stone et al., 1991). Also, due to excess nonmetabolically active weight, an obese person has to expend more energy for movement placing increased stress on the cardiovascular system. Aerobic exercise has been widely prescribed and utilized as a means of weight control and fat loss. There is also evidence indicating that strength exercise is an effective means of influencing body composition. Gettman and Pollock (1981) summarized the effects of five weight training and six circuit weight training studies on changes in body composition. The studies showed a mean decrease in body weight of 0.12kg, increase in lean body mass of 1.5kg, and a decrease in fat mass of 1.7kg.

The added benefit of strength training to an aerobic exercise program (caloric expenditure) is its effect on developing and maintaining muscle mass and metabolic rate. Metabolic rate decreases with age and a primary factor influencing this decrease is reduced fat-free mass. Campbell et al. (1995) reported that resting metabolic rate and energy intake required to maintain body weight significantly increased in older adults following 12 weeks of strength training. These data are in agreement with Pratley et al. (1994). Thus it appears that resistance exercise should be a part of a well-rounded program including aerobic endurance exercise for weight loss and controlling weight with age.

EFFECT ON CARDIOVASCULAR RISK FACTORS

There is growing evidence to indicate that strength training may also be important to risk factor intervention. Strength training exercise has been shown to increase insulin sensitivity, decrease glucose intolerance, and has a modest effect on decreasing diastolic blood pressure and may alter serum lipids.

Miller et al. (1984) reported that 10 weeks of strength training significantly reduced basal insulin levels and area under the insulin response curve following glucose ingestion. The decrease in insulin was significantly correlated with increase in lean body mass. Hurley et al. (1987) reported that insulin response to an oral glucose tolerance test was significantly lower following 16 weeks of resistance training. Smutok et al. (1993) compared the effect of endurance and strength training on responses to a glucose tolerance test. Both modalities decreased the total area under the curve for glucose levels and insulin response, and there was no difference between the two types of exercise.

Aerobic endurance exercise has been well established as a means for favorably altering high density lipoprotein cholesterol (HDL-C). The research concerning the effect of strength training is not as clear and recent studies have produced conflicting results. Studies that do show a positive result, typically involve higher volumes emphasizing multisegment exercises. Hurley et al. (1987) reported a 13% increase in HDL cholesterol following 16 weeks of heavy strength training. Wallace et al. (1989), and Johnson et al. (1982) both reported positive changes in lipid profiles, but only during the highest volumes of training. Goldberg et al. (1984) showed that a program emphasizing high volume with short rest periods increased HDL while decreasing LDL and serum triglycerides. Conversely, Kokkinos et al. (1987, 1991), Kohl et al. (1992), and Smutok et al. (1993) all reported that strength training did not significantly alter serum lipid profiles. Thus, the available evidence seems to indicate that the type of exercise performed by average strength trainers may not be sufficient to impact serum lipids.

SAFETY AND PRACTICAL APPLICATION

Data regarding the safety of strength training and testing show that it is safe if proper guidelines are followed. Gordon et al. (1995) reported no adverse cardiovascular events following maximal strength testing in 6,653 healthy men and women. Other studies have shown no excess incidence of cardiovascular events using resistance training compared to aerobic endurance training in varied populations. Muscle soreness is common in beginning exercisers but significant musculoskeletal injuries are rare. Persons with previous joint injuries are at higher risk for sustaining an injury from strength training.

An important reason why strength training is beneficial in daily life and may cause less risk in doing various lifting tasks is related to the training effect. For example, McCartney et al. (1993) showed that following 12 weeks of leg press training, maximal strength increased 24%, and that blood pressure measured during submaximal lifting decreased following the training period. Thus, strength training can decrease the stress placed on the heart during lifting tasks such as carrying groceries, snow shoveling, and lifting moderate to heavy boxes, which have been implicated as a cause of heart attacks.

CONCLUSION

The effects of resistance/strength training on muscular strength and endurance (muscle mass) and rehabilitation from musculoskeletal injury is well known. As a result, most of the major health organizations have included it as an important component of a well-rounded exercise program along with aerobic endurance and flexibility exercise. More recently, strength training has been shown to be beneficial in improving many factors associated with good health. These factors include increased function and prevention of falls, decreased pain in chronic low back pain patients, improved glucose tolerance and insulin sensitivity, increased BMD, increased basal metabolic rate (weight control), and improved quality of life. Added long-term epidemiological studies are necessary to confirm these findings. It appears that most of the above findings can be attained in strength training programs that include 8–10 exercises that are performed 2–3 days per week, using 1 set of 8–15 repetitions to fatigue.

FIGURE 14.1

Comparison of the effects of aerobic endurance training to strengthen training on health and fitness variables.

Variable	Aerobic Exercise	Resistance Exercise
Bone mineral density	↑↑	↑↑
Body composition		
%fat	↓↓	↓
LBM	↔	↑↑
Strength	↔	↑↑↑
Glucose metabolism		
Insulin response to glucose challenge	↓↓	↓↓
Basal insulin levels	↓	↓
Insulin sensitivity	↑↑	↑↑
Serum lipids		
HDL	↑↑	↑↔
LDL	↓↓	↓↔
Resting heart rate	↓↓	↔
Stroke volume	↑↑	↔
Blood pressure at rest		
Systolic	↓↓	↔
Diastolic	↓↓	↓↔
VO$_2$max	↑↑↑	↑
Endurance time	↑↑↑	↑↑
Physical function	↑↑	↑↑↑
Basal metabolism	↑	↑↑

REFERENCES

Ades, P.A., Ballor, D.L., & Ashikaga, T. et al. (1996). Weight training improves walking endurance in healthy elderly persons. *Annals of Internal Medicine, 124,* 568–572.

American College of Sports Medicine: *Guidelines for exercise testing and prescription.* (1995). Philadelphia: Williams and Wilkins, 173–193.

American College of Sports Medicine: The recommended quantity and quality of exercise for developing and maintaining cardiorespiratory and muscular fitness in healthy adults. (1990). *Medicine and Science in Sports and Exercise, 22,* 265–274.

Bendall, M.J., Bassey, E.J. & Pearson, M.B. (1989). Factors affecting walking speed in elderly people. *Age Aging, 18,* 327–332.

Braith, R.W., Mills, R.M., Welsch, M.A., et al. (1996). Resistance exercise training restores bone mineral density in heart transplant recipients. *Journal of the American College of Cardiology.*

Campbell, W.W., Crim, M.C., Young, V.R. et al. (1995). Effects of resistance training and dietary protein intake and protein metabolism in older adults. *American Journal of Physiology, 268,* E1143–E1153.

Feigenbaum, M.S., & Pollock, M.L. (1997). Strength training: rationale for current guidelines for adult fitness programs. *Phys Sports Med.*

Fiatarone, M.A., & Evans, W.J. (1993). The etiology and reversibility of muscle dysfunction in the aged. *Journal of Gerontology, 48,* 77–83.

Fiatarone, M.A., Marks, E.C., Ryan, N.D. et al. (1990). High-intensity strength training in nonagenarians. *Journal of the American Medical Association, 263,* 3029–3034.

Fiatarone, M.A., O'Neill, E.F., Doyle Ryan, N. et al. (1994). Exercise training and nutritional supplementation for physical frailty in very elderly people. *New England Journal of Medicine, 330,* 1769–1775.

Fife, D., Baranik, J.I. & Chatterjee, M.S. (1984). Northeastern Ohio trauma study: II: Injury rates by age, sex, and cause. *American Journal of Public Health, 74,* 473–478.

Fletcher, G.F., Balady, G., Froelicher, V.F., et al. (1995). Exercise standards: A statement for healthcare professionals from the American Heart Association. *Circulation, 91,* 580–615.

Gettman, L.R., & Pollock, M.L. (1981). Circuit weight training: A critical review of its physiological benefits. *Phys Sports Med, 9,* 44–60.

Goldberg, L., Elliot, D.L., Schutz, R.W. et al. (1984). Changes in lipid and lipoprotein levels after weight training. *Journal of the American Medical Association, 252,* 504–506.

Gordon, N.F., Kohl, H.W., Pollock, M.L. et al. (1995). Cardiovascular safety of maximal strength testing in healthy adults. *American Journal of Cardiology, 76,* 851–853.

Greenspan, S.L., Myers, E.R., Maitland, L.A. et al. (1994). Fall severity and bone mineral density as risk factors for hip fracture in ambulatory elderly. *Journal of the American Medical Association, 271,* 128–133.

Hamdy, R., Anderson, J., Whalen, K., & Harvill, L. (1994). Regional differences in bone density of young men involved in different exercises. *Medicine and Science in Sports and Exercise, 26,* 884–888.

Heinonen, A., Oja, P., Kannus, P. et al. (1993). Bone mineral density of female athletes in different sports. *Calcified Tissue International, 23,* 1–14.

Hickson, R.C., Rosenkoetter, M.A., & Brown, M.M. (1980). Strength training effects on aerobic power and short-term endurance. *Medicine and Science in Sports and Exercise, 12,* 336–339.

Hurley, B. (1994). Does strength training improve health status? *Journal of Strength Conditioning, 2,* 7–13.

Hurley, B.F., Hagberg, J.M., Goldberg, A.P. et al. (1987). Resistive training can reduce coronary risk factors without altering VO$_2$max or percent body fat. *Medicine and Science in Sports and Exercise, 20,* 150–154.

Johnson, C.C., Stone, M.H., Lopez, S.A. et al. (1982). Diet and exercise in middle-aged men. *Journal of the Dietetic Association, 81,* 695–701.

Karlsson, M., Johnell, O., & Obrant, K. (1993). Bone mineral density in weight lifters. *Calcified Tissue International, 52,* 212–215.

Kohl, H.W., Gordon, N.F., Scott, C.B. et al. (1992). Musculoskeletal strength and serum lipid levels in men and women. *Medicine and Science in Sports and Exercise, 24,* 1080–1087.

Kokkinos, P.F., Hurley, B.F., Smutok, M.A. et al. (1991). Strength training does not improve lipoprotein-lipid profiles in men at risk for CHD. *Medicine and Science in Sports and Exercise, 23,* 1134–1139.

Kokkinos, P.F., Hurley, B.F., Vaccaro, P. et al. (1987). Effects of low and high-repetition resistive training on lipoprotein-lipid profiles. *Medicine and Science in Sports and Exercise, 20,* 50–54.

Larsson, L.G., Grimby, G., & Karlsson, J. (1979). Muscle strength and speed of movement in relation to age and muscle morphology. *Journal of Applied Physiology, 46,* 451–456.

McCartney, N., McKelvie, R.S., Martin, J. et al. (1993). Weight-training induced attenuation of the circulatory response to weightlifting in older men. *Journal of Applied Physiology, 74,* 1056–1060.

Menkes, A., Mazel, S., Redmond, R. et al. (1993). Strength training increases regional bone mineral density and bone remodeling in middle-aged and older men. *Journal of Applied Physiology, 74,* 2478–2484.

Miller, W.J., Sherman, W.M., & Ivy, J.L. (1984). Effect of strength training on glucose tolerance and post-glucose insulin response. *Medicine and Science in Sports and Exercise, 16,* 539–543.

Mooney, V., Kron, M., Rummerfield, P. et al. (1995). The effect of workplace based strengthening on low back injury rates: A case study in the strip mining industry. *Journal of Occupational Rehabilitation, 5,* 157–167.

Nelson, B., O'Reilly, E., Miller, M. et al. (1995). The clinical effects of intensive, specific exercise on chronic low-back pain: A controlled study of 895 consecutive patients with one year follow-up. *Orthopedics, 18,* 971–981.

Nevitt, M.C., Cummings, S.R., & Hudes, E.S. (1991). Risk factors for injurious falls: a prospective study. *Journal of Gerontology, 46,* M164–170.

Pollock, M., Garzarella, L., Graves, J. et al. (1992). Effects of isolated lumbar extension resistance training on bone mineral density of the elderly. *Medicine and Science in Sports and Exercise, 24,* S66.

Pollock, M.L., Graves, J.E., Swart, D.L. et al. (1994). Exercise training and prescription for the elderly. *Southern Journal of Medicine, 87,* S88–S95.

Pollock, M.L., & Wilmore, J.H. (1990). *Exercise in health and disease: Evaluation and prescription for prevention and rehabilitation* (2nd ed.). Philadelphia: Saunders.

Prately, R., Nicklas, B., Rubin, M. et al. (1994). Strength training increases resting metabolic rate and norepinephrine levels in healthy 50- to 65-yr-old men. *Journal of Applied Physiology, 76,* 133–137.

Risch, S., Norvell, N., Pollock, M. et al. (1993). Lumbar strengthening in chronic low back pain patients: physiologic and psychological benefits. *Spine, 18,* 232–238.

Rubin, C.T., & Lanyon, L.E. (1984). Regulation of bone formation by applied dynamic loads. *Journal of Bone J Surg Am, 66,* 397–402.

Russell, G., Highland, T., Dreisenger, T. et al. (1990). Changes in isometric strength and range of motion of the isolated lumbar spine following eight weeks of clinical rehabilitation. *Presented at the North American Spine Society Annual Meeting,* Monterey, CA.

Smutok, M.A., Reece, C., Kokkinos, P.F. et al. (1993). Aerobic versus strength training for risk factor intervention in middle-aged men at high risk for coronary heart disease. *Metabolism, 42,* 177–184.

Snow-Harter, T., Going, S., Pamenter, R. et al. (1995). Effects of resistance training on regional and total bone mineral density in premenopausal women: A randomized prospective study. *Journal Bone Mineral Res, 10,* 1015–1024.

Spengler, D., Bigos, S., Martin, N. et al. (1986). Back injuries in industry: a retrospective study. 1. Overview and cost analysis. *Spine, 11,* 241–246.

Stone, M.H., Fleck, S.J., Triplett, N.T. et al. (1991). Health and performance related potential of resistance training. *Sports Medicine, 11,* 210–231.

U.S. Department of Health and Human Services, *Physical Activity and Health: A Report of the Surgeon General.* Atlanta, GA: U.S. Department of Health and Human Services, Centers for Disease Control and Prevention, National Center for Chronic Disease Prevention and Health Promotion, 1996.

Wallace, M.B., Moffatt, R.J., Haymes, E.M. et al. (1991). Acute effects of resistance exercise on parameters of lipoprotein metabolism. *Medicine and Science in Sports and Exercise, 23,* 199–204.

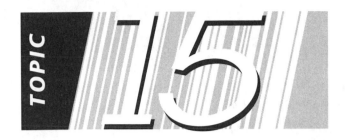

TOPIC

Exercise, Obesity, and Weight Control

Jack H. Wilmore
TEXAS A & M UNIVERSITY

INTRODUCTION

It is ironic that while millions of people are dying of starvation each year in most parts of the world, many Americans are dying as an indirect result of an overabundance of food. Further, billions of dollars are spent each year overfeeding the American public, which then leads to the spending of billions of dollars more each year on various weight loss methods. This review will investigate various aspects of overweight and obesity, and show how they are affected by physical activity. But first, we must define and differentiate between the terms *overweight* and *obesity*.

OVERWEIGHT, OBESITY AND THEIR ASSESSMENT

The terms *overweight* and *obesity* are often used interchangeably, but this is technically incorrect as they have different meanings. Overweight is defined as a body weight that exceeds the normal or standard weight for a particular person, based on his

or her height and frame size. These standards are established solely on the basis of population averages. It is quite possible to be overweight according to these standard tables and yet have a body fat content that is average or even below average. For example, almost all college and professional football players are overweight by these tables, but few are overfat. There are also people who are within the normal range of body weights for their height and frame size by the standard tables, but who have, in fact, excessive body fat.

Obesity is the condition in which the individual has an excessive amount of body fat. This means that the actual amount of body fat, or its percentage of a person's total weight, must be assessed or estimated. A number of laboratory and field assessment techniques can provide reasonably accurate estimates of a person's body composition. Exact standards for allowable fat percentages, however, have not been established. But there is general agreement among clinicians and scientists that men over 25% body fat and women over 35% should be considered obese, and that relative fat values of 20% to 25% in

ORIGINALLY PUBLISHED AS SERIES 1, NUMBER 6, OF THE PCPFS *RESEARCH DIGEST*.

Note: Parts of this review were adapted by permission from Wilmore, J., & D. Costill, 1994, *Physiology of Sport and Exercise.* (Champaign, IL: Human Kinetics), 491–504.

"Physical inactivity is certainly a major, if not the primary, cause of obesity in the United States today. A certain minimal level of activity might be necessary for us to accurately balance our caloric intake to our caloric expenditure. With too little activity, we appear to lose the fine control we normally have to maintain this incredible balance. This fine balance amounts to less than 10 kcal per day, or the equivalent of one potato chip!"

men and 30% to 35% in women should be considered borderline obese.

PREVALENCE OF OBESITY AND OVERWEIGHT

The prevalence of obesity and overweight in the United States has increased dramatically over the past 30 years. On the basis of data from a large study conducted between 1976 and 1980 by the National Center for Health Statistics (National Center for Health Statistics, 1986), 28.4% of American adults aged 25 to 74 years are overweight. Between 13% and 26% of the U.S. adolescent population, 12 to 17 years of age, are obese, depending on gender and race, and an additional 4% to 12% are superobese. This represents a 39% increase in the prevalence of obesity when compared with data collected between 1966 and 1970. Equally alarming, there has been a 54% increase in the prevalence of obesity among children 6 to 11 years of age (Gortmaker et al., 1987).

It has also been demonstrated that the average individual in this country will gain approximately one pound of additional weight each year after the age of 25 years. Such a seemingly small gain, however, results in 30 pounds of excess weight by the age of 55 years. Since the bone and muscle mass decreases by approximately one half pound per year due to reduced physical activity, fat is actually increasing by 1.5 pounds each year. This means a 45 pound gain in fat over this 30-year period! It is no wonder that weight loss is a national obsession.

THE CONTROL OF BODY WEIGHT

It is important to have a basic understanding of how body weight is controlled or regulated in order to better understand how one becomes obese. The issue of how body weight is regulated has puzzled scientists for years. It is rather remarkable that the body takes in an average of about 2,500 kcal per day, or nearly one million kcal per year. The average gain of 1.5 pounds of fat each year, which we just discussed, represents an imbalance between energy intake and expenditure of only 5,250 kcal per year (using 3,500 kcal to represent the energy equivalent of a pound of adipose tissue), or less than 15 kcal per day. Even with a weight gain of 1.5 pounds of fat, the body is able to balance the food intake to within one potato chip per day of what is expended! That is truly remarkable.

The ability of the body to balance its intake and expenditure has led scientists to propose that body weight is regulated within a narrow range similar to the way in which body temperature is regulated. There is excellent evidence for this in the animal research literature (Keesey, 1986). When animals are force-fed or starved for various periods of time, their weight will increase or decrease markedly, but they will always return to their original weight, or to the weight of the control animals (for those animals that naturally continue to increase weight throughout their life span), when allowed to go back to their normal eating patterns.

Similar results have been found in humans, although the number of studies has been limited. Subjects placed on semi-starvation diets have lost up to 25% of their body weight, but regained that weight within months of returning to a normal diet (Keys et al., 1950). In overfeeding studies of Vermont prisoners, overfeeding resulted in weight gains of 15 to 25%, yet weight returned to its original level shortly after the completion of the experiment (Sims, 1976).

How is the body able to do this? The total amount of energy expended each day can be expressed in three categories: resting metabolic rate (RMR), the thermic effect of feeding (TEF), and the thermic effect of activity (TEA). RMR is your body's metabolic rate early in the morning following an overnight fast and eight hours of sleep. The term *basal metabolic rate (BMR)* is also used, but generally implies that the person sleeps over in the clinical facility where the metabolic rate measurement will be made. Most research today uses resting metabolic rate. It accounts for 60 to 75% of the total energy expended each day.

The TEF, which represents the increase in metabolic rate that is associated with the digestion, absorption, transport, metabolism, and storage of the ingested food, accounts for approximately 10% of the total energy expended each day. There is probably also a wastage component included in the thermic effect of a mcal, where the body is able to increase its metabolic rate above that necessary for the processing and storage of the ingested food. This component may be defective in obese individuals. The TEA, which is simply the energy expended above resting metabolic rate levels necessary to accomplish a given task or activity, whether it be washing your face or taking a brisk 3-mile walk, accounts for the remainder.

The body makes very important adaptations in each of these three components of total energy expenditure when there are major increases or decreases in the energy intake. With very low calorie diets, there are decreases in the RMR, TEF, and TEA. The body appears to be attempting to conserve its energy stores. This is dramatically illustrated by the decreases reported in resting metabolic rate of 20 to 30% or more within several weeks after patients begin a very low calorie diet. Conversely, with overeating RMR, TEF, and TEA all increase to prevent the unnecessary storage of a large number of calories. It is quite possible that all of these adaptations are under the control of the sympathetic nervous system and play a major, if not the primary, role in controlling weight around a given set-point.

ETIOLOGY OF OBESITY

The results of recent medical and physiological research show that obesity can be the result of any one, or a combination of many, factors. Its etiology is not as simple or straightforward as was once believed. A number of experimental studies on animals have linked obesity to hereditary or genetic factors. Studies by Dr. Albert Stunkard at the University of Pennsylvania have shown a direct genetic influence on height, weight, and BMI (Stunkard et al., 1986a, 1986b, 1990).

A study from Laval University in Quebec, Canada, has provided possibly the strongest evidence of a significant genetic component in the establishment of obesity (Bouchard et al., 1990). With periods of overfeeding of identical monozygotic twins (1,000 kcal above maintenance levels, six out of every seven days), there was a threefold variation in the weight gained over 100 days between twin pairs, while there were relatively small differences within twin pairs. This is illustrated in Figure 15.1. Similar results were found for gains in fat mass, percentage body fat, and subcutaneous fat.

Obesity has also been experimentally and clinically linked with both physiological and psycho-

FIGURE 15.1

Similarity within twin pairs of weight gain in response to a 1,000 kcal increase in dietary intake for 84 days of a 100 day period of study. Each point represents one pair of twins (A and B). The closer the points are to the diagonal line, the more similar the twins are to each other.

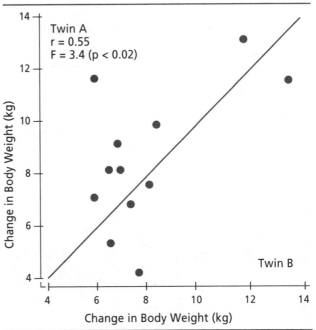

logical trauma. Hormonal imbalances, emotional trauma, and alterations in basic homeostatic mechanisms have all been shown to be either directly or indirectly related to the onset of obesity. Environmental factors, such as cultural habits, inadequate physical activity, and improper diets, also make major contributions to excessive fat gain. Thus, obesity is of complex origin, and the specific causes undoubtedly differ from one person to the next. Recognizing this fact is important both in the treatment of existing obesity and in the application of measures to prevent its onset.

HEALTH IMPLICATIONS OF OVERWEIGHT AND OBESITY

There is an increased risk for general excess mortality associated with overweight and obesity. This relationship is curvilinear as is illustrated in Figure 15.2. A large jump in risk occurs when the body mass index (BMI) exceeds a value of 30 kg/m². The BMI is a simple ratio of body weight divided by height squared, and provides an estimate of obesity. The causes of the excess mortality associated

FIGURE 15.2

Relation of body mass index to excess mortality.

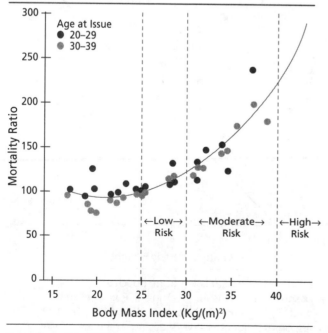

From: Bray, G.A. (1985). Obesity: definition, diagnosis and disadvantages. *Medical Journal of Australia, 142,* S2–S8.

with obesity and overweight include heart disease, hypertension, and diabetes.

It has been recognized since the 1940s that there are major gender differences in the way in which fat is stored or patterned in the body. Males tend to pattern fat in the upper regions of the body, particularly in the abdominal area, while females tend to pattern fat in the lower regions of the body, particularly in the hips, buttocks, and thighs. When obese, the male pattern is referred to as upper body, "apple-shaped," or android obesity, and the female pattern is referred to as lower body, "pear-shaped," or gynoid obesity. Research beginning in the late 1970s and early 1980s clearly established upper body obesity as a risk factor for heart disease, hypertension, stroke, elevated blood lipids, and diabetes (Björtorp et al., 1988). Further, upper body obesity appears to be more important as a risk factor for these diseases than total body fatness. With upper body obesity, the increased risk may be the result of the location of these depots in close proximity to the portal circulatory system.

GENERAL TREATMENT OF OBESITY

In theory, weight control seems to be a very simple matter. The energy consumed by the body in the form of food must equal the total energy expended, which is the sum of the RMR, TEF, and TEA. The body normally maintains a balance between caloric intake and caloric expenditure. However, when this balance is upset, a loss or gain in weight will result. It would appear that both weight losses and weight gains are largely dependent on just two factors—dietary intake and habitual physical activity This now appears to be an oversimplification considering the results of the overfeeding study of monozygotic twins discussed earlier in this paper, where there was considerable variation in the weight gained for the same amount of overfeeding (Bouchard et al., 1990). Thus, not everyone will respond the same to the same intervention. This must be considered when designing treatment programs for individuals attempting to lose weight. Also, it is important for the individual trying to lose weight to understand this fact so that he or she will not get discouraged.

Many special diets have achieved popularity over the years, including the Drinking Man's Diet, the Beverly Hills Diet, the Cambridge Diet, the California Diet, Dr. Stillman's Diet, and Dr. Adkin's Diet. Each claims to be the ultimate in terms of effectiveness and comfort in weight loss. Some of the more recent diets have been developed for use either in the hospital or at home under the supervision of a physician. These are referred to as very low calorie diets, as they allow only 350 to 500 kcal of food per day. Most of these have been formulated with a certain amount of protein and carbohydrate in order to minimize the loss of fat-free tissue. Research has shown that many of these diets are effective, but no one single diet has been shown to be any more effective than any other. Again, the important factor is the development of a caloric deficit, while maintaining a balanced diet that is complete in all respects with regard to vitamin and mineral requirements. The diet that meets these criteria and is best suited to the comfort and personality of each individual is the best diet.

Generally, improper eating habits are at least partially responsible for most weight problems, so any given diet should not be looked on as a "quick fix." The individual should be instructed to make *permanent* changes in his or her dietary habits, particularly reducing the intake of fat and simple sugars. Just eating a low fat diet will gradually bring weight down to desirable levels for most individuals without restricting the quantity of food eaten. For most individuals, reducing the total caloric intake by not more than 250 to 500 kcal per day would be sufficient to accomplish the desired weight loss goals.

Behavior modification has been proposed as one of the most effective techniques for dealing with weight problems. By changing basic behavior patterns, many associated with eating, major weight losses have been achieved. Further, these weight losses appear to be much more permanent, in that the weight is less likely to be regained. This approach appeals to most people since the techniques seem to make sense. For example, individuals might not have to reduce the amount of food they eat but simply agree that all eating will be done in one location. Or, the individual will be allowed to eat as much as he or she wants, but it must be eaten with the first helping—no second helpings! There are a number of very simple things that can be done to regulate the individual's eating behavior which can result in substantial weight loss.

Hormones and drugs have also been used to assist patients in weight loss, mainly through increasing their RMR. Surgical techniques are also used in the treatment of extreme obesity, but only as a last resort when other treatment procedures have failed and the obesity constitutes a life-threatening situation.

THE ROLE OF PHYSICAL ACTIVITY IN WEIGHT REDUCTION AND CONTROL

Inactivity is a major cause of obesity in the United States. In fact, inactivity might be a far more significant factor in the development of obesity than overeating. Thus, exercise must be recognized as an essential component in any program of weight reduction or control.

The Excess Post-Exercise Oxygen Consumption (EPOC)

It has often been stated that physical activity has only a limited influence on changing body composition, and that even exercise of a vigorous nature results in the expenditure of too few calories to lead to substantial reductions in body fat. Yet, research has conclusively demonstrated the effectiveness of exercise training in promoting major alterations in body composition. How do we account for this apparent conflict?

When estimating the energy cost of an activity, it is typical to multiply the average or steady-state rate of energy expenditure for a specific activity times the minutes engaged in that activity. However, the metabolism remains elevated following exercise. This was, at one time, referred to as the oxygen debt, but is now referred to as the excess post-exercise oxygen consumption (EPOC). The recovery of the metabolic rate back to pre-exercise levels can require several minutes for light exercise, several hours for very heavy exercise, and up to 12 to 24 hours or even longer for prolonged, exhaustive exercise.

The EPOC can add up to a substantial energy expenditure when totaled over the entire period of recovery. If the oxygen consumption following exercise remains elevated by an average of only 50 ml/min or 0.05 liter/min, this will amount to approximately 0.25 kcal/min or 15 kcal/hr. If the metabolism remains elevated for five hours, this would amount to an additional expenditure of 75 kcal that would not normally be included in the calculated total energy expenditure for that particular activity. This major source of energy expenditure, which occurs during recovery, but is directly the result of the exercise bout, is frequently ignored in most calculations of the energy cost of various activities. If the individual in this example exercised five days per week, he or she would have expended 375 kcal, or lost the equivalent of approximately 0.1 pounds of fat in one week, or 1.0 pounds in 10 weeks, just from the additional caloric expenditure during the recovery period alone.

Changes in Weight and Body Composition with Exercise Training

A number of studies have shown major changes in both weight and body composition with exercise training. In one study, the researchers investigated the changes in body composition with diet, exercise, and a combination of diet and exercise (Zuti & Golding, 1976). A caloric deficit of 500 kcal per day was maintained by each of three groups of adult women during a 16-week period of weight loss. The diet-only group reduced their normal daily intake by 500 kcal per day, but did not alter their activity levels. The exercise-only group increased their activity by 500 kcal per day, but did not alter their diet. The combination group reduced their caloric intake by 250 kcal and increased their activity by 250 kcal. While there were similar decreases in body weight, the two groups that exercised lost substantially more body fat. A major difference between the two exercise groups and the diet-only group was the gain in fat-free body mass with exercise and its loss with diet-only

In a second study, 72 mildly obese male subjects were assigned to one of several treatment programs, which included either exercise or nonexercise in combination with different dietary treatments. While the exercise and nonexercise groups lost similar amounts of weight, the exercise group lost significantly more fat weight and did not lose fat-free mass. The nonexercising group lost a significant amount of fat-free mass (Pavlou et al., 1985).

Not all studies have been able to demonstrate such dramatic changes in weight and body composition with exercise training. However, most studies have found similar trends, in that total weight decreases, fat weight and relative body fat decrease, and fat-free mass is either maintained or increases (Ballor & Keesey, 1991; Stefanick, 1993; Wilmore, 1983). While most of these studies have used aerobic training, several studies have shown impressive decreases in body fat and increases in fat-free mass with resistance training. The evidence is clear that exercise is an important part of any weight loss program. However, it is also clear that to maximize decreases in body weight and body fat, it is necessary to combine exercise with decreases in caloric intake.

Mechanisms for Change in Body Weight and Composition

In looking for ways to explain the above changes in body weight and composition with exercise, it is important to consider both sides of the energy balance equation. When evaluating energy expenditure, it is useful to consider each of the three components of energy expenditure: RMR, TEF, and TEA. When evaluating energy intake, it is also important to consider the energy that is lost in the feces (energy excreted), which is generally less than 5% of the total calories ingested.

The Energy Balance Equation

Energy Intake − Energy Excreted = RMR + TEF + TEA

It has been contended that exercise will stimulate the appetite to such an extent that food intake will be unconsciously increased to at least equal that expended during exercise. Jean Mayer, world-famous nutritionist, reported a number of years ago that animals exercising for periods of from 20 minutes up to one hour per day had a lower food intake than nonexercising control animals (Mayer et al., 1954). He concluded from this and other studies that when activity is reduced to below a certain minimum level, a corresponding decrease in food intake does not occur and the animal or human begins to accumulate body fat. This has led to the theory that a certain minimum level of physical activity is necessary before the body can precisely regulate or fine-tune food intake to balance energy expenditure. A sedentary lifestyle might reduce the ability of the fine-tuning device to control food intake precisely, resulting in a positive energy balance and a weight gain.

Exercise does, in fact, appear to be a mild appetite suppressant, at least for the first few hours following intense exercise training. Further, studies have shown that the total number of calories consumed per day does not change when one begins a training program, even with a greatly increased caloric expenditure. While some have interpreted this as evidence that exercise does not affect appetite, it might be more accurate to conclude that appetite was affected in that caloric intake did not increase in proportion to the additional caloric expenditure resulting from the exercise program. In studies conducted on rats, the food intake of male rats appears to be reduced with exercise training, while female rats tend to eat the same or even more than nonexercising control rats (Oscai, 1973). There is no obvious explanation for this gender difference, and so far similar results have not been reported in humans.

It is possible that the decrease in appetite occurs only with intense levels of exercise in which the increased catecholamine levels might suppress the appetite. It is also possible that the increased body temperature that accompanies high intensity activity, or almost any activity performed under hot and humid conditions, leads to a decreased appetite. When the weather is hot, or when there is an elevated body temperature as a result of illness, there is a loss in the desire for food. This might also explain why there is little or no desire to eat after a hard running workout, but a relatively strong craving for food following a hard swimming workout. In the pool, providing the water temperature is well below core temperature, the heat generated by exercise is lost very effectively, making it possible to better regulate core temperature.

The effect of exercise on the components of energy expenditure became a major topic of interest among researchers in the late 1980s and early 1990s. Of obvious interest is how exercise training might affect the RMR, since it represents 60% to 75% of the total number of calories expended each day. If a 25-year-old male's total caloric intake was 2,700 kcal per day, and his RMR accounted for just 60% of that total (0.60 x 2700 = 1620 kcal RMR), just a 1% increase in his RMR would be an extra 16 kcal expended each day, or 5,913 kcal per year. This small increase in RMR alone would account for the equivalent of a 1.7 pound fat loss per year!

The role of physical training in increasing RMR has not been totally resolved. Several cross-sectional studies have found that highly trained runners have higher RMRs than individuals of similar age and size who are untrained. However, other studies have not been able to confirm this (Poehlman, 1989). Few longitudinal studies have been conducted where untrained individuals are trained for a period of time and their changes in RMR are determined. Those longitudinal studies that have been conducted suggest that there might be an increase in RMR following training, but the data are not conclusive (Broeder et al., 1992). Since RMR is closely related to the fat-free mass of the body, there is now interest in the possible use of resistance training to increase the fat-free mass in an attempt to increase RMR.

A number of studies have been conducted on the role of individual bouts of exercise and exercise training in increasing the TEF. It is reasonably clear that a single bout of exercise, either before or after a meal, increases the thermic effect of that meal. Less clear is the role of exercise training on the TEF. Studies have shown increases, others have shown decreases, and still others have shown no effect of exercise training on the TEF.

With respect to the specific loss of body fat with exercise, several research studies have pointed to the possible role of human growth hormone as being responsible for the increased fatty acid mobilization during exercise. Growth hormone levels do increase sharply with exercise and remain elevated for up to several hours in the recovery period. Other research has suggested that with exercise the adipose tissue is more sensitive to the sympathetic nervous system, or to the levels of circulating catecholamines, which would result in increased lipid mobilization. More recent research suggests that a specific fat-mobilizing substance, which is highly responsive to elevated levels of activity, is responsible. Thus, it is impossible to state with certainty which factors are of greatest importance in mediating this response.

Spot Reduction, Other Myths, and Exercise Devices

Many individuals, including athletes, believe that by exercising a specific area of the body, the fat in that localized area will be utilized, thus reducing the locally stored fat. Several early research studies reported results that tended to support the concept of spot reduction. However, later research suggested that spot reduction is a myth and that exercise, even when localized, draws from all of the fat stores of the body, not just from the local depots.

One study utilized outstanding tennis players to investigate the phenomenon of spot reduction, theorizing that they would be ideal subjects for studying spot reduction since they could act as their own controls, in that the dominant arm exercises vigorously every day for several hours, while the nondominant arm is relatively sedentary (Gwinup et al., 1971). They postulated that if spot reduction was a reality, the nondominant (inactive) arm should have substantially more fat than the dominant (active) arm. In fact, while the arm girths were substantially greater in the dominant arm due to exercise-induced muscle hypertrophy, there were absolutely no differences between the arms in subcutaneous skinfold fat thicknesses. Another study reported no difference in the rate of change in fat cell diameters at the abdomen, subscapular and gluteal fat biopsy sites following a 27-day intense sit-up training program, indicating a lack of specific adaptation at the site of exercise training (Katch et al., 1984). Researchers now theorize that fat is mobilized from either those areas of highest concentration or equally from all areas, thus negating the spot reduction theory. Changes in girth, such as the abdominal girth, can occur with exercise training, but these changes are the result of increased muscle tone, not fat loss.

During the latter part of the 1980s and early 1990s, various professional exercise groups promoted low intensity aerobic exercise to increase the loss of body fat. It has been clearly established that the higher the exercise intensity, the greater the body's reliance on carbohydrate as an energy source. With high intensity aerobic exercise, carbohydrate might supply 65% or more of the body's energy needs. These groups theorized that low intensity aerobic training would allow the body to use more fat as the energy source, thus more effectively reducing the body's fat stores. While it is true that the body uses a higher percentage of fat for energy at lower intensities of exercise, the total number of calories expended from the use of fat is not different. Furthermore, there are substantially more calories expended during the higher intensity workout for the same period of time.

With the popularity of exercise increasing, there are many gimmicks and gadgets on the market. While some of these are legitimate and effective, many are of no practical value for either exercise conditioning or weight loss. Three such devices were evaluated to determine the legitimacy of their claims: the Mark II bust developer; the Astro-Trimmer exercise belt; and the Slim-Skins vacuum pants. The last two devices claimed to take inches off the abdomen, hips, buttocks, and thighs in a matter of minutes, while the first device claimed to add two to three inches to the bust within three to seven days. All three failed to produce any changes whatsoever when evaluated in tightly controlled scientific studies (Wilmore et al., 1985a, 1985b). To gain the benefits from exercise it is necessary actually to do the work!

REFERENCES

Ballor, D.L., & Keesey, R.E. (1991). A meta-analysis of the factors affecting exercise-induced changes in body mass, fat mass and fat-free mass in males and females. *International Journal of Obesity, 15,* 717–726.

Bjorntorp, P., Smith, U., & Lönnroth, P. (1988). Health implications of regional obesity. *Acta Medica Scandinavica Symposium Series* No. 4, Stockholm: Almqvist & Wiksell International.

Bouchard, C., Tremblay, A., Després, J.-P., Nadeau, A., Lupien, P.J., Thériault, G., Dussault, J., Moorjani, S., Pinault, S., & Fournier, G. (1990). The response to long-term overfeeding in identical twins. *New England Journal of Medicine, 322,* 1477–1482.

Bray, G.A. (1985). Obesity: definition, diagnosis and disadvantages. *Medical Journal of Australia, 142,* S2–S8.

Broeder, C.E., Burrhus, K.A., Svanevik, L.S., & Wilmore, J.H. (1992). The effects of either high intensity resistance or endurance training on resting metabolic rate. *American Journal of Clinical Nutrition, 55,* 802–810.

Gortmaker, S.L., Dietz, W.H., Jr., Sobol, A. M., & Wehler, C.A. (1987). Increasing pediatric obesity in the United States. *American Journal of Diseases of Children, 141,* 535–540.

Gwinup, G., Chelvam, R., & Steinberg, T. (1971). Thickness of subcutaneous fat and activity of underlying muscles. *Annals of Internal Medicine, 74,* 408–411.

Katch, F.I., Clarkson, P.M., Kroll, W., McBride, T., & Wilcox, A. (1984). Effects of sit up exercise training on adipose cell size and adiposity. *Research Quarterly for Exercise and Sport, 55,* 242–247.

Keesey, R.E. (1986). A set-point theory of obesity. In K.D. Brownell & J.P. Foreyt (Eds.), *Handbook of Eating Disorders: Physiology, Psychology, and Treatment of Obesity, Anorexia, and Bulimia* (pp. 63–87). New York: Basic Books.

Keys, A., Brozek, J., Henschel, A., Mickelsen, O., & Taylor, H.L. (1950). *The Biology of Human Starvation.* Minneapolis: University of Minnesota Press.

Mayer, J., Marshall, N.B., Vitale, J.J., Christensen, J.H., Mashayekhi, M.B., & Stare, F.J. (1954). Exercise, food intake, and body weight in normal rats and genetically obese adult mice. *American Journal of Physiology, 177,* 544–548.

National Center for Health Statistics. (1986). *Health, United States, 1986.* DHHS Publ. No. (PHS) 87-1232. Public Health Service, Washington DC: U.S. Government Printing Office, December 1986.

National Institutes of Health. (1985). Health implications of obesity: National Institutes of Health Consensus Development Conference Statement. *Annals of Internal Medicine, 103,* 1073–1077.

Oscai, L.B. (1973). The role of exercise in weight control. *Exercise and Sport Sciences Reviews, 1,* 103–123.

Pavlou, K.N., Steffee, W.P., Lerman, R.H., & Burrows, V. (1985). Effects of dieting and exercise on lean body mass, oxygen uptake, and strength. *Medicine and Science in Sports and Exercise, 17,* 466–471.

Poehlman, E.T. (1989). A review: exercise and its influence on resting energy metabolism in man. *Medicine and Science in Sports and Exercise, 21,* 515–525.

Sims, E.A.H. (1976). Experimental obesity, dietary-induced thermogenesis and their clinical implications. *Clinics in Endocrinology and Metabolism, 5,* 377–395.

Stefanick, M.L. (1993). Exercise and weight control. *Exercise and Sport Sciences Reviews, 21,* 363–396.

Stunkard, A.J., Foch, T.T., & Hrubec, Z. (1986a). A twin study of human obesity. *Journal of the American Medical Association, 256,* 51–54.

Stunkard, A.J., Harris, J. R., Pedersen, N.L., & McClearn, G.E. (1990). The body-mass index of twins who have been reared apart. *New England Journal of Medicine, 322,* 1483–1487.

Stunkard, A.J., Sorensen, T.I.A., Hanis, C., Teasdale, T.W., Chakraborty, R., Schull, W.J., & Schulsinger, F. (1986b). An adoption study of human obesity. *New England Journal of Medicine, 314,* 193–198.

Wilmore, J.H. (1983). Body composition in sport and exercise: Directions for future research. *Medicine and Science in Sports and Exercise, 15,* 21–31.

Wilmore, J.H., Atwater, A.E., Maxwell, B.D., Wilmore, D.L., Constable, S.H., & Buono, M.J. (1985a). Alterations in body size and composition consequent to Astro-Trimmer and Slim-Skins training programs. *Research Quarterly for Exercise and Sport, 56,* 90–92.

Wilmore, J.H., Atwater, A.E., Maxwell, B.D., Wilmore, D.L., Constable, S.H., & Buono, M.J. (1985b). Alterations in breast morphology consequent to a 21-day bust developer program. *Medicine and Science in Sports and Exercise, 17,* 106–112.

Zuti, W.B., & Gelding, L.A. (1976). Comparing diet and exercise as weight reduction tools. *Physician and Sportsmedicine, 4,* 49–53.

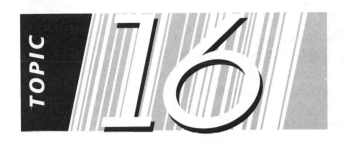
The Influence of Exercise on Mental Health

Daniel M. Landers
ARIZONA STATE UNIVERSITY

A NOTE FROM THE EDITORS

Mental health as discussed in this paper by Dr. Daniel Landers, a leading authority on this topic, focuses on conditions sometimes considered to be illness states (i.e., pathological depression) as well as conditions that limit wellness or quality of life (i.e., anxiety, low self-esteem). To aid the reader, some basic terms used in this paper are outlined in the boxes below.

Definitions

Acute.   Acute refers to something that occurs at a specific time often for a relatively short duration. For example, acute exercise refers to a bout of exercise done at a specific time for a specific amount of time. Acute anxiety is anxiety that exists in a person in response to a specific event (same as state anxiety).

Anxiety.   Anxiety is a form of negative self-appraisal characterized by worry, self-doubt, and apprehension.

Chronic.   Chronic refers to something that persists for a relatively long period of time. Chronic depression, for example, would be depression that lasts a long time. A chronic exerciser is someone who does exercise on a regular basis.

Depression.   Depression is a state of being associated with feelings of hopelessness or a sense of defeat. People with depression often feel "down" or "blue" even when circumstances would dictate otherwise. All people feel "depressed" at times, but a "depressed" person feels this way much of the time.

(continued)

ORIGINALLY PUBLISHED AS SERIES 2, NUMBER 12, OF THE PCPFS *RESEARCH DIGEST.*

Clinical depression. This is depression (see definition) that persists for a relatively long period of time or becomes so severe that a person needs special help to cope with day-to-day affairs.

Meta-analysis. A type of statistical analysis that researchers use to make sense of many different research studies done on the same topic. By analyzing findings from many different studies, conclusions can be drawn concerning the results of all studies considered together. Both unpublished and published studies can be included in this type of analysis.

Positive mood. Positive self-assessments associated with feelings of vigor, happiness, and/or other positive feelings of well-being.

State anxiety. State anxiety is anxiety present in very specific situations. For example, state sports anxiety is present when a person is anxious in a specific sports situation even if the person is not generally anxious.

Trait anxiety. Trait anxiety is the level of anxiety present in a person on a regular basis. A person with high trait anxiety is anxious much of the time while a person low in trait anxiety tends to be anxious less often and in fewer situations.

Mental Health Benefits of Physical Activity

Reduced anxiety

- Best results with "aerobic exercise"
- Best after weeks of regular exercise
- Best benefits to those who are low fit to begin with
- Best benefits for those high in anxiety to begin with

Reduced depression

- Best after weeks of regular exercise
- Best when done several times a week
- Best with more vigorous exercise
- Best for those who are more depressed (needs more research)

Benefits (anxiety and depression) similar to those for other treatments

Activity associated with positive self-esteem

Activity associated with restful sleep

Activity associated with ability to respond to stress

For some time now, it has been common knowledge that exercise is good for one's physical health. It has only been in recent years, however, that it has become commonplace to read in magazines and health newsletters that exercise can also be of value in promoting sound mental health. Although this optimistic appraisal has attracted a great deal of attention, the scientific community has been much more cautious in offering such a blanket endorsement. Consider the tentative conclusions from the Surgeon General's Report on Physical Activity and Health (*PCPFS Research Digest,* 1996) that "physical activity appears to relieve symptoms of depression and anxiety and improve mood" and that "regular physical activity may reduce the risk of developing depression, although further research is needed on this topic."

The use of carefully chosen words, such as "appears to" and "may" illustrate the caution that people in the scientific community have when it comes to claiming mental health benefits derived from exercise. Part of the problem in interpreting the scientific literature is that there are over 100 scientific studies dealing with exercise and depression or exercise and anxiety and not all of these studies show statistically significant benefits with exercise training. The paucity of clinical trial studies and the fact that a "mixed bag" of significant and nonsignificant findings exists makes it difficult for scientists to give a strong endorsement for the positive influence of exercise on mental health. There is no doubt that

HIGHLIGHT ▌▌▐ ▐▐▐▐▐▐ ▐▐ ▐▐▐▐▐▐ ▐▐ ▐▐▐▐ ▐▐▐ ▐ ▐ ▐▐▐▐▐▐ ▐▐▐▐▐▐▐▐▐▐▐ ▐ ▐ ▐▐▐ ▐▐▐ ▐▐ ▐▐ ▐▐▐▐▐ ▐▐ ▐▐▐▐▐▐ ▐▐

"We now have evidence to support the claim that exercise is related to positive mental health as indicated by relief in symptoms of depression and anxiety."

the mental health area needs more clinical trial studies. This would be particularly useful in determining if exercise "causes" improvements in variables associated with sound mental health. However, until these clinical trial studies materialize, there is still much that can be done to strengthen statements made about exercise and mental health.

What evidence would prompt some scientists to "stick their necks out" in favor of more definitive statements? One reason for greater optimism is the recent appearance of quantitative reviews (i.e., meta-analyses) of the literature on a number of mental health topics. These reviews differ in several ways from the traditional narrative reviews. A meta-analysis allows for a summary of results across studies. By including all published and unpublished studies and combining their results, statistical power is increased. Another advantage of using this type of review process is that a clearly defined sequence of steps is followed and included in the final report so that anyone can replicate the studies. Two additional advantages that meta-analysis has over other types of reviews include: (a) the use of a quantification technique that gives an objective estimate of the magnitude of the exercise treatment effect; and (b) its ability to examine potential moderating variables to determine if they influence exercise-mental health relationships. Given these advantages, this paper will focus primarily on results derived from large-scale meta-analytic reviews.

ANXIETY REDUCTION FOLLOWING EXERCISE

It is estimated that in the United States approximately 7.3% of the adult population has an anxiety disorder that necessitates some form of treatment (Regier et al., 1988). In addition, stress-related emotions, such as anxiety, are common among healthy individuals (Cohen, Tyrell, & Smith, 1991). The current interest in prevention has heightened interest in exercise as an alternative or adjunct to traditional interventions such as psychotherapy or drug therapies.

Anxiety is associated with the emergence of a negative form of cognitive appraisal typified by worry, self-doubt, and apprehension. According to Lazarus and Cohen (1977), it usually arises "... in the face of *demands that tax or exceed the resources of the system* or ... demands to which there are no readily available or automatic adaptive responses" (p. 109). Anxiety is a cognitive phenomenon and is usually measured by questionnaire instruments. These questionnaires are sometimes accompanied by physiological measures that are associated with heightened arousal/anxiety (e.g., heart rate, blood pressure, skin conductance, muscle tension). A common distinction in this literature is between state and trait questionnaire measures of anxiety. Trait anxiety is the general predisposition to respond across many situations with high levels of anxiety. State anxiety, on the other hand, is much more specific and refers to the person's anxiety at a particular moment. Although "trait" and "state" aspects of anxiety are conceptually distinct, the available operational measures show a considerable amount of overlap among these subcomponents of anxiety (Smith, 1989).

For meta-analytic reviews of this topic, the inclusion criterion has been that only studies examining anxiety measures before and after either acute or chronic exercise have been included in the review. Studies with experiment-imposed psychosocial stressors during the postexercise period have not been included since this would confound the effects of exercise with the effects of stressors (e.g., Stoop color-word test, active physical performance). The meta-analysis by Schlicht (1994), however, included some stress-reactivity studies and therefore was not interpretable.

Landers and Petruzzello (1994) examined the results of 27 narrative reviews that had been conducted between 1960 and 1991 and found that in 81% of them the authors had concluded that physical activity/fitness was related to anxiety reduction following exercise and there was little or no conflicting data presented in these reviews. For the other 19%, the authors had concluded that most of the findings were supportive of exercise being related to a reduction in anxiety, but there were some divergent results. None of these narrative reviews concluded that there was no relationship.

There have been six meta-analyses examining the relationship between exercise and anxiety reduction (Calfas & Taylor, 1994; Kugler, Seelback, & Krüskemper, 1994; Landers & Petruzzello, 1994; Long & van Stavel, 1995; McDonald & Hodgdon, 1991; Petruzzello, Landers, Hatfield, Kubitz, & Salazar, 1991). These meta-analyses ranged from 159 studies (Landers & Petruzzello, 1994; Petruzzello et al., 1991) to five studies (Calfas & Taylor, 1994) reviewed. All six of these meta-analyses found that across all studies examined, exercise was significantly related to a reduction in anxiety. These effects ranged from "small" to "moderate" in size and were consistent for trait, state, and psychophysiological measures of anxiety. The vast majority of the narrative reviews and all of the meta-analytic reviews support the conclusion that across studies published between 1960 and 1995 there is a small to moderate relationship showing that both acute and chronic exercise reduces anxiety. This reduction occurs for all types of subjects, regardless of the measures of anxiety being employed (i.e., state, trait or psychophysiological), the intensity or the duration of the exercise, the type of exercise paradigm (i.e., acute or chronic), and the scientific quality of the studies. Another meta-analysis (Kelley & Tran, 1995) of 35 clinical trial studies involving 1,076 subjects has confirmed the psychophysiological findings in showing small (−4/−3 mm Hg), but statistically significant, postexercise reductions for both systolic and diastolic blood pressure among normal normotensive adults.

In addition to these general effects, some of these meta-analyses (Landers & Petruzzello, 1994; Petruzzello et al., 1991) that examined more studies and therefore had more findings to consider were able to identify several variables that moderated the relationship between exercise and anxiety reduction. Compared to the overall conclusion noted above, which is based on hundreds of studies involving thousands of subjects, the findings for the moderating variables are based on a much smaller database. More research, therefore, is warranted to examine further the conclusions derived from the following moderating variables. The meta-analyses show that the larger effects of exercise on anxiety reduction are shown when: (a) the exercise is "aerobic" (e.g., running, swimming, cycling) as opposed to nonaerobic (e.g., handball, strength-flexibility training), (b) the length of the aerobic training program is at least 10 weeks and preferably greater than 15 weeks, and (c) subjects have initially lower levels of fitness or higher levels of anxiety. The "higher levels of anxiety" includes coronary (Kugler et al., 1994) and panic disorder patients (Meyer, Broocks, Hillmer-Vogel, Bandelow, & Rüther, 1997). In addition, there is limited evidence which suggests that the anxiety reduction is not an artifact "due more to the cessation of a potentially threatening activity than to the exercise itself" (Petruzzello, 1995, p. 109), and the time course for postexercise anxiety reduction is somewhere between four to six hours before anxiety returns to pre-exercise levels (Landers & Petruzzello, 1994). It also appears that although exercise differs from no treatment control groups, it is usually not shown to differ from other known anxiety-reducing treatments (e.g., relaxation training). The finding that exercise can produce an anxiety reduction similar in magnitude to other commonly employed anxiety treatments is noteworthy since exercise can be considered at least as good as these techniques, but in addition, it has many other physical benefits.

EXERCISE AND DEPRESSION

Depression is a prevalent problem in today's society. Clinical depression affects 2–5% of Americans each year (Kessler et al., 1994) and it is estimated that patients suffering from clinical depression make up 6–8% of general medical practices (Katon & Schulberg, 1992). Depression is also costly to the health care system in that depressed individuals annually spend 1.5 times more on health care than nondepressed individuals, and those being treated with antidepressants spend three times more on outpatient pharmacy costs than those not on drug therapy (Simon, VonKorff, & Barlow, 1995). These costs have led to increased governmental pressure to reduce health care costs in America. If available and effective, alternative low-cost therapies that do not have negative side effects need to be incorporated into treatment plans. Exercise has been proposed as an alternative or adjunct to more traditional approaches for treating depression (Hales & Travis, 1987; Martinsen, 1987, 1990).

The research on exercise and depression has a long history of investigators (Franz & Hamilton, 1905; Vaux, 1926) suggesting a relationship between exercise and decreased depression. Since the early 1900s, there have been over 100 studies examining this relationship, and many narrative reviews on this topic have also been conducted. During the 1990s there have been at least five meta-analytic reviews (Craft, 1997; Calfas & Taylor, 1994; Kugler et al., 1994; McDonald & Hodgdon, 1991; North, McCullagh, & Tran, 1990) that have examined studies ranging from as few as nine (Calfas & Taylor, 1994) to as many as 80 (North et al., 1990). Across these five meta-analytic reviews, the results consistently show that both acute and chronic exercise are related to a significant reduction in depression. These effects are generally "moderate" in magnitude (i.e., larger than the anxiety-reducing effects noted earlier) and occur for subjects who were classified as nondepressed, clinically depressed, or mentally ill. The findings indicate that the antidepressant effect of exercise begins as early as the first session of exercise and persists beyond the end of the exercise program (Craft, 1997; North et al., 1990). These effects are also consistent across age, gender, exercise group size, and type of depression inventory.

Exercise was shown to produce larger antidepressant effects when: (a) the exercise training program was longer than nine weeks and involved more sessions (Craft, 1997; North et al., 1990); (b) exercise was of longer duration, higher intensity, and performed a greater number of days per week (Craft, 1997); and (c) subjects were classified as medical rehabilitation patients (North et al., 1991) and, based on questionnaire instruments, were classified as moderately/severely depressed compared to mildly/moderately depressed (Craft, 1997). The latter effect is limited since only one study used individuals who were classified as severely depressed and only two studies used individuals who were classified as moderately to severely depressed. Although limited at this time, this finding calls into question the conclusions of several narrative reviews (Gleser & Mendelberg, 1990; Martinsen, 1987, 1993, 1994), which indicate that exercise has antidepressant effects only for those who are initially mild to moderately depressed.

The meta-analyses are inconsistent when comparing exercise to the more traditional treatments for depression, such as psychotherapy and behavioral interventions (e.g., relaxation, meditation), and this may be related to the types of subjects employed. In examining all types of subjects, North et al. (1990) found that exercise decreased depression more than relaxation training or engaging in enjoy-able activities, but did not produce effects that were different from psychotherapy. Craft (1997), using only clinically depressed subjects, found that exercise produced the same effects as psychotherapy, behavioral interventions, and social contact. Exercise used in combination with individual psychotherapy or exercise together with drug therapy produced the largest effects; however, these effects were not significantly different from the effect produced by exercise alone (Craft, 1997).

That exercise is at least as effective as more traditional therapies is encouraging, especially considering the time and cost involved with treatments like psychotherapy. Exercise may be a positive adjunct for the treatment of depression since exercise provides additional health benefits (e.g., increase in muscle tone and decreased incidence of heart disease and obesity) that behavioral interventions do not. Thus, since exercise is cost effective, has positive health benefits, and is effective in alleviating depression, it is a viable adjunct or alternative to many of the more traditional therapies. Future research also needs to examine the possibility of systematically lowering antidepressant medication dosages while concurrently supplementing treatment with exercise.

OTHER VARIABLES ASSOCIATED WITH MENTAL HEALTH

Positive mood. The Surgeon General's Report also mentions the possibility of exercise improving mood. Unfortunately the area of increased positive mood as a result of acute and chronic exercise has only recently been investigated and therefore there are no meta-analytic reviews in this area. Many investigators are currently examining this subject and many of the preliminary results have been encouraging. It remains to be seen if the additive effects of these studies will result in conclusions that are as encouraging as the relationship between exercise and the alleviation of negative mood states like anxiety and depression.

Self-esteem. Related to the area of positive mood states is the area of physical activity and self-esteem. Although narrative reviews exist in the area of physical activity and enhancement of self-esteem, there are currently four meta-analytic reviews on this topic (Calfas & Taylor, 1994; Gruber, 1986; McDonald &

Hodgdon, 1991; Spence, Poon, & Dyck, 1997). The number of studies in these meta-analyses ranged from 10 studies (Calfas & Taylor, 1994) to 51 studies (Spence et al., 1997). All four of the reviews found that physical activity/exercise brought about small, but statistically significant, increases in physical self-concept or self-esteem. These effects generalized across gender and age groups. In comparing self-esteem scores in children, Gruber (1986) found that aerobic fitness produced much larger effects on self-esteem scores than other types of physical education class activities (e.g., learning sports skills or perceptual-motor skills). Gruber (1986) also found that the effect of physical activity was larger for handicapped compared to nonhandicapped children.

Restful sleep. Another area associated with positive mental health is the relationship between exercise and restful sleep. Two meta-analyses have been conducted on this topic (Kubitz, Landers, Petruzzello, & Han, 1996; O'Connor & Youngstedt, 1995). The studies reviewed have primarily examined sleep duration and total sleep time as well as measures derived from electroencephalographic (EEG) activity while subjects are in various stages of sleep. Operationally, sleep researchers have predicted that sleep duration, total sleep time, and the amount of high amplitude, slow wave EEG activity would be higher in physically fit individuals than those who are unfit (i.e., chronic effect) and higher on nights following exercise (i.e., acute effect). This prediction is based on the "compensatory" position, which posits that "fatiguing daytime activity (e.g., exercise) would probably result in a compensatory increase in the need for and depth of nighttime sleep, thereby facilitating recuperative, restorative and/or energy conservation processes" (Kubitz et al., p. 278).

The sleep meta-analyses by O'Connor and Youngstedt (1995) and Kubitz et al. (1996) show support for this prediction. Both reviews show that exercise significantly increases total sleep time and aerobic exercise decreases rapid eye movement (REM) sleep. REM sleep is a paradoxical form in that it is a deep sleep, but it is not as restful as slow wave sleep (i.e., stages 3 and 4 sleep). Kubitz et al. (1996) found that acute and chronic exercise was related to an increase in slow wave sleep and total sleep time, but was also related to a decrease in sleep onset latency and REM sleep. These findings support the compensatory position in that trained subjects and those engaging in an acute bout of ex-

ercise went to sleep more quickly, slept longer, and had a more restful sleep than untrained subjects or subjects who did not exercise. There were moderating variables influencing these results. Exercise had the biggest impact on sleep when: (a) the individuals were female, low fit, or older; (b) the exercise was longer in duration; and (c) the exercise was completed earlier in the day (Kubitz et al., 1996).

SUMMARY

The research literature suggests that for many variables there is now ample evidence that a definite relationship exists between exercise and improved mental health. This is particularly evident in the case of a reduction of anxiety and depression. For these topics, there is now considerable evidence derived from over hundreds of studies with thousands of subjects to support the claim that "exercise is related to a relief in symptoms of depression and anxiety." Obviously, more research is needed to determine if this overall relationship is "causal," and there is also a need to examine further some of the variables that are believed to moderate the overall relationship.

For many of the other variables related to mental health, the initial meta-analyses have shown evidence that is promising. Compared to the area of depression and anxiety, however, there is either a need for more research on these topics or more quantitative reviews of the expansive research that already exists. For example, the relatively new research into the influence of exercise on positive mood states is in need of more research studies, whereas the area of exercise and self-esteem needs quantitative reviews of the expansive research literature that already exists. At the present time, it appears that aerobic exercise enhances physical self-concept and self-esteem, but more research needs to be done to confirm these initial findings. Exercise is related not only to a relief in symptoms of depression and anxiety but it also seems to be beneficial in enhancing self-esteem, producing more restful sleep, and helping people recover more quickly from psychosocial stressors. None of these relationships is the result of a single study. They are based on most, if not all, of the available research in the English language at the time the meta-analytic review was published. The overall positive patterns of the meta-analytic findings for these variables lends greater confidence that exercise has an important role to play in promoting sound mental health.

REFERENCES

Calfas, K.J., & Taylor, W.C. (1994). Effects of physical activity on psychological variables in adolescents. *Pediatric Exercise Science, 6,* 406–423.

Cohen, S., Tyrell, D.A.J., & Smith, A.P. (1991). Psychological stress and susceptibility to the common cold. *New England Journal of Medicine, 325,* 606–612.

Corbin, C., & Pangrazi, B. (Eds.) (1996). What you need to know about the Surgeon General's Report on Physical Activity and Health. *Physical Activity and Fitness Research Digest,* July, Series 2(6), p. 4.

Craft, L.L. (1997). *The effect of exercise on clinical depression and depression resulting from mental illness: A meta-analysis.* Unpublished master's thesis, Arizona State University, Tempe.

Franz, S.I., & Hamilton, G.V. (1905). The effects of exercise upon retardation in conditions of depression. *American Journal of Insanity, 62,* 239–256.

Gleser, J., & Mendelberg, H. (1990). Exercise and sport in mental health: A review of the literature. *Israel Journal of Psychiatry and Related Sciences, 27,* 99–112.

Gruber, J.J. (1986). Physical activity and self-esteem development in children. In G.A. Stull & H.M. Eckert (Eds.), *Effects of physical activity and self-esteem development in children.* (The Academy Papers No 19, pp. 30–48). Champaign, IL: Human Kinetics Publishers.

Hales, R., & Travis, T.W. (1987). Exercise as a treatment option for anxiety and depressive disorders. *Military Medicine, 152,* 299–302.

Katon, W., & Schulberg, H. (1992). Epidemiology of depression in primary care. *General Hospital Psychiatry, 14,* 237–247.

Kelley, G., & Tran, Z.V. (1995). Aerobic exercise and normotensive adults: A meta-analysis. *Medicine and Science in Sports and Exercise, 27(10),* 1371–1377.

Kessler, R.C., McGonagle, K.A., Zhao, S., Nelson, C.B., Hughes, M., Eshelman, S., Wittchen, H.U., & Kendler, K.S. (1994). Lifetime and 12-month prevalence of DSM-III-R psychiatric disorders in the United States: Results from the National Co-morbidity Survey. *Archives of General Psychiatry, 51,* 8–19.

Kubitz, K.K., Landers, D.M., Petruzzello, S.J., & Han, M.W. (1996). The effects of acute and chronic exercise on sleep. *Sports Medicine, 21(4),* 277–291.

Kugler, J., Seelback, H., & Krüskemper, G.M. (1994). Effects of rehabilitation exercise programmes on anxiety and depression in coronary patients: A meta-analysis. *British Journal of Clinical Psychology, 33,* 401–410.

Landers, D.M., & Petruzzello, S.J. (1994). Physical activity, fitness, and anxiety. In C. Bouchard, R.J. Shephard, & T. Stevens (Eds.), *Physical activity, fitness, and health.* Champaign, IL: Human Kinetics Publishers.

Lazarus, R.S., & Cohen, J.P. (1977). Environmental stress. In I. Altman & J.F. Wohlwill (Eds.), *Human behavior and the environment: Current theory and research.* New York: Plenum Press.

Long, B.C., & van Stavel, R. (1995). Effects of exercise training on anxiety: A meta-analysis. *Journal of Applied Sport Psychology, 7,* 167–189.

Martinsen, E.W. (1987). The role of aerobic exercise in the treatment of depression. *Stress Medicine, 3,* 93–100.

Martinsen, E.W. (1990). Benefits of exercise for the treatment of depression. *Stress Medicine, 9,* 380–389.

Martinsen, E.W. (1993). Therapeutic implications of exercise for clinically anxious and depressed patients. *International Journal of Sport Psychology, 24,* 185–199.

Martinsen, E.W. (1994). Physical activity and depression: Clinical experience. *Acta Psychiatrica Scandinavica, 377,* 23–27.

McDonald, D.G., & Hodgdon, J.A. (1991). *The psychological effects of aerobic fitness training: Research and theory.* New York: Springer-Verlag.

Meyer, T., Broocks, A., Hillmer-Vogel, U., Bandelow, B., & Rüther, E. (1997). Spiroergometric testing of panic patients: Fitness level, trainability and indices for clinical improvement. *Medicine & Science in Sports and Exercise* (Abstract), 29(5), S270.

North, T.C., McCullagh, P., & Tran, Z.V. (1990). Effect of exercise on depression. *Exercise and Sport Science Reviews, 18,* 379–415.

O'Connor, P.J., & Youngstedt, M.A. (1995). Influence of exercise on human sleep. *Exercise and Sport Science Reviews, 23,* 105–134.

Petruzzello, S.J. (1995). Anxiety reduction following exercise: Methodological artifact or "real" phenomenon? *Journal of Sport and Exercise Psychology, 17,* 105–111.

Petruzzello, S.J., Landers, D.M., Hatfield, B.D., Kubitz, K.A., & Salazar, W. (1991). A meta-analysis on the anxiety-reducing effects of acute and chronic exercise. *Sports Medicine, 11(3),* 143–182.

Regier, D.A., Boyd, J.H., Burke, J.D., Rae, D.S., Myers, J.K., Kramer, M., Robins, L.N., George, L.K., Karno, M., & Locke, B.Z. (1988). One-month prevalence of mental disorders in the United States. *Archives of General Psychiatry, 45,* 977–986.

Schlicht, W. (1994). Does physical exercise reduce anxious emotions: A meta-analysis. *Anxiety, Stress, and Coping, 6,* 275–288.

Simon, G.E., VonKorff, M., & Barlow, W. (1995). Health care costs of primary care patients with recognized depression. *Archives of General Psychiatry, 52,* 850–856.

Smith, R.E. (1989). Conceptual and statistical issues in research involving multidimensional anxiety scales. *Journal of Sport and Exercise Psychology, 11,* 452–457.

Spence, J.C., Poon, P., Dyck, P. (1997). The effect of physical-activity participation on self-concept: A meta-analysis (Abstract). *Journal of Sport and Exercise Psychology, 19,* S109.

Vaux, C.L. (1926). A discussion of physical exercise and recreation. *Occupational Therapy and Rehabilitation, 6,* 30–33.

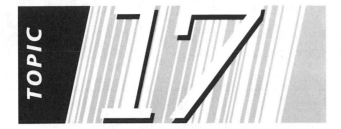

Economic Benefits of Physical Activity

Larry R. Gettman
NATIONAL HEALTH CALL CENTER GROUP

A NOTE FROM THE EDITORS

Many of the papers in this volume have focused on the health benefits of physical activity. For example, a previous issue summarized the many health benefits reported in the Surgeon General's Report on Physical Activity and Health. It is health benefits that led public health experts to include a national health goal for the year 2000 relating to employee worksite physical activity and fitness programs. Though health benefits are the principal reason why employees benefit from such programs, there are other benefits that come to employers who establish worksite physical activity programs for their employees. Specifically, data are now available to show that employee physical activity programs can save employers money. In this paper, Larry Gettman, one of the leading authorities on the economic benefits of worksite physical activity and wellness programs, summarizes the literature relating to the economic benefits of physical activity programs. This information can be useful in persuading employers to establish programs and meet national health objectives by increasing the availability of worksite activity programs.

ORIGINALLY PUBLISHED AS SERIES 2, NUMBER 7, OF THE PCPFS *RESEARCH DIGEST*.

INTRODUCTION

Because health care costs in this country have increased at alarming rates in recent years, with the estimate that they will exceed $1 trillion by the year 2000, there is a concern by corporations, government, and individuals in controlling these costs. One way to cut costs is to influence how health care is delivered—the treatment side of the equation. The other way to cut costs is to *prevent* health problems before they arise thus avoiding the treatment costs in the first place. This is where physical activity and health promotion fit into the prevention formula. And therefore the question naturally arises, "Is physical activity economically beneficial?"

THE ECONOMIC BENEFITS OF PHYSICAL ACTIVITY

The most widely used measure of the economic benefits of physical activity programs is the benefit/cost ratio. The benefit is expressed in amount of dollars saved from lower medical costs, less absenteeism, or reduced disability expenses. The costs in

"Published research investigating the economics of physical activity has reported improved health and lower health care costs, absenteeism, and disability associated with exercise and fitness programs."

the equation refer to the cost of the physical activity program. The ratio is money saved divided by the money spent. For example, a benefit/cost ratio of 3.43 would mean that $3.43 were saved for each $1.00 spent. Benefit/cost ratios reported in the literature for physical activity programs range from .76 to 3.43 (see Table 17.1).

Of course, physical activity is just one part of worksite health promotion, which may also include health risk assessment and behavior modification strategies for nutrition and weight control, stress management, stop smoking, blood pressure control, etc. There are many other studies reporting positive benefit/cost ratios ranging from 1.15 to 5.52 for a variety of health promotion programs (Messer & Stone, 1995). Some of those benefit/cost studies were conducted on comprehensive health promotion programs that included physical activity along with stress management, weight control, nutrition education, stop smoking, etc. These studies were not included in Table 17.1 because the specific benefit/cost ratio for isolated physical activity was not reported. It should be noted as a reminder, though, that all benefit/cost ratios reported for comprehensive health promotion programs are positive, meaning that the benefits of health promotion outweigh the costs of the program.

In addition to benefit/cost studies, there are health risk appraisal publications that have reported lower annual medical claims costs for exercising individuals (low risk) compared to sedentary (high risk) individuals (see Table 17.2). However, the differences between the high risk and low risk medical costs reported by Bertera (1991) and Yen et al. (1991) in Table 17.2 are statistically non-significant.

INFLUENCING HEALTH CARE COSTS WITH FITNESS INTERVENTIONS

Additional information is provided in this section to supplement the evidence cited in Tables 17.1 and 17.2.

- In a study that spanned 14 years, Cady (1985) showed that the fittest employees had only one-eighth as many injuries as the least fit employees and that unfit employees incurred twice the amount of injury cost.
- Baun (1986) showed that exercisers in a Tenneco fitness program had $553 lower health care costs per person compared to non-exercisers.
- Gettman (1986) found that physically active employees at Mesa Petroleum Co. spent $217 per person less on medical claims and had 21 hours per person less of sick time than sedentary employees.
- Describing an Army staff project, Karch (1988) noted that participants who logged the most hours of exercise had the greatest decrease in the number of health services used.
- Tsai et al. (1988) showed that injury rates and costs associated with injuries decrease as physical activity levels increase.
- Shore et al. (1989) reported that back fitness improved in municipal workers after six months of exercising and that injury-related absences dropped 0.25 day while nonparticipant absences increased 3.1 days.
- Shephard (1992) reported a zero increase in medical costs for a company with a fitness program and a 35% increase in medical costs for a company with no fitness program.
- Connors (1992) reported that GE Aircraft employees who were members of the fitness center for three years lowered their average annual health care costs from $1044 to $757 per individual. In contrast, nonmembers increased their average annual health care costs from $773 to $941 per person.

It has been established that physical inactivity increases the risk for several health problems and diseases (Blair et al., 1992). Logic tells us that if a person is inactive (sedentary) and develops more health problems than an active person, the sedentary, unhealthy, or diseased person is going to spend more

TABLE 17.1 ||█| |█|█|█ █|█ |█|█|█| || █|█ █|█ | █|█|█| █|█|█|█|█| | | |█ █ |█ █ || █ ███|█ ███|█|█|█|█ ||| █

Worksite fitness programs and benefit/cost evaluations.

Study/Author(s)/Year	Purpose	Benefit/Cost Ratio
Canada Life Shephard, 1992	Compare medical costs in a company with a fitness program to a control company with no fitness program.	3.43
Toronto Municipality Shore et al., 1989	Evaluate a fitness program designed to reduce job-related injuries and absenteeism.	1.41
Mesa Petroleum Gettman, 1986	Examine relationship between physical activity level and medical costs and absenteeism.	0.76 (1982) 1.07 (1983)
Prudential Fitness Bowne et al., 1984	Evaluate effects of worksite fitness program on health care and disability costs.	1.93

dollars on health care than the healthy, active person. Therefore, physical activity that leads to healthier living will be economically beneficial because fewer dollars will be spent on health problems.

A CONSERVATIVE CONSENSUS STATEMENT

The consensus statement published by the Association of Worksite Health Promotion indicates that worksite health promotion, including physical activity, *may* produce health care cost savings making the programs economically beneficial (Kaman, 1995). This conservative statement is based on criticism directed at past health promotion research. Despite the consistent finding that worksite health promotion is effective, critics claim that weak research methods were used. Study groups have been self-selected and biased, and there has been a lack of control groups and a lack of random selection in

TABLE 17.2 ||█|█| █|█|█|█|█|█| | | █|█ |██ || █ █|█|█|█|█ ███|█| |█|

Association between annual medical claims costs per person and the sedentary risk factor.

Study/ Author(s)/ Year	Sedentary High Risk Cost	Active Low Risk Cost	Difference
Du Pont Co. Bertera, 1991	$3335	$3205	$130 ns
Steelcase employees Yen et al., 1991	$ 870	$ 479	$391 ns
Milliman & Robertson Business & Health, 1995	$1248	$1152	$ 96

comparison groups. In addition, there are other factors besides health promotion that may reduce health care costs, and research is needed to identify the specific independent influence that health promotion has on health care costs.

While some of this criticism may be warranted and while research on any topic can always be improved, we cannot negate the consistent findings of the wide variety of investigative approaches that have reported the positive economics of worksite health promotion, including physical activity. R.J. Shephard, a pioneer in worksite fitness research and one of the most respected professionals in the field, states that "large, randomized, double-blind, controlled experiments are not feasible in the context of worksite exercise programs" (Shephard, 1996). And, as an additional point, randomly selecting individuals into groups for research purposes raises some sensitive ethical questions. For example, randomly selecting a person into a sedentary control group and then asking that person to remain sedentary for the sake of good research denies that person the opportunity to change behavior, become active, and reap the rewards of a healthier lifestyle. Most of the past research conducted on the economics of physical activity have used observational methods and descriptive statistics. In the opinion of this author, it is not weak research to observe what happens in a group of people over time and then report the descriptive statistics.

CONCLUSION

Considering the evidence presented through a wide variety of studies, it is concluded that physical activity is economically beneficial. Future research should continue to document the specific relationship between physical activity and the economic costs related to health care and sick time.

MAJOR SOURCES OF INFORMATION

Acknowledgment is given to five excellent review documents that summarize the research related to the general topic of health promotion and its associated economics. The reader is strongly encouraged to review these documents.

■ Shephard (1996) examined the methodology of 52 studies on worksite fitness and exercise programs and concluded that participants in these programs show improvements in health-related fitness, a reduction of cardiac risk factors, and a containment of illness. Health promotion practitioners should encourage the development of fitness and exercise programs for both large and small companies and foster employee participation. Researchers should explore further the association between changes in fitness and the economic benefits to the employer.

■ Messer and Stone (1995) provided a thorough review and analysis of the studies reporting positive benefit/cost ratios for worksite fitness and health promotion programs. The state of the art in benefit/cost analysis is increasingly rigorous and defensible. Ultimately, benefit/cost analysis may provide the framework for establishing the economic viability of worksite fitness.

■ Kaman (1995) edited the second major volume on the topic of worksite health promotion economics sponsored by the Association for Worksite Health Promotion. The consensus statement in this book details the current knowledge on the impact of health promotion on health care costs.

■ Opatz (1994) edited the first major volume on the economics of worksite health promotion sponsored by the Association for Worksite Health Promotion. Part I of the book addresses the problems in trying to measure the costs and benefits of health promotion; Part II describes the proper techniques for evaluating programs; and Part III profiles programs at specific worksites.

■ Pelletier (1993) published the second in his series of articles that summarize the impact of health promotion programs on health and cost. From 1980 to 1991 there were 24 published studies indicating positive health benefits and economic results and from 1991 to 1993, another 23 studies indicated the same. Pelletier states, "When anyone cavalierly dismisses [these] studies with the glib dismissal of 'there is no evidence,' they are simply ignorant of more than 13 years of increasingly sophisticated research with documentation of both health and cost outcomes."

REFERENCES

Baun, W.B., Bernacki, E.J., & Tsai, S.P. (1986). A preliminary investigation: Effect of a corporate fitness program on absenteeism and health care cost. *Journal of Occupational Medicine, 28,* 18–22.

Bertera, R.L. (1991). The effects of behavioral risks on absenteeism and health-care costs in the workplace. *Journal of Occupational Medicine, 33,* 1119–1124.

Blair, S.N., Kohl, H.W., III, Gordon, N.F., & Paffenbarger, Jr., R.S. (1992). How much physical activity is good for health? *Annual Review of Public Health, 13,* 99–126.

Bowne, D.W., Russell, M.L., Morgan, J.L., Optenberg, S.A., & Clarke, A.E. (1984). Reduced disability and health-care costs in an industrial fitness program. *Journal of Occupational Medicine, 26,* 809–816.

Cady, L.D. (1985). Programs for increasing health and physical fitness of firefighters. *Journal of Occupational Medicine, 27,* 110–114.

Connors, N. (1992, March). Wellness promotes healthier employees. *Business & Health,* 66–71.

Gettman, L.R. (1986). Cost-benefit analysis of a corporate fitness program. *Fitness in Business, 1,* 11–17.

Kaman, R.L. (Ed.) (1995). *Worksite health promotion economics: Consensus and analysis.* Champaign, IL: Human Kinetics Publishers.

Karch, R.C., Newton, D.L., Schaeffer, M.A., Zoltick, J.M., Zajtchuk, R., & Rumbaugh, J.H. (1988). *Cost-benefit and cost-effectiveness measures of health promotion in a military-civilian staff.* Washington, DC: American University, National Center for Health Fitness.

Messer, J., & Stone, W. (1995). Worksite fitness and health promotion benefit/cost analysis: A tutorial, review of literature, and assessment of the state of the art. AWHP's *Worksite Health, 2,* 34–43.

Milliman & Robertson, Inc. (1995). The cost of unhealthy behavior. (In *Workplace prevention: The state of the nation.*) *Business & Health, Vol. 13 Supplement,* 20–25.

Opatz, J.P. (Ed.) (1994). *Economic impact of worksite health promotion.* Champaign, IL: Human Kinetics Publishers.

Pelletier, K.R. (1993). A review and analysis of the health and cost-effective outcome studies of comprehensive health promotion and disease prevention programs at the worksite: 1991–1993 update. *American Journal of Health Promotion, 8,* 50–62.

Shephard, R.J. (1992). Twelve years experience of a fitness program for the salaried employees of a Toronto life assurance company. *American Journal of Health Promotion, 6,* 292–301.

Shephard, R.J. (1996). Worksite fitness and exercise programs: A review of methodology and health impact. *American Journal of Health Promotion, 10,* 436–452.

Shore, G., Prasad, P., & Zrobak, M. (1989). Metrofit: A cost-effective fitness program. *Fitness in Business, 4,* 147–153.

Tsai, S.P., Bernacki, E.J., & Baun, W.B. (1988). Injury prevalence and associated costs among participants of an employee fitness program. *Preventive Medicine, 17,* 475–482.

Yen, L.T., Edington, D.W., & Witting, P. (1991). Associations between health risk appraisal scores and employee medical claims costs in a manufacturing company. *American Journal of Health Promotion, 6,* 46–54.

Physical Activity and Children

Because risks to health are easiest to document among adults, the preponderance of research has been done using adult subjects. Recently, attention has started to shift to children because childhood and adolescent activity may track to adulthood and offer lifelong benefits. In this section, Charles Corbin, Robert Pangrazi, and Greg Welk make a case for using different activity models for children than we use for adults. Oded Bar-Or presents information concerning the health benefits of physical activity for children and adolescents. Vern Seefeldt and Martha Ewing offer an overview of youth sports in America. The final paper, by Linda Bunker, is a review of girls in the sports arena.

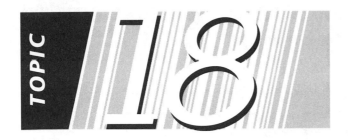

TOPIC 18

Toward an Understanding of Appropriate Physical Activity Levels for Youth

Charles B. Corbin, Robert P Pangrazi, ARIZONA STATE UNIVERSITY

Greg J. Welk, COOPER INSTITUTE FOR AEROBICS RESEARCH

OVERVIEW

In the not so distant past, children were protected from vigorous physical activity. Even leading educators felt that children were incapable of exercise that caused high heart rates. In the last half century science has found that children can safely perform high intensity exercise. However, many of the guidelines for physical activity for children formulated in the last 30 years have been based on what is often called the Exercise Prescription Model (EPM), an approach developed primarily for adults. Since 1985, there has been a shift from the EPM to a Lifetime Physical Activity Model (LPAM) as the basis for establishing activity guidelines for adults. This model suggests that moderate daily lifetime exercise such as walking results in an energy expenditure of 3 to 4 kcal/kg/day (1000 to 2000 calories per week), which is sufficient to produce health benefits. Because high intensity activity is a deterrent to some, this model is offered as a "new strategy" for health risk reduction through physical activity.

Just as the LPAM is more appropriate for many adults than the EPM, the LPAM is better suited for

children than the EPM. Like many adults, children often do not respond well to high intensity physical activity. The LPAM standards for minimal activity requirements necessary to gain the health benefits of physical activity (3 to 4 kcal/kg/day) provide the basis for a child-specific physical activity model called the Children's Lifetime Physical Activity Model (C-LPAM). This model suggests that children should, as a minimum, expend the same number of kcal/kg/day as adults. However, it also suggests that optimally, children should be encouraged to do additional physical activity (6 to 8 kcal/kg/day) because children have different needs than adults and it is during childhood that lifetime activity patterns are developed.

PHYSICAL ACTIVITY AND CHILDREN

In 1879 a German physician named Behnke warned of the danger of vigorous physical activity among children (Karpovich, 1937). He cautioned adults to restrict activity among children because of the "natural disharmony" between the development

---

ORIGINALLY PUBLISHED AS SERIES 1, NUMBER 8, OF THE PCPFS *RESEARCH DIGEST.*

HIGHLIGHT

Children's Lifetime Physical Activity Model (C-LPAM)

The Health Standard: A Minimum Activity Standard

Frequency   Daily. Frequent activity sessions (3 or more) each day.

Intensity   Moderate. Alternating bouts of activity with rest periods as needed or moderate activity such as walking or riding a bike to school.

Time   Duration of activity necessary to expend at least 3 to 4 kcal/kg/day. Equal to calorie expenditure in 30 minutes or more of active play or moderate sustained activity which may be distributed over 3 or more activity sessions.

The Optimal Functioning Standard: A Goal for All Children

Frequency   Daily. Frequent activity sessions (3 or more) each day.

Intensity   Moderate to vigorous. Alternating bouts of activity with rest periods as needed or moderate activity such as walking or riding a bike to school.

Time   Duration of activity necessary to expend at least 6 to 8 kcal/kg/day. Equal to calorie expenditure in 60 minutes or more of active play or moderate sustained activity which may be distributed over 3 or more activity sessions.

---

of the size of the heart muscle and the size of the large vessels. He suggested that the blood vessels develop at a relatively slower rate than the heart muscle, making the vessels unable to accommodate the faster growing heart. He concluded that there would be "grave danger" for the exercising child because of high blood pressure and accompanying circulatory problems.

Physical and health educators (Van Hagen, Dexter, & Williams, 1951; Young, 1923) perpetuated this myth as did "experts" in child growth and development (Hurlock, 1967). A widely used textbook in elementary school physical education warned that ". . . the heart increases greatly in size during this growth period (11–14 years), with veins and arteries developing much more slowly. The heart, therefore, should not be overtaxed with heavy and too continuous activity" (Van Hagen et al., 1951, p. 52). As late as 1967 Hurlock's text on adolescent development indicated that until late adolescence, when the size of the blood vessels catches up with the size of the heart, ". . . too strenuous exercise may cause an enlargement of the heart and result in valvular disease" (Hurlock, 1967, p. 47). Apparently these experts had cited other experts, each of whom had relied on Behnke or other uninformed sources.

The myth of children being unable to perform vigorous exercise persisted in the literature well into

the 1960s even though published data had been presented in 1937 debunking the ideas of Behnke. Karpovich (1937) reexamined Behnke's data and showed that a simple mathematical error had been made. Though the circumference of the artery of children is proportionally small compared to the size of the heart, the blood-carrying capacity of the artery is proportional to increases in heart size. Behnke assumed that the blood-carrying capacity of the artery could be measured using the circumference of the artery when in fact it is the cross-sectional area of the interior of the artery that is critical. Karpovich was not the only one to debunk the "child's heart" myth. Another researcher, Boas (1931), conducted studies with exercising children that led him to conclude that during vigorous exercise the muscles will "flag" so that the child will "collapse before the heart is called for its last ounce of effort."

Even though research discredited the notion that children were incapable of vigorous exercise, many educators were skeptical about prescribing strenuous activity for children well into the 1960s. Texts for elementary school physical educators began to include sections documenting the cardiovascular capabilities of children (Corbin, 1969) and repudiating earlier incorrect statements. Still, not all physical educators were convinced of the capabilities of children as evidenced by the fact that the

600 yard run/walk (introduced in 1958) continued as the measure of cardiovascular fitness for children in the 1965 and 1975 national youth fitness battery (AAHPERD, 1980). Many physical educators continued to believe that children were not physically able to run long distances or to perform endurance activities and thought it was dangerous for them to do so.

Further evidence about the concern for exercising children was the resistance researchers experienced from human subjects committees that were just being organized in the 1960s and early 1970s. An example was an initial rejection by a human subjects committee for a study of the heart rates of children using telemetry during various distance runs (Corbin, 1972). The committee felt that children should be stopped from running if heart rates exceeded 170 bpm and if distances exceeded 600 yards. It was necessary to educate the committee members, including medical doctors. The study was ultimately approved even though heart rates often exceeded 200 bpm and distances were as long as 800 yards.

It was not until 1978 that an American Academy on Pediatrics position paper (cited in AAP, 1991) noted that many children who had previously been screened out of physical education were capable of "full and active" participation. In 1980 longer runs became part of national physical fitness test batteries for children (AAHPERD, 1980).

THE EXERCISE PRESCRIPTION MODEL

The health fitness movement for adults began to gain momentum in the 1960s. Paul Dudley White, physician for President Eisenhower during the 1950s, emphasized the health value of physical activity (Pomroy & White, 1958) and his national visibility brought attention to the health benefits of activity. The classic study of Morris, Hady, Raffle, Roberts, and Parks (1953) of London transportation workers was published, providing good evidence for the health value of physical activity. By the early 1960s, Taylor and colleagues (1962) had added to the body of literature supporting the value of physical activity for health. Rehabilitation programs for cardiac patients using physical activity were gaining credibility due to the work of pioneers such as Hellerstein and Wolffe. The exercise prescription model (EPM) was developed and served as the

basis for most cardiovascular exercise for the next two decades.

During the late 1950s and 1960s, considerable work was conducted regarding the EPM in an attempt to define the intensity and frequency of short duration exercise required to promote gains in cardiovascular fitness as measured by VO_2max. Karvonen's classic research (1959) identified the threshold of training and provided a basis for the EPM. By 1966, widely used exercise physiology texts cited Karvonen's formula for fitness development. DeVries (1966), for example, cited the work of Karvonen and noted that exercise must be performed at 60% of heart rate reserve. This guideline was similar to "rules of thumb" advocated for performance improvement by swimming and track coaches of the era. Whatever the original reasons for research concerning the EPM and the related concepts of threshold of training and target zone heart rates, the major emphasis in exercise prescription was on physiological VO_2max and performance improvement.

By the 1970s, the EPM and its focus on higher intensity and shorter duration activity (using percentage of maximum heart rate or O_2 consumption as the criterion for intensity) was firmly established for adults. In 1972, the American Heart Association published an exercise testing and training handbook (AHA, 1972) and by 1978 the emerging American College of Sports Medicine (ACSM, 1978) published its first position statement outlining the frequency, intensity, duration, and mode of exercise prescription necessary to produce cardiovascular fitness gains for the adult population. This statement was updated in 1990 (ACSM, 1990).

The EPM and the exercise guidelines developed based on this model have been useful and effective. For young adults of Western cultures, exercise programs based on the EPM are useful because cardiovascular fitness can be achieved without a major time commitment. Improved fitness can be accomplished by performing continuous exercise in as few as three days per week. This allows busy people to fit moderate to high intensity exercise into their otherwise sedentary lifestyles. In addition, the EPM is particularly effective for athletes and those interested in optimal physical performance.

Ironically, the model for prescribing adult physical activity that gained the greatest attention (EPM) was quite different than the type of activity that seemed effective for public health promotion. Although the epidemiological literature suggested exercise of longer duration and relatively low intensity reduced heart disease risk (Morris et al., 1953; Taylor et al., 1962), the type of exercise prescription gaining notoriety was shorter in duration and of higher intensity.

Because improvement in cardiovascular fitness (rather than the reduction of health risk) was central to the EPM, measures of cardiovascular fitness were of particular importance. The 12-minute run developed by Cooper to test the cardiovascular fitness of military personnel was popularized for the general public in the book *Aerobics* (Cooper, 1968). Shorter runs were developed for children, and in 1980, the health-related physical fitness test which included a mile run was adopted by AAHPERD (1980). By 1985, all of the major national fitness tests included a distance run of at least a mile in length. The capability of children to perform vigorous physical activity was acknowledged. In the absence of specific research to guide recommendations, the EPM was used to design exercise programs for children. Professionals had come full circle. Instead of fearing for the health of children who participated in vigorous exercise, they developed guidelines for physical activity similar to those designed for adults.

A LIFESTYLE PHYSICAL ACTIVITY MODEL: THE NEW STRATEGY*

In July of 1992 the American College of Sports Medicine and the Centers for Disease Prevention and Control (CDC), in cooperation with the President's Council on Physical Fitness and Sports, issued a statement acknowledging the importance of lifestyle physical activity as a means of reducing disease risk. The new recommendation is to accumulate throughout the day a minimum of 30 minutes of moderate intensity physical activity over the course of most days of the week. Examples of such activities are ". . . walking up stairs (instead of taking the elevator), gardening, raking leaves, dancing, and walking all or part of the way to work. Activity can also come from planned exercise or recreation such as jogging, playing tennis, swimming, and cycling" (CDC & ACSM, 1994, p. 7). Another example of lifestyle exercise that can be used to meet CDC/ACSM guidelines is a two-mile walk daily.

Blair and colleagues have called this "new strategy" the Lifestyle Exercise Model (Blair, Kohl, & Gordon, 1992). Haskell (1994), in his Wolffe lecture to the American College of Sports Medicine, also advocated the adoption of a lifestyle exercise model he calls the Physical Activity Health Paradigm. In this article, this model is referred to as the Lifetime Physical Activity Model (LPAM). Strong scientific evidence exists to support the LPAM (Haskell, 1994). The work of Paffenbarger and colleagues (Paffenbarger, Hyde, Wing, & Hsueh, 1986; Paffenbarger, Hyde, Wing, & Steenmetz, 1984; Paffenbarger, Wing, & Hyde, 1978) showed that the expenditure of 2000 kcals per week resulted in a significant reduction in morbidity and mortality among Harvard alumni. Those who expended 2,000 to 3,500 kcal per week attained the optimal value from their exercise. The studies of Harvard men showed that lifestyle activities such as climbing stairs, walking, doing physically active household activities and participating in active sports helped reduce disease risk not only for heart disease but for cancer and other types of hypokinetic conditions. Leon and colleagues (1987), studying a different group of adults, found that a 1,500 kcal per week expenditure through moderate intensity physical activity produced similar health benefits to those found for the Harvard alums. Haskell (1985), based on a literature review, suggested 150 kcal per day (1,050 kcal per week) as the minimum threshold for lifestyle exercise. These studies have demonstrated that health benefits accrue from lower intensity, longer duration exercise.

Blair et al. (1992), based on research at the Cooper Institute for Aerobics Research, have proposed that adults expend 3 kilocalories per kilogram of body weight per day (kcal/kg/day) in physical activity to achieve the benefits of regular physical activity. This standard is similar to the one used by previous researchers to classify people as "very active" (Montoye, 1987) and amounts to approximately 200 kcal per day for a 150-pound person, or 1,400 kcal per week. The kcal/kg/day standard allows individuals to calculate the caloric expenditure (based on their body weight) required to obtain health benefits. The physical activity necessary to expend 1,000 to 2,000 calories per week or 3 kcal/kg/day is the basis on which the CDC/ACSM guidelines for lifestyle physical activity were developed.

---

*For comprehensive coverage of the scientific basis for the LPAM, readers are referred to articles by Blair (1993), Blair et al. (1992), and Haskell (1994). See References.

The LPAM differs from the EPM in several ways. First, the LPAM focuses on the amount of physical activity necessary to produce health benefits as associated with reduced morbidity and mortality rather than fitness and performance benefits. While the LPAM promotes fitness as it relates to good health, it does not focus on fitness performance as does the EPM. Moderate to high intensity exercise of shorter duration as outlined by the EPM was designed to promote changes on fitness tests such as VO$_2$max. Second, the LPAM recognizes the value of a wide range of physical activities that expend calories throughout the day rather than requiring continuous moderate to vigorous physical activity done in one exercise bout. Finally, the LPAM acknowledges that some activity is better than none at all, and that up to a point, progressively increasing amounts of physical activity provide added health benefits.

The shift to the LPAM from the EPM does not mean, however, that the EPM is no longer a useful model. For young adults with limited amounts of time, moderate to vigorous physical activity is still an effective approach to achieving health benefits. For those who are interested in enhancing fitness for relatively high-level performance such as sport involvement or active careers (law enforcement, military, etc.), the EPM is also an effective model. However, the type of exercise prescribed in the EPM is not necessarily the best approach for the general population that wants to receive substantial health benefits.

CHILDREN AND THE EPM

Just as most physical activity recommendations for adults have been based on the EPM for the past 20 to 30 years, recommendations for children have been based principally on guidelines evolving from the EPM. Rowland (1985) concluded that children need to follow the same exercise prescription as adults to achieve cardiovascular fitness. Using Karvonen's heart rate reserve method for calculating target heart rates, Sady (1986) estimated a heart rate of 159 as the threshold for aerobic exercise for most children. These results and the findings of other studies have served as the basis for recommendations suggesting that children need to perform 20 to 30 minutes of continuous moderate to vigorous physical activity (MVPA) at least three times a week. Typically heart rate standards are used as the indicator of MVPA. Recommendations vary but, in general, heart rates advocated are 140 bpm and higher.

Using heart rate standards as indicators has caused several researchers to conclude that many, if not most, children are inactive. Some examples illustrate the point. Using heart rates above 140 for 20 minutes of continuous exercise as the criterion of MVPA, Armstrong and Bray (1990) studied children and found 77% of boys and 88% of girls to be inactive by this measure. In a subsequent study of younger children, Armstrong, Balding, Gentle, and Kirby (1991) found 61% of boys and 66% of girls to be inactive. Using observation techniques to assess 20 minutes of MVPA as the standard, Sleap and Warburton (1992) found 86% of children to be inactive, and Baranowski, Hooks, Tsong, Cieslik, and Nader (1987) found 89.6% of children to be inactive. In another study involving 177 trials of day-long monitoring of children averaging 703 minutes a day, Welk (1994) found 17% of children to have heart rates above 140 bpm for 20 consecutive minutes. If EPM were used to evaluate activity, it would be easy to conclude that most children are inactive.

Using data from the same studies but applying standards that are more consistent with the LPAM, a different conclusion is reached. When minutes of physical activity during the day are determined for these same studies, the data of Armstrong and Bray (1990) show that on the average boys were active 45 minutes and girls 31 minutes of each day (above 140 but not consecutive minutes). A second study (Armstrong & Bray, 1991) found younger boys were active 68 minutes and girls 59 minutes each day. Similarly, children studied by Baranowski, Hooks, Tsong, Cieslik, and Nader (1987) performed 60 to 70 minutes of activity per day even though 89% would be classified as inactive by the EPM standard. Eighty-six percent of the children Sleap and Warburton (1992) studied were inactive in terms of EPM exercise yet, on average, they participated in 88 minutes of activity. Data from Welk's study (1994) using activity and heart rate monitors at the same time showed that 99% of boys and 98% of girls exceeded an energy expenditure of 4 kcal/kg/day, a standard that is slightly higher than the 3 kcal/kg/day advocated by proponents of the LPAM.

It is apparent that the same children who fail to meet activity standards based on the EPM generally

TABLE 18.1

Physical activity and children: Basic concepts.

Concept	Implication
Young animals, including humans, are inherently active.	Children will be active if given encouragement and opportunity.
Children are concrete rather than abstract thinkers.	Children are often unwilling to persist in activity if they see no concrete reason to do so.
The relationship between activity and fitness is weak among children.	Children may receive little feedback for their efforts in some activities.
Childhood activity is often intermittent and sporadic in nature.	Children will not likely do prolonged exercise without rest periods.
Total volume is a good indicator of childhood activity.	Given the opportunity, many children will perform relatively large volumes of intermittent physical activity.
Physical activity patterns vary with children of different developmental and ability levels.	Young children are not attracted to high intensity exercise but highly skilled older children may see its value for enhancing performance in sports.

meet standards established for the LPAM. Rather than judge children as inactive based on MVPA data, it seems more reasonable to suggest the EPM is an inappropriate model for judging activity levels of most children. Children are sporadic exercisers who alternate between vigorous activity and rest. They are high volume exercisers who generally do not engage in continuous high intensity exercise. See Table 18.1 for a listing of concepts and implications concerning physical activity and children.

THE CHILDREN'S LIFETIME PHYSICAL ACTIVITY MODEL (C-LPAM)

Evidence suggests that among adults 3 to 4 kcal/kg/day is a good minimum standard for producing the health benefits of physical activity. A similar minimum standard for children (3 to 4 kcal/kg/day) seems appropriate in light of recent evidence that shows active children have a more beneficial coronary risk profile than their sedentary counterparts (Raitakara, Porkka, Taimela, Telama, Rasanen, & Viikari, 1994) and that many children already meet this standard (Blair, Clarke, Cureton, & Powell, 1989; Welk, 1994). Also, it is a standard that inactive children, those who need activity the most, can achieve with a modest commitment to childhood games and activities or lifestyle activities appropriate for children such as walking or riding a bicycle to school and performing physical tasks around the home.

It is not unreasonable, however, to establish a goal for children of expending 6 to 8 kcal/kg/day. Unlike adults, children have the time and energy for activity above the minimum standards if they see a reason to be active. There are at least five reasons why this goal of higher energy expenditure is appropriate.

1. During childhood children learn basic motor skills that provide the basis for lifetime activity. Proper skill development requires substantial practice time and energy expenditure. If motor skills are not learned early in life such skills may never be developed and the opportunities for lifetime activity will be limited.

2. Lifetime physical activities learned early in life (such as walking, riding bicycles, and doing active physical tasks around home) contribute to active lifestyles and help obese children maintain healthy body fat levels later in life (Epstein, Wing, Koeske, Ossip, & Beck, 1982).

3. Children need activity for the development of all parts of health-related physical fitness including aerobic fitness, muscle strength and endurance, flexibility, and desirable level of body fatness, as well as activity to promote a high peak bone density. To promote fitness development and to learn appropriate activities for development of these fitness parts, physical activity is essential.

4. Given the opportunity and encouragement, most children will choose to be active. This is especially true if time is provided for activity.

5. People who do no physical activity are at increased risk of disease and death compared to those who are physically active. The largest decrease in risk is associated with the expenditure of approximately 3 to 4 kcal/kg/day. Additional risk reduction is associated with increased amounts of physical activity (6 to 8 kcal/kg/day). To a point, activity beyond 6 to 8 kcal/kg/day produces additional benefits, but the relative benefits decrease as more activity is performed. The 6 to 8 kcal/kg/day standard seems a reasonable one for children. Evidence suggests that people become less active as they grow older (Rowland, 1990) and that people who are active when they are young are more likely to be active in later life (Raitakara et al., 1994). This being the case, meeting a higher caloric expenditure as a child may interpret into greater activity as an adult.

For a summary of activity recommendations, see the section below, "Activity Recommendations for Children."

HIGH PERFORMANCE STANDARDS

As children grow older the EPM may become more important, especially if students make personal choices to perform high intensity physical activity designed to achieve optimal levels of fitness. For example, adolescents may wish to do EPM exercise to increase their chances of success in school or community sports. As noted earlier, children can participate in high intensity activity safely. However, the effort/benefit ratio (Fox & Biddle, 1988) for children is not good. To ensure persistence in physical activity, children must believe the benefits of the activity are equal to or greater than the amount of effort expended. Because children are concrete thinkers they often see little benefit to high intensity training, which makes their perception of effort high. Thus EPM exercise often produces a poor effort/benefit ratio.

Some children express a personal interest in EPM training. If their interest is strong and they perceive the benefits as great enough, they may successfully use the EPM exercise formula. However, because response to training is less in childhood compared to adolescence, there is some danger that children may lose interest in high intensity exercise. This is because of the lack of feedback from performance improvements. Learning skills through phys-

ical practice is often more rewarding and likely to enhance effort/benefit ratios for children. Generally, EPM physical activity designed to enhance high-level performance in fitness is more appropriate and successful for adolescents and young adults than for children. Interestingly, evidence exists to suggest that the relationship between physical activity and aerobic fitness is not strong among children (Pate, Dowda, & Ross, 1990) or adolescents (Morrow & Freedson, 1995).

IMPLICATIONS

Determining Activity Levels of Children

The best evidence suggests that children are among the most active segment of the population. Yet, using adult EPM standards, some have concluded that large numbers of children are inactive. This occurs in spite of the fact that the same children usually meet adult health standards for activity based on the scientifically documented LPAM. The C-LPAM is proposed as a more suitable model for judging the activity of children. National studies of the activity levels of children are needed, especially in an attempt to determine if children are meeting appropriate standards.

Activity Recommendations for Children

As is inevitably the case, guidelines that gain national acceptance provide the basis for recommendations to be used in schools and other programs. In the case of physical activity, EPM guidelines have provided the basis for recommendations for children in schools as well as in community sports programs. Following the lead of scholars who have applied EPM guidelines to children, some professionals have advocated implementing programs that elevate heart rates of children to 140 or higher for 20 or more consecutive minutes. In some cases, heart rate monitors have been recommended to ensure that exercise intensity levels are achieved among children (Strand & Reeder, 1993a; Strand & Reeder, 1993b).

Although programs using continuous high intensity (high heart rate) activity are not physiologically harmful to children, they are not the most appropriate for children. It is possible, given what we know about effort/benefit ratios and developmental needs of children that such activity can decrease rather than increase motivation for future activity. A more reasonable recommendation is that children perform C-LPAM activity as outlined here. In physical education programs, youth sports programs, or any other program designed to encourage current and lifetime activity for children, there are five guidelines that seem important:

1. Activity for children should focus on high volume and moderate intensity that includes sporadic activities such as active play performed in several activity sessions daily.

2. Lifestyle activity such as walking or riding bikes to and from school or performing active physical tasks at home (e.g., yardwork) should be encouraged.

3. Opportunities to learn basic motor skills and develop all parts of health-related physical fitness through appropriate moderate intensity activity should be included in the activity program.

4. Children should be afforded opportunities to begin developing behavioral skills that lead to lifetime activity.

5. EPM guidelines can be applied to individuals who are especially interested in high-level physical performance, but only when it is developmentally appropriate.

REFERENCES

American Academy of Pediatrics. (1991). *Sports medicine: Health care for young athletes* (2nd ed.). Elk Grove Village, IL: American Academy of Pediatrics.

American Alliance of Health, Physical Education, Recreation, and Dance. (1980). *Health related physical fitness test manual*. Reston, VA: American Alliance of Health, Physical Education, Recreation, and Dance.

American Association of Health, Physical Education, and Recreation. (1958). *Youth fitness testing manual*. Washington, DC: American Association of Health, Physical Education, and Recreation.

American College of Sports Medicine. (1978). The recommended quantity and quality of exercise for developing and maintaining cardiorespiratory and muscular fitness of healthy adults. *Medicine and Science in Sports and Exercise, 10*, vi–ix.

American College of Sports Medicine. (1990). The recommended quantity and quality of exercise for developing and maintaining fitness of healthy adults. *Medicine and Science in Sports and Exercise, 22*, 265–274.

American Heart Association. (1972). *Exercise testing and training of apparently healthy individuals: A handbook for physicians*. Dallas: American Heart Association.

American Heart Association. (1992). Medical/scientific statement on exercise: Benefits and recommendations for physical activity programs for all Americans. *Circulation, 86(1)*, 2726–2730.

Armstrong, N., Balding, J., Gentle, P., & Kirby, S. (1990). Patterns of physical activity among 11–16-year-old British children. *British Medical Journal, 301*, 203–205.

Armstrong, N., & Bray, S. (1991). Physical activity patterns defined by continuous heart rate monitoring. *Archives of Disease in Children, 66*, 245–247.

Baranowski, T., Hooks, P., Tsong, Y., Cieslik, C., & Nader, P.R. (1987). Aerobic physical activity among third to sixth grade children. *Developmental and Behavioral Pediatrics, 8(4)*, 203–206.

Blair, S.N. (1993). C.H. McCloy Research Lecture: Physical activity, physical fitness, and health. *Research Quarterly for Exercise and Sport, 64(4)*, 365–376.

Blair, S.N., Clarke, D.G., Cureton, K.J., & Powell, K.E. (1989). Exercise and fitness in childhood: Implications for a lifetime of health. In C.V. Gisolfi and Lamb, D.V. (Eds.), *Perspectives in Exercise. Science and Sports Medicine, Volume 2, Youth Exercise and Sport* (pp. 401–430). Indianapolis: Benchmark Press.

Blair, S.N., Kohl, H.W. III, & Gordon, N.F. (1992). Physical activity and health: A lifestyle approach. *Medicine, Exercise, Nutrition, and Health, 1, 54–57*.

Blair, S.N., Kohl, H.W. III, Paffenbarger, R.S., Clark, D.B., Cooper, K.H., & Gibbons, L.W. (1989). Physical fitness and allcause mortality. *Journal of the American Medical Association, 262*, 2395–2401.

Boas, E.P. (1931). The heart rate of boys during and after exhausting exercise. *Journal of Clinical Investigation, 10*, 145–147.

Cooper, K.H. (1968). *Aerobics*. New York: M. Evans.

Corbin, C.B. (1969). *Becoming physically educated in the elementary school*. Philadelphia: Lea & Febiger.

Corbin, C.B. (1972). Relationships between PWC and running performance of young boys. *Research Quarterly, 43*, 235–238.

DeVries, H.A. (1966). *Physiology of exercise for physical education and athletics*. Dubuque, IA: W.C. Brown.

Epstein, L.H., Wing, R.R., Koeske, R., Ossip, D., & Beck, S. (1982). A comparison of lifestyle change and programmed aerobic exercise on weight loss in obese children. *Behavior Therapy, 13*, 651–665.

Fox, K., & Biddle, S. (1988). Children's participation motives. *British Journal of Physical Education, 19*, 34–38.

Haskell, W.L. (1985). Physical activity and health: Need to define the required stimulus. *American Journal of Cardiology, 5*, 4D–9D.

Haskell, W.L. (1994). Health consequences of physical activity: Understanding and challenges regarding dose response. *Medicine and Science in Sports and Exercise, 26(6),* 649–660.

Hurlock, E.B. (1967). *Adolescent development.* New York: McGraw-Hill.

Karpovich, P.V. (1937). Textbook fallacies regarding the development of the child's heart. *Research Quarterly, 8,* 33.

Karvonen, M.J. (1959). The effects of vigorous exercise on the heart. In Rosenbaum, F.F., & Belknap, E.L. (Eds.), *Work and the heart.* New York: P.B. Hoebner.

Leon, A.S., Connett, J., Jacobs, D.R., & Rauramaa, R. (1987). Leisuretime physical activity levels and risk of coronary heart disease and death. *Journal of the American Medical Association, 258,* 2388–2395.

Montoye, H.J. (1987). How active are modern populations? *The Academy Papers, 21,* 34–45.

Morris, J.N., Hady, J.A., Raffle, P.A., Roberts, C.B., & Parks, J.W. (1953). Coronary heart disease and physical activity of work. *Lancet, 2,* 1053–1057, 1111–1120.

Morrow, J.R., & Freedson, P.S. (1995). Relationship between habitual physical activity and aerobic fitness in adolescents. *Pediatric Exercise Science.*

Paffenbarger, R.S., Hyde, R.T., Wing, A.L., & Hsueh, R.T. (1986). Physical activity, allcause mortality, and longevity of college alumni. *New England Journal of Medicine, 314,* 605–613.

Paffenbarger, R.S., Hyde, P.T., Wing, A.L., & Steenmetz, C.H. (1984). A natural history of athleticism and cardiovascular health. *Journal of the American Medical Association, 252,* 491–495.

Paffenbarger, R.S., Wing, A.L., & Hyde, R.T. (1978). Physical activity as an index of heart attack risk in college alumni. *American Journal of Epidemiology, 108,* 161–175.

Pate, R.R., Dowda, M., & Ross, J.G. (1990). Associations between physical activity and physical fitness in American children. *American Journal of Diseases in Children, 144,* 1123–1129.

Pomroy, W.C., & White, P.D. (1958). Coronary heart disease in former football players. *Journal of the American Medical Association, 167,* 711–714.

Raitakari, O.T., Porkka, K.V.K., Taimela, S., Telama, R., Rasanen, L., & Viikari, J.S.A. (1994). Effects of persistent physical activity and inactivity on coronary risk factors in children and young adults. *American Journal of Epidemiology, 140(3),* 195–205.

Rowland, T.W. (1985). Aerobic response to endurance training in prepubescent children: A critical analysis. *Medicine and Science in Sports and Exercise, 17,* 493–497.

Rowland, T.W. (1990). *Exercise and children's health.* Champaign, IL: Human Kinetics Publishers.

Sady, S.P. (1986). Cardiorespiratory exercise training in children. *Clinics in Sports Medicine,* 493–514.

Sleap, M., & Waburton, P. (1992). Physical activity levels of 5–11-year-old children in England as determined by continuous observation. *Research Quarterly for Exercise and Sport, 63(3),* 238–245.

Strand, B., & Reeder, S. (1993a). Analysis of heart rate levels during middle school physical education activities. *Journal of Physical Education, Recreation, and Dance, 64(3),* 85–91.

Strand, B., & Reeder, S. (1993b). Physical education with a heartbeat. *Journal of Physical Education, Recreation, and Dance, 64(3),* 81–84.

Taylor, H.L., et al. (1962). Death rates among physically active and sedentary employees of the railway industry. *American Journal of Public Health, 52,* 1697–1707.

U.S. Centers for Disease Control & Prevention and American College of Sports Medicine. (1994). Summary statement: Workshop on physical activity and public health. *Sports Medicine Bulletin, 28(4),* 7.

Van Hagen, W.V., Dexter, G., & Williams, J.F. (1951). Physical education in the elementary school. Sacramento, CA: California State Department of Education.

Welk, G.J. (1994). A comparison of methods for the assessment of physical activity in children. Unpublished doctoral dissertation, Arizona State University, Tempe, AZ.

Young, E. (1923). *Hygiene in the schools.* Philadelphia: W.B. Saunders.

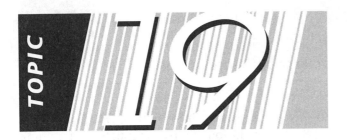

Health Benefits of Physical Activity During Childhood and Adolescence

Oded Bar-Or

MCMASTER UNIVERSITY

INTRODUCTION

The beneficial effects to health of enhanced physical activity (PA) during adult years are numerous. There is mounting evidence that such benefits include a reduction in morbidity and mortality from diseases of several body systems (Bouchard et al., 1994). Much less evidence is available regarding the effects of an active lifestyle during childhood and adolescence on adult health.

The main reason for the paucity of information on the possible carryover of benefits from childhood to adulthood is the lack of longitudinal studies that have followed the same individuals over many years. Ideally, one would need randomly to assign children into those who are given enhanced PA programs and those who remain sedentary over years and then observe the long-term effects of PA or of inactivity. On ethical grounds, such studies are hard to justify (it is unethical to demand that children not engage in PA for an extended period of time). In addition, they are extremely expensive and logistically most complicated. A second-best alternative would be to conduct controlled intervention studies that last shorter periods and include several groups of sub-

jects who span a wide age range (from childhood to middle age). Such "mixed longitudinal" studies are feasible, but have yet to be launched. Another approach is to identify adults with and without diseases and question them about their PA during earlier years. Such "retrospective" studies are easier to perform, but their outcome depends on the ability of people to correctly remember and report their PA behavior during earlier years. Conclusions derived from retrospective studies are less valid than those derived from longitudinal interventions.

The purpose of this article is to examine briefly the current evidence that enhanced PA during childhood and adolescence imparts immediate health benefits, or reduces risk for adult chronic disease. Emphasis will be given to the following conditions: obesity, hypertension, abnormal plasma lipoprotein profile, and osteoporosis. Table 19.1 summarizes the evidence attesting to such benefits.

SHORT-TERM BENEFITS

Before analyzing the carryover effects of childhood PA, one should identify the *immediate* effects of a training program (or an active lifestyle) on health-

ORIGINALLY PUBLISHED AS SERIES 2, NUMBER 4, OF THE PCPFS *RESEARCH DIGEST.*

related risk factors. These are measured while the program is still in progress, or immediately upon its conclusion. Evidence for such benefits has been sought from intervention training programs that last a few weeks or several months at the most. An alternative approach has been cross-sectional studies that compare children (or youth) who habitually engage in athletic pursuit with those who lead a sedentary lifestyle. The drawback of the latter approach is that differences in health-related risk between groups might not be a result of the physical activity per se. They may instead reflect heredity or events that took place before the child became physically active.

Body fatness. (See Bar-Or & Baranowski, 1994, for a review.) Many, although not all, cross-sectional studies suggest that obese children and youth are less active than their leaner peers. There is only scant evidence, though, that inactivity is *a cause of* juvenile obesity (Roberts, 1993). Training studies with nonobese youth have shown little or no reduction in body adiposity (Wilmore, 1983). However, enhanced PA with or without a low-calorie diet, did reduce % body fat or excess body weight in obese children and youth.

Blood pressure. (See Alpert & Wilmore, 1994, for a review.) Some cross-sectional studies show a slightly higher resting blood pressure among sedentary adolescents compared with their active peers. Most studies, however, do not show such a difference, particularly if the groups have the same adiposity level. Training of healthy, previously inactive children or adolescents who have a normal blood pressure induces little (1-6 mmHg) or no drop in blood pressure. However, in adolescents with hypertension, training over several months does induce a reduction of both systolic and diastolic blood pressure. Even though such a reduction is modest (around 10 mmHg), it may be beneficial for some individuals with mild hypertension who otherwise may require medication to control their blood pressure. The training programs that induced a decline in blood pressure were comprised mostly of aerobic activities. In one study (Hagberg et al., 1984), the inclusion of a five-month weight training regimen following a six-month aerobic program further reduced the blood pressure of adolescents with hypertension. Such beneficial effects of exercise disappear within several months of termination of the program.

Blood lipids. (See Armstrong & Simons-Morton, 1994, for a review.) Based on some cross-sectional studies, children and adolescents who are physically active, or whose aerobic fitness is high, have a more favorable blood lipid profile than their sedentary, or less fit, peers. This difference is particularly apparent in high-density lipoprotein cholesterol (HDL-C = the "good" cholesterol), which is higher in the active groups. Other cross-sectional comparisons, however, do not reveal such differences. In most of the cross-sectional studies it is impossible to separate a high activity level from a high fitness level.

Training studies of several weeks' duration have failed to show any beneficial effect on the blood lipid profile in healthy children or adolescents. More beneficial responses have been shown for groups who have a high coronary risk. These include children and adolescents with insulin-dependent diabetes mellitus, obesity, or with at least one parent who has three or more coronary risk factors.

Skeletal health. (See Bailey & Martin, 1994, for a review.) The possible link between skeletal health and PA has received attention in recent years with the finding that physically active postmenopausal women, and elderly populations in general, have a higher bone mineral density (BMD) and less osteoporosis than less active controls. One of the determinants of bone health in old age is the "peak" BMD reached by young adulthood. Bone mass and BMD subsequently (and inevitably) decline with the years, until the bones become fragile.

This topic has an important pediatric relevance, because the great majority of bone build-up occurs during adolescence. A question of major public health relevance is whether enhanced PA during childhood and adolescence will result in a higher peak BMD.

Cross-sectional comparisons have shown that young athletes in weight-bearing sports such as gymnastics, soccer and volleyball (but not in non-weight-bearing sports such as swimming) have a higher BMD than do nonathletes. Likewise, bones of the dominant limb in "asymmetrical" sports, such as tennis or little-league pitching, have a higher BMD than the nondominant limb. Conversely, bones of a limb immobilized for several weeks or months had a lower BMD than in the contralateral, nonimmobilized limb.

Retrospective studies, in which adults were asked about their PA during childhood, suggest that women who had been physically active during childhood had a higher BMD in the third and fourth decades of life than women who had been less active as children.

Longitudinal results of weight-bearing training programs are equivocal. Most controlled interventions yielded little or no increase in BMD or bone mass of exercising adolescents (e.g., Blimkie et al., 1993).

CARRYOVER TO ADULT LIFE

There are several models that may explain a possible link between an adult person's health and her or his activity behavior in earlier years. As suggested by Blair et al. (1989) there are conceivably three avenues by which an enhanced PA level during childhood might improve adult health:

1. Childhood activity improves child health which, in turn, is beneficial to adult health.

2. An active lifestyle during childhood has a direct benefit to health in later years.

3. An active child becomes an active adult who, in turn, has a lower risk for disease than an inactive adult.

Research provides no proof, or disproof, for any of these links. However, because a sedentary lifestyle in adults has been proven to entail a high risk for several chronic diseases (Bouchard et al., 1994), the most plausible link is that an active lifestyle during childhood and adolescence would be carried over through adulthood which, in turn,

would reduce risk for disease. There are, however, no prospective studies that have tracked activity patterns from childhood to adulthood. Even though activity patterns and attitudes toward PA remain quite stable during late adolescence (but less so around age 10–12 years) (Malina, 1990), there is a low relationship between the two.

HOW MUCH PHYSICAL ACTIVITY?

There are practically no data as to the *optimal dose* of PA during childhood and adolescence that might maintain and/or enhance health. However, a group of experts from various countries has recently generated a consensus statement (Sallis & Patrick, 1994), which includes the following guidelines for adolescents:

1. *All adolescents should be physically active daily, or nearly every day,* as part of play, games, sports, work, transportation, recreation, physical education, or planned exercise; in the context of family, school, and community activities.

2. Adolescents should engage in *three or more sessions per week* of activities that last 20 minutes or more at a time and that require *moderate to vigorous* levels of exertion.

There is no formal consensus statement for preadolescents although Corbin, Pangrazi, and Welk (1994) have made recommendations for physical activity levels for this group in a previous issue of the *President's Council on Physical Fitness and Sports Physical Activity and Fitness Research Digest.*

CONCLUSION

Based on current information, no long-term studies exist that support or reject the notion that physical activity during childhood and adolescence is beneficial to adult health. There is, however, some evidence for short-term benefits of enhanced PA during the early years, particularly among children and youth who are at a high risk for chronic illness in later years. Much more research is needed to study this important issue further. In particular, it is essential to identify means of keeping young people motivated to maintain an active lifestyle as they reach young adulthood and middle age.

TABLE 19.1 ||█| |||████ ██ |████| || █||| ██| | █ |||██|| |████████|| | | ||██ |██ || |█████ ██ ████|| |█|

Possible effects of enhanced physical activity during childhood and adolescence on risk for chronic disease.

Observed Variable/Risk	Cross-Sectional Comparisons	Short-Term Effects of Intervention Programs	Carryover to Adult Life
Adiposity/ Obesity	Obesity is associated with hypoactivity.	*General Population:* Little or not reduction in % fat *Obese:* reduction in % fat	*General Population:* No information *Obese:* % fat returns to pretraining levels in most patients
Resting Blood Pressure/ Hypertension	Less active groups have similar or slightly higher BP compared with active groups.	*General Population:* Little or no reduction in blood pressure *Hypertensives:* 5–12 mmHg reduction in SBP and less in DBP	*General Population:* No information *Hypertensives:* BP returns to pretraining values within weeks
Blood Lipid Profile	Young athletes sometimes have a better profile than sedentary controls (mostly in HDL-cholesterol).	*General Population:* No improvement in profile *High-risk Population:* Improved profile	*General Population:* No information *High-risk Population:* No information
Bone Mineral Density/ Osteoporosis	Athletes (weight-bearing activities) have higher BMD than nonathletes.	Immobility induces loss of BMD. Training over several months induces no increase in BMD.	Retrospective data suggest a possible carryover.

BMD = bone mineral density; BP = blood pressure; DBP = diastolic blood pressure; HDL = high-density lipoprotein; SBP = systolic blood pressure.

The contrast between cross-sectional data and those generated through training studies is intriguing. The former suggest favorable health characteristics among active children and youth, compared with sedentary controls. Training studies, on the other hand, show little or no beneficial effect of training among healthy children and youth. This contrast may reflect a preselection of those who become active, and are healthier to start with, versus those who choose to pursue a sedentary lifestyle. It is possible, though, that interventions more vigorous than those commonly used in research would yield greater effects. It has been shown, for example, that army recruits who undergo an intense eight hours per day training regimen for several months respond with an increase in bone mineral content (Margulies et al., 1986) and an improved lipid profile (Rubinstein et al., 1995). Likewise, it is possible that longer interventions (e.g., 1–2 years) than those used in most studies would yield more positive training-induced results.

REFERENCES

Alpert, B.S., & Wilmore, J.H. (1994). Physical activity and blood pressure in adolescents. *Pediatric Exercise Science, 6,* 361–380.

Armstrong, N., & Simons-Morton, B. (1994). Physical activity and blood lipids in adolescents. *Pediatric Exercise Science, 6,* 381–405.

Bailey, D.A., & Martin, D.A. (1994). Physical activity and skeletal health in adolescents. *Pediatric Exercise Science, 6,* 330–347.

Bar-Or, O. (1994). Childhood and adolescent physical activity and fitness and adult risk profile. In C. Bouchard, R.J. Shephard, & T. Stephens (Eds.), *Physical activity, fitness, and health. International proceedings and consensus statement* (pp. 931–942). Champaign, IL: Human Kinetics Publishers.

Bar-Or, O., & Baranowski, T. (1994). Physical activity, adiposity, and obesity among adolescents. *Pediatric Exercise Science, 6,* 348–360.

Bar-Or, O., & Malina, R.M. (1995). Exercise during childhood and adolescence. In L.W.Y. Cheung & J.B. Richmond (Eds.), *Child health, nutrition, and physical activity* (pp. 79–123). Champaign, IL: Human Kinetics Publishers.

Blair, S.N., Clark, D.B., & Cureton, K.J. (1989). Exercise and fitness in childhood: Implications for a lifetime of health. In C.V. Gisolfi & D.L. Lamb (Eds.), *Perspectives in exercise science and sports medicine, Vol 2. Youth, exercise and sport* (pp. 401–430). Indianapolis: Benchmark Press.

Blimkie, C., Rice, S., Webber, C., Martin, J., Levy, D., & Gordon, C. (1993). Effects of resistance training on bone mass and density in females. *Medicine and Science in Sports & Exercise, 25,* S48.

Bouchard, C., Shephard, R.J., & Stephens, T. (Eds.) (1994). *Physical activity, fitness and health.* International proceedings and consensus statement. Champaign, IL: Human Kinetics Publishers.

Calfas, K.J., & Taylor, W.C. (1994). Effects of physical activity on psychological variables in adolescents. *Pediatric Exercise Science, 6,* 406–423.

Corbin, C.B., Pangrazi, R.P., & Welk, G.J. (1994). Toward an understanding of appropriate physical activity levels for youth. *President's Council on Physical Fitness and Sports Physical Activity and Fitness Research Digest, 1(8),* 1–8.

Hagberg, J.M., Ehsani, A.A., Goldring, D., Hernandez, A., Sinacore, D.R., & Holloszy, J.O. (1984). Effect of weight training on blood pressure and hemodynamics in hypertensive adolescents. *Journal of Pediatrics, 104,* 147–151.

Malina, R.M. (1990). Growth, exercise, fitness and later outcomes. In C. Bouchard, R.J. Shephard, T. Stephens, J.R. Sutton, & B.D. McPherson (Eds.), *Exercise, fitness and health: A consensus of current knowledge* (pp. 637–653). Champaign, IL: Human Kinetics Publishers.

Margulies, J.Y., Simkin, A., Leichter, I., Bivas, A., Steinberg, R., Giladi, M., Stein, M., Kashtan, H., & Milgrom, C. (1986). Effect of intense physical activity on the bone-mineral content in the lower limbs of young adults. *Journal of Bone and Joint Surgery, 68,* 1090–1093.

Roberts, S.B. (1993). Energy expenditure and the development of early obesity. *Annals of the New York Academy of Medicine, 699,* 18–25.

Rubinstein, A., Burstein, R., Lubin, F., Chetrit, A., Dann, E.J., Levtov, O., Geter, R., Deuster, P.A., & Dolev, E. (1995). Lipoprotein profile changes during intense training of Israeli military recruits. *Medicine and Science in Sports and Exercise, 27,* 480–484.

Sallis, J.F., & Patrick, K. (1994). Physical activity guidelines for adolescents: Consensus statement. *Pediatric Exercise Science, 6,* 302–314.

Wilmore, J.H. (1983). The 1983 C.H. McCloy Research Lecture. Appetite and body composition consequent to physical activity. *Research Quarterly of Exercise and Sport, 54,* 415–425.

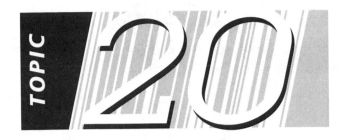

Youth Sports in America: An Overview*

Vern D. Seefeldt, Martha E. Ewing
MICHIGAN STATE UNIVERSITY

INTRODUCTION

Participation in organized sports has become a common rite of childhood in the United States. In the early part of the twentieth century, agencies began sponsoring sports and recreational activities to provide wholesome leisuretime pursuits, initially designed to keep boys out of trouble. Schools sponsored intramural sports programs to provide instruction in sports skills, plus an opportunity to engage in controlled, competitive activities. Although educators, parents, child welfare workers, and leaders of agency-sponsored sports programs do not always agree about the benefits and the objectives of youth sports programs, the notion of providing wholesome, character-building activities to occupy the leisure time of children and youth, to enable them to make the transition from childhood to adulthood (Berryman, 1996), has become an accepted view.

Prior to 1954, most of the organized sports experiences for children and youth occurred within social agencies such as the YMCAs/YWCAs, Boys and Girls Clubs, and Boy Scouts and Girl Scouts (LeUnes & Nation, 1989). Since 1954, the opportunities for youth to participate in sports have moved from social agencies and activities organized by the youth themselves to adult-organized programs. This movement towards adult-organized sports activities for youth was associated with the advent of Little League Baseball by Carl Statz in 1954 (Hale, 1956) with approximately 70,000 participants (Skubic, 1955). By 1989, there were 2.5 million children, aged eight to twelve, playing baseball on more than 42,000 teams in 28 countries.

While the number of youth involved in organized sports programs is impressive, the opportunities to engage in sports programs are unequal across genders and social classes. Greater opportunities exist among the children who grow up in middle and upper classes where resources enable adults to sponsor, organize, and administer programs for their children (Ponessa, 1992).

The rise of organized sports opportunities for girls has increased dramatically since the passage of

ORIGINALLY PUBLISHED AS SERIES 2, NUMBER 11, OF THE PCPFS *RESEARCH DIGEST.*

*This overview is a condensation of materials contained in a monograph entitled *Role of Organized Sport in the Education and Health of American Children and Youth,* commissioned by the Carnegie Corporation of New York in 1996. Authors were Martha Ewing, Vern Seefeldt, and Tempie Brown.

"Although sports are not viewed as a panacea for society's ills, sports participation that emphasizes skill-building and socially acceptable responses to personal relations has proven to be a popular aid in the education of youth."

Title IX in 1972. Although still fewer in overall participation, the number of female participants continues to rise as variables such as opportunity for involvement, valuing of sports as part of total development and overall fitness for girls and women has increased.

The association between the involvement of children and youth in organized sports and their health and academic achievements are placed in perspective by a brief overview of youth sports in America, the characteristics of current youth sports programs, and an account of the participation and attrition patterns in sports programs of American youth. The paper concludes with recommendations regarding the sponsorship and implementation of youth sports programs so that more children and youth are able to benefit from the programs' ultimate potential.

PARTICIPATION IN ORGANIZED YOUTH SPORTS IN AMERICA

Types of Youth Sports Programs

The term *youth sports* in American culture has been applied to any of the various athletic programs that provide a systematic sequence of practices and contests for children and youth (Seefeldt, Ewing, & Walk, 1991). In reality, these sports experiences differ greatly in competitive level, length of season, cost to competitors, qualifications of coaches and officials, and skill levels of athletes. For the purpose of this paper, six categories of youth sports programs have been defined: namely, *agency-sponsored programs, national youth service organizations, club sports, recreation programs, intramural programs, and interscholastic programs*. Of these six categories, four are community-based and two are conducted within the schools.

Brief definitions of the various categories of youth sports are described under the category descriptions in Table 20.1. Also displayed in Table 20.1 are the estimated percent and number of par-

ticipants in each of the six categories. Note that by far the largest percent of participants are enrolled in agency-sponsored programs (45%), followed by enrollees in recreational programs (30%). These two categories of involvement also represent the fastest growing segments of the youth sports scene.

Participation Rates

Projections from the National Center for Education Statistics (1989) indicated a slight increase by 1995 in the potential number of 5–13-year-old youth sports participants and a slight decline in the potential number of 14–17-year-old participants. These data suggest that any increases in youth sports participation are due to changes within a relatively stable pool. Potential explanations are that the increase is due to one of the following: (1) a shift from participation in the less competitive recreational programs to the agency-sponsored programs that have national affiliations, and wherein participants are more likely to be counted in reports of participation; (2) greater recruitment and involvement of the younger-aged clients; or (3) program sponsors are providing greater accessibility to youth sports, resulting in the participation of a higher proportion of the potential enrollees. Quite likely, each of these possibilities has contributed to the greater involvement of youth in agency-sponsored sports programs.

Gender Equity in Youth Sports

Among the many forms of sexism in sports, perhaps the most pervasive and devastating is the lack of equal opportunities for girls to compete in programs similar to those offered for boys. Despite the tremendous gains in sports participation made by girls and women during the last 30 years, there is still a persistent gap in the enrollment figures between males and females. Data at the interscholastic level (see Table 20.2) indicate that the total

TABLE 20.1 ▮▮▮ ▮▮▮▮▮▮ ▮▮ ▮▮▮▮▮ ▮▮ ▮▮▮▮ ▮▮▮ ▮ ▮ ▮▮▮▮▮ ▮▮▮▮▮▮▮▮▮▮ ▮ ▮ ▮▮▮▮ ▮▮▮ ▮▮ ▮▮ ▮▮▮▮▮▮ ▮▮ ▮▮▮▮▮ ▮▮

Estimated percent of youth enrolled in specific categories of youth sports.*

Category of Activity	Percent of All Eligible Enrollees[a]	Approximate Number of Participants
Agency-Sponsored Sports (i.e., Little League baseball, Pop Warner football)	45	22,000,000
Club Sports (i.e., pay for services, as in gymnastics, ice skating, swimming)	5	2,368,700
Recreational Sports Programs (everyone plays—sponsored by recreational departments)	30	14,512,200
Intramural Sports (middle, junior, senior high schools)	10	451,000
Interscholastic Sports (middle, junior, senior high schools)	12[b]	1,741,200
	40[c]	5,776,820

* Total population of eligible participants in the 5–17-year age category in (1995) was estimated to be 48,374,000 by the National Center for Education Statistics, U.S. Department of Education, 1989.

(a) Total does not equal 100 percent because of multiple-category by some athletes.

(b) Percent of total population aged 5–17 years.

(c) Percent of total high-school-aged population (N=14,510,000).

participation of girls is currently only 39% of the total participation in interscholastic athletics. The encouraging news is that there has been a slow but steady climb toward equity in the percent of female participants, from 32% of the males' participation in 1973–74 to 63% in 1994–95.

The gains in participation by girls at the interscholastic level since 1972 seem to be a direct reflection of participation rates in nonschool, agency-sponsored sports. A survey of nonschool sports participation (N = 94,500) in 1978 (Michigan Joint Legislative Study on Youth Sports) reported that the ratio of girls to boys was 3:5. In a nationwide sample involving 26,600 participants (Ewing & Seefeldt, 1989), the ratio of girls to boys was also 3:5. Some of the disparity in participation is attributable to a later entry of girls into organized sports. The average age for initial participation on an organized sports team for boys was age eight, while the mean age of entry for girls was 10. Moreover, the dropout rate of girls at younger ages was higher than that of boys, especially when co-ed composition of teams was mandated.

The greatest disparity in the youth sports scene is in the ratio of women to men who coach these young athletes. In 1978 (Michigan Joint Legislative Study on Youth Sports), the female-to-male ratio of coaches in Michigan was 1:9. Although figures for the gender of coaches in agency-sponsored sports are not available at the national level, there is no reason to believe that this is a local occurrence. At the interscholastic and intercollegiate levels, where the motto once was "women coaches for girls' and women's sports," the percent of women who coach girls' sports has dropped dramatically from 90% in 1972 to 50% in 1987 (Women's Sports Foundation, 1989). These data indicate that the lack of women coaches to serve as role models, counselors, and mentors of young girls in sports may be a subtle but formidable barrier to the entry and continued participation of girls in organized sports.

OTHER BARRIERS TO PARTICIPATION

Restricted Sports Offerings

The suggestion that barriers to participation in youth sports constitute a national dilemma may seem like a paradox to the casual observer of the national scene. Newspapers, journals, radio, and television constantly remind us of America's obsession with sports. However, closer scrutiny reveals that sports in America represent a highly exclusionary process, with only the elite performers accorded a share of the spotlight. The headlines fail to ac-

TABLE 20.2

Athletics participation survey, 1994–95.

Year	Boy Participants	Year	Girl Participants	Total	Percent of Boys Total
1971–72	3,666,917	1971–72	294,015	3,960,932	1
1972–73	3,770,621	1972–73	817,073	4,587,694	2
1973–74	4,070,125	1973–74	1,300,169	5,370,294	32
1975–76	4,109,021	1975–76	1,645,039	5,754,060	40
1977–78	4,367,442	1977–78	2,083,040	6,450,482	48
1978–79	3,709,512	1978–79	1,854,400	5,563,912	50
1979–80	3,517,829	1979–80	1,750,264	5,268,093	50
1980–81	3,503,124	1980–81	1,853,789	5,356,913	53
1981–82	3,409,081	1981–82	1,810,671	5,219,752	53
1982–83	3,355,558	1982–83	1,779,972	5,135,530	53
1983–84	3,303,599	1983–84	1,747,346	5,050,945	53
1984–85	3,354,284	1984–85	1,757,884	5,112,168	52
1985–86	3,344,275	1985–86	1,807,121	5,151,396	54
1986–87	3,364,082	1986–87	1,836,356	5,200,438	55
1987–88	3,425,777	1987–88	1,849,684	5,275,461	54
1988–89	3,416,844	1988–89	1,839,352	5,256,196	54
1989–90	3,398,192	1989–90	1,858,659	5,256,851	55
1990–91	3,406,355	1990–91	1,892,316	5,298,671	56
1991–92	3,426,853	1991–92	1,940,801	5,367,654	57
1992–93	3,416,389	1992–93	1,997,489	5,413,878	58
1993–94	[a]3,478,530	1993–94	[a]2,124,755	5,603,285	61
1994–95	[b]3,536,359	1994–95	[b]2,240,461	5,776,820	63

Source: National Federation of State High School Associations, Kansas City, MO, 1995.

(a) Total does not include 11,698 participants in coeducational sports.

(b) Total does not include 17,609 participants in coeducational sports.

count for the millions of young people who seek to participate or who would continue in organized sports were it not for the restrictions that are inherent in the adult version of highly organized competitive sports for children. In fairness to the several million adults who annually volunteer to coach youth sports, it is only through the efforts of these volunteers that youth sports are able to record their annual record-breaking participation rates.

One aspect of the youth sports scene that is obscured by the impressive enrollment figures are the players known as "dropouts." Those who cease their participation before the season ends, for whatever reason, disappear from the statistics on youth sports unless someone makes a concerted attempt to determine why they left their specific sports affiliation. Such an investigation was conducted by Ewing and Seefeldt (1989), who determined the percent of individuals who had stopped their enrollment in a specific sport during the previous year. The percent of attrition, by sports, as shown in Table 20.3, reveals that the attrition was well underway at age 10 and reached its peak at ages 14–15. The highest rates of early dropout occurred in gymnastics and the latest rate occurred in football. These data are cross-sectional in nature and reflect only attrition from a single sport, per student. Data about the athlete's subsequent sports participation after he/she ceased to participate in the sports of reference were not obtained nor did the investigators learn how many other sports were played by the athletes who "dropped out" of the specific sports.

Another barrier corroborated by these figures is that the restrictions of team membership and sports

TABLE 20.3

Percent of participants, by age, who indicated that they will not play next year, a sport they played this year.

Sport	Age								
	10	11	12	13	14	15	16	17	18
Baseball	8.5	12.5	14.9	14.0	13.9	13.8	9.7	6.6	2.7
Basketball	5.0	6.8	11.5	13.8	19.4	18.6	11.5	8.3	3.3
Football	3.3	8.1	9.6	12.1	14.8	17.7	13.4	13.3	5.6
Gymnastics	10.6	17.1	17.1	15.0	13.2	11.9	5.7	3.9	1.7
Softball	6.3	11.1	13.5	12.5	15.8	16.9	10.0	8.2	2.7
Swimming	9.7	14.7	12.8	12.1	14.1	11.3	10.9	8.3	2.5
Tennis	6.0	12.0	11.6	14.6	12.3	16.0	10.5	8.8	5.3
Volleyball	2.9	5.4	10.0	12.6	22.2	18.5	13.4	10.2	2.9
Wrestling	6.2	7.6	9.2	9.7	12.9	17.7	12.9	15.2	6.6
Ice Hockey	2.9	6.7	11.5	19.2	15.4	10.6	15.4	12.2	4.8

Source: Ewing, W. & Seefeldt, V. (1989). Participation and Attrition in American Youth Sports. Report to the Sporting Goods Manufacturers Association, North Palm Beach, Florida.

offerings per season at the interscholastic level reduce the total number of participants in youth sports by at least 50% from their previous involvement at the pre-interscholastic level. This reduction of sports activity, per capita, is especially apparent in large high schools, where membership in some sports is limited by rules, budget, space, and personnel. Thus, smaller schools are likely to have a much higher percent of their student body involved in athletics than the larger schools.

Scrutiny of the events that are associated with enrollments of youth in sports reveals that the organizational structure of sports in the United States—and not a lack of interest on the part of potential enrollees—is primarily responsible for the reduction in participation at age 14 and beyond. Data from several studies reveal that membership on a sports team remains a highly desirable aspiration (Carnegie Council on Adolescent Development, 1990; Duda, 1985) throughout the high school years. Paradoxically, the prestige associated with team membership at the interscholastic level may dissuade those who fail to "make the team" from participating in less prominent activities such as intramural or recreational leagues.

Competence of Volunteer Coaches

Approximately 2.5 million adults annually volunteer their time as coaches of youth sports teams (Martens, 1984). Most of these coaches are adults who leave coaching as soon as their children cease to be interested or eligible for additional sports competition. Impressive as this volunteer workforce is in its dedication to the needs of youth, it is insufficient in magnitude and competence to provide the knowledge, skills, and supervision required by the estimated 38 million youths whose sports participation depends on volunteer coaches.

There is common agreement that the quality of the youth sports experience depends on the competence of the adult leaders; most specifically, the coach. Thus, educational programs for volunteer coaches would seem to be in demand, but such is not the case. At least four generic programs for coaches exist at the national level and numerous other sports-specific programs are in existence through sports with national affiliations (Campbell, 1993; Feigley, 1988). Yet, the vast majority of youth sports coaches, estimated to be as high as 90%, have no formal education in coaching techniques, first aid, injury prevention, or emergency care (Kimiecki, 1988; Milne, 1990; Partlow, 1995; Seefeldt, 1992; Sieget & Newhof, 1992). Clearly, the mandatory education of coaches to meet at least the first level of competency as stated in the *National Standards for Athletic Coaches* (National Association for Sports and Physical Education, 1995) will have an immediate, beneficial effect on the sports experiences of millions of children.

TABLE 20.4
Pronouncements of professional organizations regarding youth sports.

Organization	Year	Title	Purpose/Focus
American Academy of Pediatrics	1989	Organized Athletics for Pre-Adolescent Children	Lists the safeguards that should accompany children's sports.
American Academy of Pediatrics	1988	Recommendations for Participation in Competitive Sports	Lists medical conditions that would disqualify children from athletic competition.
American Academy Pediatrics	1983	Weight Training and Weight Lifting: Information for the Pediatrician	A conservative assessment of the benefits and risks of weight lifting and weight training.
American Academy of Pediatrics	1982	Climatic Heat Stress and the Exercising Child	Documents the special problems of children when exercising in hot-humid environment.
American Academy of Pediatrics	1982	Risks of Long-Distance Running for Children	Provides guidelines for involving children in long-distance running.
American Academy of Pediatrics	1981	Competitive Sports for Children of Elementary School Age	An update of their position statement in 1968.
American Academy of Pediatrics	1981	Injuries to Young Athletes	Presents the special problems of young athletes in competitive sports.
American Academy of Pediatrics	1973	Athletic Activities for Children with Skeletal Abnormalities	Outlines the conditions under which children with specific conditions can and should not be involved in athletics.
American College of Sports Medicine	1996	Exercise and Fluid Replacement	Reviews the effects of dehydration and hydration on human performance.
American College of Sports Medicine and American College of Cardiology	1994	Recommendations for Determining Eligibility for Competition in Athletes with Cardiovascular Abnormalities	Provides an extensive set of papers that review the various abnormalities and makes recommendations to physicians.
American College of Sports Medicine	1993	The Prevention of Sports Injuries of Children and Adolescents	Suggests that 50% of current injuries could be prevented with proper techniques.
American College of Sports Medicine	1984	The Use of Anabolic-Androgenic Steroids in Sports	Documents the adverse effects of anabolic steroids on the human body.
American College of Sports Medicine	1982	The Use of Alcohol in Sports	Reviews the literature on the influence of alcohol on human performance.
American College of Sports Medicine	1979	The Participation of the Female Athlete in Long-Distance Running	Documents that female athletes should not be denied opportunities for long-distance running.
American College of Sports Medicine	1976	Weight Loss in Wrestlers	Warns of the dangers of personal health when excessive weight loss is incurred.
American Heart Association	1986	Coronary Risk Factor Modification in Children: Exercise	Reviews ways to combat the sedentary lifestyles of children.
American Medical Association	1975	Female Athletes	An early and outdated version of athletic competition for girls and women.
International Federation of Sports Medicine	1991	Excessive Physical Training in Children and Adolescents	Provides guidelines and examples of activities that are to be avoided in children's training for athletic competition.
Michigan Governor's Council on Physical Fitness, Health and Sports	1995	The Importance of Physical Activity for Children and Youth (Pivarnik)	Provides the scientific basis for physical activity in childhood and adolescence; advocates policies for families, communities, public health, and schools.
National Strength and Conditioning Association	1985	Prepubescent Strength Training	Documents the benefits and risks of strength training for prepubescent children. Provides guidelines for parents and coaches.

Overzealous Promoters

The problems of overzealous coaches and parents are so prevalent in youth sports that dozens of books and countless articles have been written to counteract this undue influence. The list of books ranges from teaching coaches and parents how to assess talent (Arnot & Gaines, 1986), to teaching pediatricians about youth sports injuries (Micheli, 1984), to information about the epidemiology of sports injuries (Caine, Caine, & Lindner, 1996). In addition, no fewer than 20 position statements (see Table 20.4) have been issued by professional organizations, addressing precautions that should apply to the sports participation of children and youth.

The rationale for the increased intensity of training and the extended duration of seasons in youth sports stems from the assumption that optimal performance can only be achieved after prolonged periods of practice. However, the data on burnout (Coakley, 1992; Rowland, 1986; Ward, 1982) and attrition (Burton, 1988; Gould, 1987) support the contention that for almost all of the youthful aspirants, these periods of intensive training have no justifiable physiological, psychological, or educational basis (International Federation of Sports Medicine, 1991). Even those who survive these rigorous sessions and go on to Olympic fame may have long-lasting physical and psychological consequences resulting from intensive training (Coakley, 1992).

There is common agreement that sports programs for children and youth can enhance motoric, physical, and social growth. However, when training sessions become so intensive that they result in social isolation, disempowerment, and permanent injuries (Coakley, 1992) then one must question their motives and tactics. Ironically, there are child labor laws in many countries that forbid stereotype work movements and excessive loading (International Federation of Sports Medicine, 1991; Roberts, 1995), but these same restrictions do not apply to children's sports. Fortunately, the numerous position statements by such organizations as the American Academy of Pediatrics (1981a, 1981b, 1982a, 1982b, 1983, 1988, 1989) and the American College of Sports Medicine (1984, 1988, 1993) have provided guidance to parents and promoters of sports for children regarding unacceptable practices. Recommendations designed to obtain desirable outcomes accompany the statements of objectionable practice.

BENEFITS OF YOUTH SPORTS PARTICIPATION

Youth Sports and Health

The Surgeon General's Report on Physical Activity and Health (1996) clearly documents the benefits of regular physical activity to the health of adults and youth alike. Because sports is a major type of activity in which youth are involved, it can be considered a viable method of promoting good health. Sports that are considered to be "lifetime" in nature are especially important in meeting national health objectives. In March of 1997 the Centers for Disease Control and Prevention (CDC) published "Guidelines for Schools and Communities for Promoting Lifelong Physical Activity." The guidelines note the benefits of regular physical activity in childhood and adolescence: improves strength and endurance, helps build healthy bones and muscles, helps control weight, reduces anxiety and stress, increases self-esteem, and may improve blood pressure and cholesterol levels. The guidelines also indicate that community sports and recreation program coordinators can help increase physical activity among youth in a variety of ways including providing a "mix of competitive team and non competitive, lifelong fitness and recreational activities," increase public facilities, and ensure coaches are competent.

Though youth sports programs can provide a role in increasing physical activity and in contributing to the health of youth, others have to be involved. The CDC guidelines suggest roles for groups other than sports programs. Parents, school administrators, teachers, coaches, and the general public all can play a role. Prominent in the report is the role of physical education in the promotion of active lifestyles among children and adolescents. While the numbers of youth involved in sports are relatively constant, the same cannot be said for school physical education programs. Physical education programs are being eroded or eliminated to make room for curricular offerings that are deemed to be more useful especially for high school students—a level at which participation is especially low compared to other age levels (Seefeldt, 1996). Although many parents regard youth sports as a suitable substitute for physical education classes, there are major differences in offerings, instruction, outcomes, and inclusion of participants. Ideally, the physical education programs should provide the basis of fundamental movement skills, appropriate physical activity behavioral development, and physical fitness attributes so students can pursue a wide variety of physical interests, including various sports.

Lack of a motor basis from which to compete successfully with peers in organized sports relegates all but the motorically gifted and physically fit aspirants to the sidelines (Pivarnik, 1995; Tyler, 1991). If the discretionary time of young individuals is not devoted to positive skill-building activities, including the abilities to participate in the games, dances, and sports of one's culture, then the potential for involvement in numerous socially unacceptable behaviors is increased (Farrell, 1990; Hechinger, 1992; Robbins, 1991; Takanishi, 1993). The inability or unwillingness of adults to provide for constructive experiences in sports during the leisure hours of youth looms as a formidable barrier, but it must be addressed in order to provide a more positive environment for children to learn the skills of a diverse society (Seefeldt, 1995).

Youth sports can play a significant public health role, as a provider of physical activity for children and adolescents alike. However, as noted above, youth sports cannot be the sole contributor to this effort. It will take the efforts of many programs, including regular school physical education programs if all youth are to benefit from the health benefits that regular physical activity can provide.

Sports and Social Development

Sports can provide excellent educational opportunities for social development because many of the social and moral requirements for participation in sports are parallels to how individuals must function in a law-abiding society. Because sports are so highly valued in the American culture, many parents believe that children should be exposed to organized sports at an early age. Participation in sports alone does not result in the development of positive social and emotional characteristics. The positive development of youth in organized sports can only be derived through sports experiences that foster positive experiences and minimize negative experiences.

Psychological readiness for competition occurs when children have the desire to compare skills with others and thereby acquire information about themselves, which is a primary attraction of sports

participation for youngsters (Passer, 1988; Roberts, 1980). A second aspect of psychological readiness occurs when a child reaches a level of cognitive maturity that allows her or him to understand the competitive process (Passer, 1988). Understanding the competitive process entails an appreciation of the social nature of competition, particularly with regard to the cooperative and strategic aspects of sports and an awareness of the nature of individual roles within a cooperating group (Brustad, 1993). Coakley (1986) stated that children are generally attracted by the excitement of sports before they have developed a mature conception of sports.

With respect to the readiness to compare skills with others, children do not generally begin actively to compare their abilities with others until they are at least five or six years old. However, until the age of eight or nine, children lack the cognitive ability to use information about an experience to make sophisticated comparisons. Until the age of eight or nine, children tend to rely on objective outcomes, such as winning or losing, and upon adult feedback to provide them with information about personal ability in sports (Horn & Hasbrook, 1986, 1987; Horn & Weiss, 1991). Research also indicates that prior to adolescence, there is only a very weak correlation between children's perceptions of competence and their actual competence as assessed by teachers or coaches (Horn & Weiss, 1991; Nicholls, 1978).

Psychological readiness also involves the mature conception of the social nature of competition. Coakley (1986) argued that children couldn't fully benefit from competitive situations until they have the capacity to understand their roles in relation to the roles of others within this context. Selman (1971, 1976) suggested that it is not until the age of eight to ten years that children develop the necessary role-taking abilities to allow them to understand another person's point of view. This ability to understand another's point of view is necessary for one to cooperate effectively with others.

Premature sports involvement may result in undesirable emotional consequences for children. The limited capacity of children to develop accurate conceptions of ability may result in inappropriate aspirations and achievement goals (Passer, 1988). When expectations for performance are too high, children are likely to experience frustration, discouragement, and low self-esteem (Brustad, 1993). Roberts (1980) contended that children are not able to develop realistic achievement goals until they can make appropriate attributions for outcomes. A mature attributional capacity will not be present until children can differentiate between ability, task difficulty, and effort in influencing performance.

Youth Sports and Moral Development

Whether participation in sports contributes to moral development remains unresolved. Shields and Bredemeier (1995) suggested that the physical behaviors of sports are not in themselves moral or immoral. In addition, the experiences that children have in sports are far from uniform. The physical act of performing sports skills will not teach moral action. However, the potential does exist to enhance moral development through the social interactions associated with involvement in sports. The evidence for and against sports as contributing to moral development will focus on the areas of delinquency and aggression.

Delinquency. In what has now become a classic work on adolescents, Coleman (1965) wrote that "if it were not for interscholastic athletics or something like it, the rebellion against school, the rate of drop-out, and the delinquency of boys might be far worse than they presently are" (pp. 44–45). Considerable evidence has been presented that sports participants are less likely than nonparticipants to engage in delinquent behavior (Donnelly, 1981; Hastad, Segrave, Pangrazi, & Peterson, 1984; Melnick, Vanfossen, & Sabo, 1988; Segrave, 1983; Segrave & Hastad, 1982). The negative relationship between sports participation and delinquency tends to be stronger among lower-class youth (Buhrman & Bratton, 1978; Schafer, 1969; Segrave & Chu, 1978) and athletes in minor sports (Segrave & Hastad, 1982). Unfortunately, the reason for this negative correlation is unclear.

Many attempts have been made to try to explain why the negative relationship exists between delinquency and sports involvement. Sports may deter delinquency by encouraging less frequent, shorter, or less intense interaction with deviant others (Hastad et. al., 1984; Segrave & Hastad, 1982). Schafer (1971) proposed that the values emphasized in the sports context—such as teamwork, effort, and achievement—tend toward conventionality and, therefore, may discourage the legitimization of delinquent behavior. The fact that sports involvement reduces the amount of unstructured time and that sports fosters a belief that hard work can lead to just rewards may also influence the negative relationship.

Being labeled an athlete may contribute to the decrease in delinquency, but not necessarily in a positive way. Purdy and Richard (1983) reported that athletes who engage in the same delinquent behavior as nonathletes may escape the negative label of "delinquent," may be treated less harshly by the courts and may have sufficient alternative positive labels to escape self-labeling as "delinquent."

Participation in sport has been used as a treatment for delinquency with some success. Trulson (1986) matched 34 delinquent teenage boys on age, socioeconomic background and test scores on aggression and personality adjustment and then divided the youth into three groups. One group received traditional Tae Kwon Do training, which combined philosophical reflection, meditation, and physical practice of the martial arts techniques. The second group received "modern" martial arts training, emphasizing only fighting and self-defense techniques. The third group ran and played basketball and football. These groups met for one hour three times a week for six months. Results revealed that members of the Tae Kwon Do group were classified as normal rather than delinquent, scored below normal on aggression and exhibited less anxiety, increased their self-esteem, and improved their social skills. The modern martial arts group scored higher on delinquency and aggression and was less well adjusted than when the experiment began. The traditional sports group showed little change on delinquency and personality measures, but their self-esteem and social skills improved. The findings support the notion that whatever advantages or liabilities are associated with sport involvement, they do not come from sport per se, but from the particular blend of social interactions and physical activities that comprise the totality of the sport experience.

Aggression. The debate continues as to whether sports contributes to increased aggression among athletes and spectators or whether sports provides an arena for the release of aggression in a socially acceptable outlet. The debate may actually be a moot one as the incidences and intensity of learned aggression vary considerably between sports, and, within a given sport, from one region of the country to another, and from one level of competition to another (M.D. Smith, 1983). Most of the research supports the notion that aggression in sports is learned.

Two generalizations should be made before discussing the concepts of moral action and aggression. First, male athletes are generally found to be more aggressive than female athletes (Bredemeier, 1984; Silva, 1983; M.D. Smith, 1983). In addition, males tend to express and accept more aggression than females (Hyde, 1986). Again, these data would suggest that aggression in sports, as well as controlling one's aggression, is a learned behavior.

The relationship of moral action to aggression has received very limited attention. The work of Bredemeier and Shields is particularly noteworthy in this area. Bredemeier (1985) reported that athletes with more mature moral reasoning were less approving of aggressive tactics than those with less mature moral reasoning. In addition, athletes with "principled" moral reasoning scores were rated as significantly less aggressive by their coaches (Bredemeier & Shields, 1986). Finally, in a study of sports camp participants, Bredemeier, Weiss, Shields, and Cooper (1987) showed children slides of potentially injurious sports acts and asked the children questions designed to reveal their perceptions of legitimacy. Results revealed that children with less mature moral reasoning judged a significantly greater number of aggressive acts to be legitimate than their more mature peers. Bredemeier et al. concluded that children who perceive an act as injurious are probably more likely to engage in it than children who judge it to be illegitimate. The findings support the notion that aggression is a learned behavior and that if one teaches youth about moral reasoning, one could reduce instances of aggression.

Youth Sports as a Deterrent to Negative Behavior

Along with the positive outcomes of learning sports skills and enhanced personal characteristics, youth sports can also act as a deterrent to negative behavior. The role of sports as a safe alternative activity to violence and intimidation is gaining interest due to increasing concern with flourishing gang membership. Youth sports, specifically, may be considered a venue for reflecting or shaping society's acceptance or disapproval for violence and aggres-

sion. There has been an abundance of research on the causes of aggression and violence in sports. At the heart of the debate is whether sports can offer a socially acceptable arena for aggressive behavior or whether the aggressive nature of sports fosters violent behavior.

Participation in sports by youth is a highly desirable alternative for gang membership. Society's current attention on the destructive nature of youth gang involvement has prompted much research over the past two decades. Historically, conditions for the foundation of gangs have been familiar to the inner city: poverty, racial division, broken families, and high unemployment (Stover, 1986). Current information on gangs has involved the identification of other conditions for gang membership such as age (Parks, 1995) and inter-/intrapersonal conflicts (Curry, 1992). Furthermore, gang activity is no longer isolated in the inner city, but has infiltrated many suburban and rural communities. For example, Los Angeles reported 200,000 gang members in 1991, Chicago spent $7 million on anti-gang efforts, and gangs have infiltrated Albuquerque, Phoenix, and Milwaukee. What is more alarming is that contemporary gangs are more violent than earlier gangs were (Evans, 1995) indicating that the problem is getting worse and more dangerous. Where gangs of the 1960s were more concerned with fist fights over "turf," contemporary gangs are involved in drug trafficking and the use of weapons, including an arsenal of assault rifles.

Reasons identified for initial gang membership include a combination of family, school, and personal conflicts as reported by juvenile delinquents (Clark, 1992; Fukada, 1991). Alienation from family and peers included lack of companionship, support, or social interaction. Reported problems in school were poor grades and discipline issues. Personal struggles included low self-esteem and self-worth. Furthermore, the lack of a positive role model was a differentiating factor of gang and non-gang members (Wang, 1994) indicating the importance of positive role models in the lives of youth. Nongang members were three times more likely to mention a teacher or parent as a role model. Furthermore, the absence of a role model was the best predictor of gang membership, which corroborates other research suggesting that intrafamilial socialization and parental support are among the most significant determinants of gang membership (Johnstone, 1983).

The reasons for continued membership in a gang have also been well documented. Gang membership provides affiliation, self-worth, companionship, and excitement (Clark, 1992). The gang fills a void in a youth's life that was created by the environmental and inter-/intrapersonal conflicts discussed above. Once in a gang, the youth develops a responsibility to the other members, as well as a duty to help the gang prosper. The gang also provides a self-identity or valued role that is reinforced by the group, such as the provider, whose "job" is to obtain money for gang use by burglary or drug dealing (Vigil, 1988). No gender or racial discrimination has been shown in gang membership (Fiqueira-McDonough, 1986), dispelling the widely held notion that gangs are comprised largely of African-American males. An increasing number of females, as well as Hispanics, Asians, and Caucasians are now involved in gang membership.

Youth sport participation is a practical substitute for gang membership. Initiation into sports at a young age allows for a positive filling of the void in a youth's life at a critical stage. Early intervention is recommended as a tool to curb delinquent behavior, which would most likely continue over a lifetime (Laub, 1994). The highest rate of criminal offenders with chronic antisocial behavior began involvement in crime at an earlier age than offenders with shorter and lower incidence careers. Continued intervention is crucial in the lives of youth who are facing a pivotal choice about whether or not to join a gang. Delinquent behavior by gang members was shown to be lower before and after gang membership, showing the positives for decreasing criminal activity outside of the gang (Thornberry, 1993). The focus has been on prevention and intervention strategies; however, once in a gang, getting out may not be the easiest task to achieve. However, leaving the gang is a consideration of many members (Hochhaus & Sousa, 1988). Peer pressure was identified by current gang members as the most important reason for not leaving a gang. Some members expressed dissonance when asked to take part in stealing, drug dealing, or violence, but the peer pressure outweighed the guilt. The desire to leave is the most promising of avenues for youth sports to reach young people who have already joined the gang. Offering an alternate activity that provides the same qualities as gang membership should become part of the recruitment strategy for youth sports.

SUMMARY

Within this paper, the number of children and adolescents participating in sports, difference in gender among participants, barriers to participation, and many of the benefits of sports participation have been documented. It is clear that participation in youth sports can have many benefits for the individual and for our society in general. It is also clear that sports is a double-edge sword in that negative consequences may result if programs are not well run. Proper education of coaches, limiting the influence of overzealous promoters, and paying attention to important guidelines outlined by various professional associations are all factors that can help sports programs have optimal benefits for youth. Based on the information presented in this paper, and our extensive experience working with youth sports programs, some recommendations are proposed in an effort to enhance the potential for youth sports in meeting the needs of *all* youth, regardless of age, gender, ethnicity, or ability.

Recommendations

- Children should be exposed to a broad array of sports opportunities during their elementary years.
- When possible, youth should be exposed to sports that have potential for lifetime use.
- Early childhood involvement in sports should emphasize instruction more than competition.
- Sports programs must reevaluate their programs and institute equitable programs that will meet the needs of all youth.
- Coaches must be encouraged to teach young athletes responsibility, independence, and leadership so that they are better prepared for everyday life.

(continued)

- Sports organizations can provide an alternative to gang membership and violence by providing opportunities for more youth to be involved and thereby benefit from being a member of a prosocial team.

- Sports organizations should make a commitment to increasing the number of women and minority coaches in youth sports programs.

- Public policy makers must become educated about the significance of youth sports in the non-school lives of youth. Dedicated revenues for sports programs are an uncommon, but necessary, means to avoid the fluctuations in funding by private and public funders.

- Programs must be designed so that they revitalize communities as partners in the delivery of sports programs.

- Communities must improve the condition and maintenance of facilities and sites so that they are attractive and safe for children and families.

- A broad-based organization that unites the public/private sector of a city should be established to plan, develop, coordinate, maintain, and evaluate the municipality's comprehensive youth sports program.

- Sports organizations should provide educational programs for all coaches of youth sports teams.

- Sports organizations should provide education to parents about the roles of parents of youth sports participants, the use of appropriate feedback, and the positive and potentially negative aspects of participation in sports.

REFERENCES

American Academy of Pediatrics. (1981a). Competitive sports for children of elementary school age. *The Physician and Sportsmedicine, 9,* 140–142.

American Academy of Pediatrics. (1981b). Injuries to young athletes. *The Physician and Sportsmedicine, 9,* 107–110.

American Academy of Pediatrics. (1982a). Climatic heat stress and the exercising child. *Pediatrics, 69,* 808–809.

American Academy of Pediatrics. (1982b). Risks of long-distance running for children. *Pediatric News and Comment, 33,* 11.

American Academy of Pediatrics. (1983). Weight training and weight lifting: Information for the pediatrician. *The Physician and Sportsmedicine, 11,* 157–162.

American Academy of Pediatrics. (1988). Recommendations for participation in competitive sports. *Pediatrics, 81,* 737–739.

American Academy of Pediatrics. (1989). Organized athletics for pre-adolescent children. *Pediatrics, 84,* 583–584.

American College of Sports Medicine. (1984). The use of anabolic-androgenic steroids in sports. *Sports Medicine Bulletin,* 13–18.

American College of Sports Medicine. (1988). Physical fitness in children and youth. *Medicine and Science in Sports and Exercise, 20,* 422–423.

American College of Sports Medicine. (1993). The prevention of sports injuries of children and adolescents. *Medicine and Science in Exercise and Sports, 25,* S1–S7.

Arnot, R., & Gaines, C. (1986). *Sports talent.* New York: Penguin Books.

Berryman, J. (1996). The rise of boys' sports in the United States, 1900 to 1970. In F. Smoll & R. Smith (Eds.), *Children and youth in sports: A biopsychosocial perspective.* Dubuque, IA: Brown and Benchmark.

Bredemeier, B.J. (1984). Sports, gender and moral growth. In J.M. Silva & R.S. Weinberg (Eds.) *Psychological foundations for sports* (pp. 400–413). Champaign, IL: Human Kinetics Publishers.

Bredemeier, B.J. (1985). Moral reasoning and the perceived legitimacy of intentionally injurious sports acts. *Journal of Sports Psychology, 7,* 110–124.

Bredemeier, B.J., & Shields, D.L. (1986). Athletic aggression: An issue of contextual morality. *Sociology of Sports Journal, 3,* 15–28.

Bredemeier, B.J., Weiss, M.R., Shields, D.L., & Cooper, B. (1987). The relationship between children's legitimacy judgments and their moral reasoning, aggression tendencies and sport involvement. *Sociology of Sport Journal, 4,* 48–60.

Brustad, R.J. (1993). Youth in sports: Psychological considerations. In R.N. Singer, M. Murphey, & L.K. Tennant (Eds.), *Handbook of research on sports psychology* (pp. 695–717). New York: Macmillan.

Buhrman, H.G., & Bratton, R. (1978). Athletic participation and status of Alberta high school girls. *International Review of Sports Psychology, 12,* 57–67.

Burton, D. (1988). The dropout dilemma in youth sports: Documenting the problem and identifying the solutions. In R. Malina (Ed.), *Young athletes: Biological, psychological and education perspectives* (pp. 245–266). Champaign, IL: Human Kinetics Publishers.

Caine, D., Caine, C., & Lindner, K. (Eds.) (1996). *Epidemiology of sports injuries.* Champaign, IL: Human Kinetics Publishers.

Campbell, S. (1993). Coaching education around the world. *Sports Science Review, 2,* 62–74.

Carnegie Council on Adolescent Development. (1990). *A matter of time: Risk and opportunity in the nonschool hours. Executive summary.* New York: Carnegie Corporation of New York.

Clark, C.M. (1992). Deviant adolescent subcultures: Assessment strategies and clinical interventions. *Adolescence, 27(106),* 283–293.

Coakley, J. (1986).When should children begin competing? A sociological perspective. In M.R. Weiss & D. Gould (Eds.), *Sports for children and youths* (pp. 59–63). Champaign, IL: Human Kinetics Publishers.

Coakley, J. (1992). Burnout among adolescent athletes: A personal failure or social problem? *Sociology of Sports Journal, 9,* 271–285.

Coleman, J.S. (1965). *Adolescents in the schools.* New York: Basic Books.

Curry, G.D. (1992). Gang involvement and delinquency among Hispanic and African American adolescent males. *Journal of Research in Crime & Delinquency, 29(3),* 273–291.

Donnelly, P. (1981). Athletes and juvenile delinquents: A comparative analysis based on a review of the literature. *Adolescence, 16,* 415–431.

Duda, J.L. (1985). Goals and achievement orientations of Anglo and Mexican-American adolescents in sports and the classroom. *International Journal of Intercultural Relations, 9,* 131–150.

Evans, J.P. (1995). Understanding violence in contemporary and earlier gangs: An exploratory application of the theory of reasoned action. *Journal of Black Psychology, 21(1),* 71–81.

Ewing, M.E., & Seefeldt, V. (1996). Participation and attrition patterns in American agency-sponsored youth sports. In F.L. Smoll & R.E. Smith (Eds.), *Children and youth in sports: A biopsychosocial perspective* (pp. 31–46). Dubuque, IA: Brown and Benchmark.

Farrell, E. (1990). *Hanging in and dropping out.* New York: Teachers' College Press, Columbia University.

Feigley, D. (1988). *Comparative analysis of youth sports educational programs.* New Brunswick, NJ: Rutgers Youth Sports Research Council.

Fiqueira-McDonough, J. (1986). School context, gender, and delinquency. *Journal of Youth and Adolescence, 15,* 79–88.

Fukada, J. (1991). The relation between family functioning and the independence of juvenile delinquents. *Japanese Journal of Criminal Psychology, 29(1),* 19–36.

Gortmaker, S., Dietz, W., & Cheung, L. (1990). Inactivity, diet and the fattening of America. *Journal of the American Dietetic Association, 90,* 1247–1252.

Gould, D. (1987). Understanding attrition in children's sports. In D. Gould & M. Weiss (Eds.), *Advances in pediatric sports science* (pp. 61–86). Champaign, IL: Human Kinetics Publishers.

Halc, C.J. (1956). Physiological maturity of Little League baseball players. *Research Quarterly, 27,* 276–284.

Haskell, W.L. (1995). Physical activity in the prevention and management of coronary heart disease. *Physical Activity and Fitness Research Digest,* 1–7. President's Council on Physical Fitness and Sports, Washington, DC.

Hastad, D.N., Segrave, J.O., Pangrazi, R., & Peterson, G. (1984). Youth sports participation and deviant behavior. *Sociology of Sports Journal, 1,* 366–373.

Hechinger, F. (1992). *Fateful choices: Healthy youth for the 21st century.* New York: Hill & Wang.

Hochhaus, C., & Sousa, F. (1988). Why children belong to gangs. *The High School Journal, 71(2),* 74–77.

Horn, T.S., & Hasbrook, C.A. (1986). Information components influencing children's perceptions of their physical competence. In M.R. Weiss & D. Gould (Eds.), *Sports for children and youths* (pp. 81–88). Champaign, IL: Human Kinetics Publishers.

Horn, T.S., & Hasbrook, C.A. (1987). Psychological characteristics and the criteria children use for self-evaluation. *Journal of Sports Psychology, 9,* 208–221.

Horn, T.S., & Weiss, M.R. (1991). A developmental analysis of children's self-ability judgments in the physical domain. *Pediatric Exercise Science, 3,* 310–326.

Hyde, J.S. (1986). Gender differences in aggression. In J.S. Hyde & M.C. Linn (Eds.), *The psychology of gender: Advances through meta-analysis* (pp. 51–66). Baltimore: Johns Hopkins University Press.

International Federation of Sports Medicine. (1991). Position statement: Excessive physical training of children and adolescents. *Clinic Journal of Sports Medicine, 1,* 262–264.

Johnstone, J.W. (1983). Recruitment to a youth gang. *Youth and Society, 14,* 281–300.

Kimiecki, J. (1988). Who needs coaches' education: U.S. coaches do. *The Physician and Sportsmedicine, 16,* 124–136.

Kuntzleman, C.T., & Reiff, G. (1992). The decline of American children's fitness levels. *Research Quarterly for Exercise and Sports, 63,* 107–111.

Laub, J.H. (1994). The precursors of criminal offending across the life course. *Federal Probation, 58(3),* 51–57.

LeUnes, A.D., & Nation, J.R. (1989). *Sports psychology: An introduction.* Chicago: Nelson-Hall.

Malina, R. (1995). Physical activity and fitness of children and youth: Questions and implications. *Medicine, Exercise Nutrition and Health, 4,* 123–135.

Martens, R. (1984). Youth sports in the U.S.A. In M. Weiss & D. Gould (Eds.), *Sports for children and youth* (Chapter 5, pp. 27–33). Champaign, IL: Human Kinetics Publishers.

Melnick, M.J., Vanfossen, B.E., & Sabo, D.F. (1988). Developmental effects of athletic participation among high school girls. *Sociology of Sports Journal, 5,* 22–36.

Micheli, L. (1984). Sports injuries in the young athlete: Questions and controversies. In L. Micheli (Ed.), *Pediatric and adolescent sports medicine.* Boston: Little, Brown & Co. *Michigan Joint Legislative Study on Youth Sports.* (1978). State of Michigan, Lansing, MI.

Milne, C. (1990). High education for coaches: Preparation survey results. *Journal for Physical Education, Recreation and Dance, 61,* 44–46.

National Association for Sports and Physical Education. (1995). *National standards for athletic coaches.* Reston, VA: National Association for Sports and Physical Education.

National Center for Education Statistics. (1989). *Projections of educational statistics to 2000.* Washington, DC: U.S. Department of Education.

Parks, C.P. (1995). Gang behavior in the schools: Reality or myth? *Educational Psychology Review, 7(1),* 41–60.

Partlow, K. (1995). *Interscholastic coaching: From accidental occupation to profession.* Champaign, IL: American Sports Education Programs.

Passer, M.W. (1988). Psychological issues in determining children's age-readiness for competition. In F.L. Smoll, R.A. Magill, & M.J. Ash (Eds.), *Children in sports* (3rd ed., pp. 203–227). Champaign, IL: Human Kinetics Publishers.

Pivarnik, J. (1995). *The importance of physical activity for children and youth.* Lansing, MI: Michigan Governor's Council on Physical Fitness, Health and Sports.

Ponessa, J. (1992). Student access to extracurricular activities. *Public Affairs Focus, 23,* 1–8. Princeton, NJ: Public Affairs Research Institute.

Purdy, D.A., & Richard, S.F. (1983). Sport and juvenile delinquency: An examination and assessment of four major theories. *Journal of Sport Behavior, 6,* 179–193.

Robbins, D. (1991). *The future by design.* (DHHS Publication No [ASM] 91-1760. Washington, DC: U.S. Printing Office, Superintendent of Documents.

Roberts, G.C. (1980). Children in competition: A theoretical perspective and recommendations for practice. *Motor Skills: Theory into Practice, 4,* 37–50.

Roberts, L. (1995). Child labour: A form of modern slavery. In *The way forward: Conference on human rights* (pp. 35–42). Verbier, Switzerland.

Rowland, T. (1986). Exercise fatigue in adolescents: Diagnosis of athlete burnout. *The Physician and Sportsmedicine, 14,* 69–72.

Schafer, W.E. (1969). Participation in interscholastic athletics and delinquency: A preliminary study. *Social Problems, 17,* 40–47.

Schafer, W.E. (1971). *Sports, socialization, and the school: Toward maturity of enculturation.* Paper presented at the Third International Symposium on the Sociology of Sports, Waterloo, ON.

Seefeldt, V. (1992). Coaching certification: An essential step for the revival of a faltering profession. *Journal for Physical Education, Recreation and Dance, 63,* 29–30.

Seefeldt, V. (1995). *Recreating recreation and sports in Detroit, Hamtramck and Highland Park: Final report to the Skillman Foundation.* Detroit, MI: The Skillman Foundation.

Seefeldt, V. (1996). Physical activity is no substitute for physical education. *Journal for Physical Education, Recreation and Dance, 67,* 10–11.

Seefeldt, V., Ewing, M.E., & Walk, S. (1991). *Overview of youth sports in the United States.* Paper commissioned by the Carnegie Council on Adolescent Development.

Segrave, J.O. (1983). Sports and juvenile delinquency. In R. Terjung (Ed.), *Exercise and sports sciences review, 2,* 161–209.

Segrave, J.O., & Chu, D.B. (1978). Athletics and juvenile delinquency. *Review of Sports and Leisure, 3,* 1–24.

Segrave, J.O., & Hastad, D. (1982). Delinquent behavior and interscholastic participation. *Journal of Sports Behavior, 5,* 96–111.

Selman, R.L. (1971). Taking another's perspective: Role-taking development in early childhood. *Child Development, 42,* 1721–1734.

Selman, R.L. (1976). Social-cognitive understanding: A guide to educational and clinical practice. In T. Lickona (Ed.), *Moral development and behavior* (pp. 299–316). New York: Holt, Rinehart & Winston.

Shields, D.L., & Bredemeier, B.J. (1995). *Character development and physical activity.* Champaign, IL: Human Kinetics Publishers.

Siegel, D., & Newhof, C. (1992). What should it take to be a coach? *Journal for Physical Education, Recreation and Dance, 63,* 60–63.

Silva, J.M. (1983). The perceived legitimacy of rule violating behavior in sports. *Journal of Sports Psychology, 5,* 438–448.

Skubic, E. (1955). Emotional responses of boys to Little League and Middle League competitive baseball. *Research Quarterly, 26,* 342–352.

Smith, M.D. (1983). *Violence and sports.* Toronto: Butterworths.

Stover, D. (1986). A new breed of youth gang is on the prowl and a bigger threat than ever. *American School Board Journal, 69,* 19–21.

Takanishi, R. (1993). *Adolescence in the 1990s: Risk and opportunity,* New York: Teachers' College Press.

Thornberry, T.P. (1993). The role of juvenile gangs in facilitating delinquent behavior. *Journal of Research in Crime & Delinquency, 30(1),* 55–87.

Trulson, M.E. (1986). Martial arts training: A novel "cure" for juvenile delinquency. *Human Relations, 39,* 1131–1140.

Tyler, J. (1991). *The serious business of play: A focus on recreation in the Milwaukee agenda.* Public Policy Forum, 633 W. Wisconsin Avenue, Milwaukee, WI.

Vigil, J.D. (1988). Group processes and street identity: Adolescent Chicano gang members. *Ethos, 16(4),* 421–445.

Wang, A.Y. (1994). Pride and prejudice in high school gang members. *Adolescence, 29(114),* 279–291.

Ward, D. (1982). Burned out. *Sports and Athletes, 5,* 48–51.

Women's Sports Foundation. (1989). *The Women's Sports Foundation Report: Minorities in sports.* New York: Women's Sports Foundation.

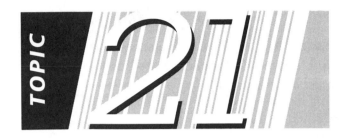
Psycho-Physiological Contributions of Physical Activity and Sports for Girls

Linda K. Bunker
UNIVERSITY OF VIRGINIA

A NOTE FROM THE EDITORS

Participation in sport and exercise contributes not only to the physical development of children, but also to their social and emotional development. There is a great deal of information available about the importance of sport experiences for males, but far less research and even fewer advocates for parallel experiences for girls (Berryman, 1996). In an effort to synthesize what we know about the benefits of physical activity, the President's Council on Physical Fitness and Sports (1997a) issued a report entitled *Physical Activity and Sport in the Lives of Girls: Physical and Mental Health Dimensions from an Interdisciplinary Approach.* Linda Bunker, a well-known researcher, author and advocate of sports and physical activity for girls and women served as the content editor for this report. We asked Linda to summarize some of the contributions of physical activity and sports for girls. We encourage you to seek additional information in the special President's Council on Physical Fitness and Sports volume noted above and cited in the references.

INTRODUCTION

Maintaining physical fitness and developing good fundamental movement skills by actively participating in daily activity contributes to happier and healthier lives by facilitating both physical and emotional health. Since the passing of Title IX of the Educational Amendments Act in 1972, appropriately more emphasis has been placed on providing opportunities for both girls and boys to participate in physical activities and youth sport. There are now over 2.25 million young women participating in sport at the high school level, with one in three now participating compared to one in 27 in 1972. Today, girls comprise almost 37 percent of all high school athletes (National Federation of State High Schools Association, 1995–1996).

In the Executive Summary of the recent monograph entitled *Physical Activity and Sport in the Lives of Girls,* the President's Council of Physical Fitness and Sport (1997b) suggested that

> Physical activity and sport are not simply things young girls do *in addition* to the rest of their lives, but rather, they comprise an interdependent set of physiological, psychological and social processes

ORIGINALLY PUBLISHED AS SERIES 3, NUMBER 1, OF THE PCPFS *RESEARCH DIGEST.*

"Involvement in sport and physical activity contributes to the physical movement capacities of girls, the health status of their bodies, the values and ethical behaviors they develop and their personal, unique identity. Physical activity must be an integral part of everyday life, not an "add-on!"

that can influence, and, in varying degrees, sustain girls' growth and development. (pg.18)

Involvement in sport and physical activity contributes to the physical movement capacities of girls, the health status of their bodies, the values and ethical behaviors they develop and their personal development of a unique identity. Though it would be impossible to cover all of these aspects in this article, an overview of contributions and issues (potential challenges) related to physiological dimensions, and psycho-social development is provided.

PHYSIOLOGICAL DIMENSIONS

Childhood activities related to sport and physical activity should include opportunities for girls to develop fundamental fitness, and to acquire the motor skills necessary for life-long learning and leisure time activities. All children need a reasonable level of motor skill in order to participate in activities that facilitate good immune system functioning, build physical fitness, and maintain appropriate body weight.

Motor Skill Development

One of the most basic benefits of physical activity is the development of motor skills. Once acquired, motor skills enhance one's abilities to perform leisure activities and to function effectively in movement situations. As noted above, an indirect benefit of learning motor skills is that skilled people are more likely to be active and fit than those who lack confidence in their abilities in sports and recreational activities. It is through regular involvement in regular physical activities that allow practice that motor skills are learned. Providing these opportunities to learn these skills is important for all people, including *all* girls and women.

Physical Fitness

Though maturation and heredity have considerable effect on the fitness of youth, regular physical activity can contribute significantly in this area. All areas of fitness are affected by regular exercise but three that seem to be especially impacted by regular physical activity are muscular fitness, cardiovascular fitness (aerobic fitness), and anaerobic power. Benefits in muscular fitness including muscle strength and endurance as a result of physical activity and sport are well documented for both girls and boys. For most girls, muscular fitness increases at a linear rate until about age 14, but for sedentary girls it may slow more rapidly or even decrease (Blimkie, 1989). However, systematic physical activity including both short-term training programs (Sale, 1989) and regular physical activity programs can produce marked improvement in strength for girls, generally thought to be due to improved motor unit activation (Sewall & Micheli, 1986).

Cardiovascular fitness and anaerobic power influence the ability of the body to do work in a specific amount of time. Cardiovascular or aerobic performances (which occur over longer periods of time) and anaerobic performances (which occur over shorter bursts such as sprinting) are both enhanced by regular physical activity. In general, aerobic power impacts one's ability to do endurance or repeated activities, and increases with growth prior to adolescence, but seems to decline for girls (relative to body mass) while it is maintained in boys (Armstrong & Weisman, 1994). This may be a function of both less physical activity and the increase in body fat, but fortunately, both short-term and long-term training programs have been shown to be beneficial in reversing this trend in both anaerobic and aerobic power (Bar-Or & Malina, 1995). It appears that the primary advantage of training is an increase in oxygen uptake (aerobic fitness) and improved efficiency of movement (e.g., running, jumping).

Body Composition

One of the primary advantages of active physical participation for children seems to be directly linked to lower body fat and a better ratio of lean to fat mass. Children with above average levels of body fat generally have higher total cholesterol, and LDL cholesterol and often-associated elevated blood pressure (Williams et al., 1992). Elevated levels of cholesterol in children are very important because children who have higher levels of cholesterol are almost three times more likely than other children to have high cholesterol levels as adults (National Cholesterol Education Program, 1991). The best strategy for lowering cholesterol in children is a combination of exercise and diet which may also lead to lowered blood pressure, and other benefits thought to be brought about because of decreased cardiac output, decreased peripheral resistance, and reduced risk of blood clotting (Blair et al., 1996).

Exercise and sport experiences can also be beneficial in maintaining appropriate body weight, or the balance between energy expenditure and caloric intake (especially the relative proportion of fat intake in terms of the percent of total calories. The problem of juvenile obesity is twice as great today as it was in the 1960s (Blair et al., 1996), and a particular problem for juvenile girls. For most young girls, normal daily activity provides an adequate balance of intake and expenditures, but for females with weight problems, maintaining regular exercise levels is an important adjunct in weight control because of its role in facilitating fat-free mass and promoting the loss of fat (Wells, 1991). It is also thought to be important in reducing the risk of non-insulin dependent diabetes which is one of the ten most prevalent causes of death in the United States (Blair et al., 1996).

Reproductive Functioning and Increased Bone Density

Another impact of exercise unique to females is the impact of exercise on reproductive functioning and menarche. There are many anecdotal reports of more regular menstrual cycles and less physical distress associated with moderate physical activity. However, there are also reports of delayed onset of the menstrual cycle (menarche) in athletes that may be either a cause or effect of athletic participation.

For example, it is possible that young girls who mature earlier are socialized away from sport, and that girls who have less body fat and longer limb to trunk ratios (characterized by pre-pubescence) may have an advantage in sport and therefore self-select (Stager, Wigglesworth & Hatler, 1990; Wells, 1991).

Extremely high levels of training/exercise or other physiological stressors have been associated with the absence of regular menstrual cycles (amenorrhea) and parallel reduction in circulating levels of estrogen. This reduction in estrogen can be a factor in reduced bone density (osteoporosis) which could negatively impact skeletal development and maintenance (Fehily, Coles, Evans & Elwood, 1992). On the other hand, the increased levels of exercise which may reduce obesity and delay the onset of menarche have also been shown to be an advantage in reducing the risk for estrogen dependent cancers (primarily breast and ovarian cancer) (Kramer & Wells, 1996).

In later life women are especially at risk of osteoporosis (low bone density). One major advantage of physical activity for girls is that it increases "peak bone mass." Peak bone mass is the level of bone mass at its highest point—usually occurring in the teens or early 20s. High peak bone mass can be viewed much as a bank savings account where withdrawals can be made later in life when needed. The higher the peak mass, the less likely that losses later in life will result in low bone mass or osteoporosis.

Recent popular literature has contained reference to the "Female Athlete Triad" which seems to impact girls who are training at high levels. The triad refers to three areas of behavior that may be deleterious to female athletes: osteoporosis, amenorrhea, and disordered eating. The foundation of these problems is thought to be a preoccupation with body weight and maintaining an "ideal body physique" or body composition (ratio of lean to fat body weight). This preoccupation can affect many female athletes, especially those participating in "style" athletics such as gymnastics, diving, ice skating, cheerleading or other sports where they are either formally or informally judged on how they look (Gill, 1995; Plaisted, 1995; Reel & Gill, 1996). When children practice behaviors of undereating, underconsumption of calories, and overexercise, it may produce undesirable effects—whether related to sport and exercise or acting in school plays or singing.

Immune System Functioning

Extensive research has emerged in the last ten years which supports the contention that regular exercise (at a moderate level) facilitates the body's ability to fight infection (e.g. upper respiratory infection (Nieman, 1994)) and disease through increased immune system function (Freedson & Bunker, 1997). This increased ability to maintain health appears to be related to increases in levels of interleukin-1 and interferon and increased numbers of natural killer cells, circulating lymphocytes, granulocytes, and other protective bodies (Kramer & Wells, 1996). It appears that increases in monocyte and macrophage function help to retard diseases caused by viruses such as common colds and influenza and may even serve to help retard aberrant cells such as cancer (Newsholme & Parry-Billings, 1994). It may be necessary to temper enthusiasm about reducing the chances of illness due to regular exercise. There is some evidence that children who participate in group activities (such as sport, band, church) or strenuous exercise have decreased NK cell activity at rest and some immune suppression (Nieman, 1994) and may acquire more infections perhaps due to increased exposure rates (Shephard, 1984).

PSYCHO-SOCIAL DIMENSIONS

The involvement of girls in sport is largely impacted by the attitudes of parents and other role models (teachers, family). Unlike the involvement of boys that is largely impacted by their peer role models and social pressure, girls are subject to many influences both positive and negative. If parents support their involvement and encourage it rather than dampening it because of inappropriate cultural stereotypes (e.g., "tomboy"), then girls can benefit in many positive ways from sport and physical activity.

Self-Concept

Involvement in sport and physical activity directly affects the development of a child's self-concept and perception of self-esteem and competence. Physical activities provide a wonderful arena for girls to test their abilities to solve problems, learn new skills, and find ways to account for success and failure. They are a fundamental source of opportunities to challenge oneself, take risks and develop skills that may lead to higher self-esteem (Jaffee & Wu, 1996).

Most girls participate in sport to have fun, improve skills, be with friends and become physically fit while enjoying the challenges and being successful (Weiss & Petlichkoff, 1989). In particular, when motivation to participate in sport was examined, Gill (1992) found three different reasons: competitiveness, win orientation and goal orientation. Girls seem to be higher in goal orientation or the desire to achieve personal goals while boys seem to be more motivated by winning. Girls accomplish these goals by learning to cooperate with one another (Garcia, 1994) and therefore probably continue to foster an intrinsic motivation toward participation (Gill, 1992).

The motivation to cooperate in learning skills and developing physical fitness presents an interesting challenge to organized sport and physical education. Many girls prefer activities which allow them to work together to improve, or to function cooperatively to accomplish goals (Jaffee & Manzer, 1992), rather than competitive activities such as physical fitness testing (Wiese-Björnstal, 1997). It is therefore important to structure daily physical education experiences to provide motivation for children who have both goal and win orientations.

There appears to be a strong interaction between how girls perceive their success in sport and how others influence that perception. During early years, both boys and girls are about equal in terms of physical skills and rely on adult comments (especially parents) to help them judge their competency until about age 10 (Weiss & Ebbeck, 1996).

Between 10 and 14 years of age peers become the primary source of validation for their perception of personal skill. During adolescence there appears to emerge a gender difference such that girls rely on adults and their own self-comparisons, while boys seem to rely more on competitive outcomes, their ability to learn new skills and their own egocentric judgments of physical competence (Weiss & Ebbeck, 1996). These differences suggest the important role of parents, teachers and coaches in influencing girls' attitudes toward participation, and the concomitant psychological benefits they receive from participation in sport and physical activity.

Emotional Well-Being

Participation in sport and physical exercise has a positive effect on emotional well-being. Children who are depressed or having emotional problems benefit from increased levels of physical activity (Biddle, 1995), with benefits reported to lower levels of depression (Morgan, 1994) and general anxiety (Landers & Petruzzello, 1994). The effects of participation in an active lifestyle may have both a beneficial treatment effect, and also a palliative or buffering effect prior to any onset of emotional problems (Wiese-Björnstal, 1997).

We know that most children are healthiest and happiest when they have a sense of optimism and self-control. Sport and physical activity provide one medium for enhancing positive feelings about oneself, reducing depression (Biddle, 1995), increasing alertness, and decreasing tension and anxiety (Singer, 1992). The following are among the conclusions of the International Society of Sport Psychology and are based on examining the research literature regarding the influence of exercise on depression and anxiety (Singer, 1992):

- Exercise can help reduce anxiety
- Exercise can help decrease mild to moderate depression
- Long-term exercise can help reduce neuroticism and anxiety
- Exercise can help reduce various types of stress
- Exercise can have a beneficial emotional effect

The reasons for these benefits are very complex and may include both psycho-social effects (North, McCullogh & Tran, 1990) and biochemical mechanisms such as increased norepinephrine, serotonin or endogenous opioids (Greenberg & Oglesby, 1997), or the simple movement of large muscles which may be inconsistent with depression (Greist & Jefferson, 1992). In addition, regular exercise and its body composition benefits may also result in increased energy and improved sleep patterns (Martinsen & Stephens, 1994) and a general feeling of self-accomplishment for sticking to goals and developing new skills (Koniak-Griffin, 1994), which would reduce the sense of loss of control (often linked to depression). It has also been found that athletic participation in females reduces "some high-risk behaviors in adolescents, particularly suicide ideation" (Oler et al., 1994; p.784).

Caution should be taken if a "more is better" attitude is employed and involvement in physical activity is at an extreme. The incidence of burn-out in young athletes who participate in sport and physical activity to the exclusion of other aspects of their lives is alarming. When children are very competitively oriented, and place excess stress on themselves relative to winning or being successful (in other people's eyes), the stress and anxiety may rise to the point of withdrawal from the activity. This often happens when children feel that the demands are too great, and they lose the joy of participation which was their initial motivation. Gould (1993) has suggested that this may occur when there is constant or intense competition, too much adult pressure, high training demands (time and intensity) and competitive pressure, and the loss of personal control in making decisions about participation or training. In addition, children often place undue pressures on themselves and may become perfectionistic or overly concerned about pleasing others.

Social Competence

For children, understanding the social nature of life, learning to balance "pleasing others" with acting in your own best interests and respecting the rights of others are important aspects of maturing. Sport and exercise can provide a great venue for exploring strategies to resolve conflicts, act fairly, plan proactively, and to generally develop a moral code of behavior. Opportunities exist for children to experience their own decision-making and to observe other role models such as parents, coaches and other athletes and to get feedback about their own ethical behaviors (Martens, 1993). There are many opportunities for good moral development through sport and physical activity, especially when these opportunities are provided under adult guidance and structured to support positive growth and avoid the potential negative impact of antisocial behaviors (cheating, aggression and intimidation) that accompany some inappropriately competitive activities (Gibbons, Ebbeck & Weiss, 1995). Sport can be a great avenue for developing more mature moral reasoning skills that are characterized by more assertion and less aggression, and more compliance with rules and fair play (Stephens & Bredemeier, 1996). Some children love low levels of competition while others are psychologically ready for higher levels of competition when they want to compare their skills with others and when they can understand the competitive process (Passer, 1988).

In a thoughtful review of social development issues related to sport and physical activity, Wiese-Björnstal (1996) emphasized that one key to positive experiences for children is "the provision of quality, adult leadership that places high priority on the development of prosocial or ethical behavior in sport and physical activity settings" (p. 24) and develops reasonable expectations for children which leads to appropriate levels of challenge (and sometimes frustration) while building self-esteem and the capacity to meet new challenges (Brustad, 1993). Such leadership not only reinforces the positive benefits of sport participation, but can also reduce the negative influences which girls often feel toward their emerging gender identity.

As both girls and boys enter adolescence, they struggle with their own personal self-concept and gender identity. Most children are given social status by their peers by virtue of their skills (at sport, music, academics) but girls have historically also been subjected to social criteria related to physical appearance and their ability to interact with boys (Thorne, 1993). There is some hope that this is changing as all children learn to accept one another for their unique talents and as parents and other adults understand the important role of physical fitness and motor skills in the development of children. For example, high school girls who are athletes are beginning to perceive themselves as equally as popular as non-athletes in 83% of the cases (Women's Sports Foundation, 1989) and 87% of the parents are shifting to recognize the equal importance of sport participation for both girls and boys.

SUMMARY

Physical activity and sports involvement are important developmental opportunities for both boys and girls as they "learn to move and move to learn" about themselves, their bodies and their social contexts. Contributions include increased strength and power, better cardiovascular functioning, enhanced immune system responses, opportunities to develop moral reasoning, positive self-concepts and social interaction skills. There are, however, unique dimensions of the sport experience for girls in terms of physiological and psychological/emotional development and the challenges which sometimes exist between socially influenced expectations (i.e., idealized body physique) and the health benefits of regular exercise (body composition, body weight, menstrual functioning, etc.).

RECOMMENDATIONS AND CONCLUSIONS

- Children should participate in regular physical activity and sport experiences, especially in quality, adult supervised activities and daily physical education in schools.

- Opportunities should be provided which include both health-related fitness activities and skill building to enhance physical competence and life-long participation.

- A wide range of activities should be available, including both individual and group experiences and cooperative vs. competitive ones.

- Excessive exercise and training should be carefully monitored because it may be linked to amenorrhea, while excess emphasis on body physique may lead to disordered eating—the signs of these problems should be carefully attended to by adults.

- Moderate and regular physical activity can promote psychological and emotional well-being, including reduced depression.

- Equal and safe opportunities should be provided for both boys and girls to participate in a full range of physical fitness and sport activities.

REFERENCES

Armstrong. N., &Weissman, J.R. (1994). Assessment and interpretation of aerobic fitness in children and adolescents. In J.E. Holloszy (Ed.), *Exercise and Sport Science Review* (pp. 435–476). Philadelphia: Williams and Wilkins.

Bar-Or, O. & Malina, R.M. (1995). Activity, fitness, and heath of children and adolescents. In L.W. Y. Cheung & J.B. Richmond (Eds.), *Child health, nutrition, and physical activity* (pp. 79–123). Champaign, IL: Human Kinetics Publishers.

Berryman, J. (1996). The rise of boys sports in the United States, 1900–1970 In F. Smoll & R. Smith (Eds.). *Children and Youth in Sports: A Biopsychosocial Perspective*. Dubuque, IA: Brown and Benchmark.

Biddle, S. (1995). Exercise and psychosocial health. *Research Quarterly for Exercise and Sport, 66(4),* 292–297.

Blair, S. N., Horton, E., Leon, A.S., Lee. I. M., Drinkwater, B.L., Dishman, R.D., Mackey, M., & Keinholz, M.L. (1996). Physical activity, nutrition and chronic disease. *Medicine and Science in Sports and Exercise, 28,* 335–349.

Blimkie, C.J.R. (1989). Age and sex associated variation in strength during childhood: Anthropometric, morphologic, neurologic, biomechanical, endocrinologic, and physical activity correlates. In C.V. Gisolfi & D.R. Lamb (Eds.), *Perspectives in exercise science and sports medicine, 2: Youth exercise and sport* (pp. 99–163). Indianapolis: Benchmark.

Brustad, R.J. (1993). Youth in sports: Psychological considerations. In R.N. Singer, Murphey & L.K. Tenneant (Eds.) *Handbook of research on sports psychology.* (695–717). New York: Macmillan.

Fehily, A.M., Coles, R.J., Evans, W.D., Elwood, P.C. (1992). Factors affecting bone density in young adults, *American Journal of Clinical Nutrition, 56*: 579–586.

Freedson, P. & Bunker, L.K. (1997). Section I: Physiological dimensions. In the President's Council on Physical Fitness and Sport, *Physical Activity and Sport in the Lives of Girls* (pp. 1–16). Washington, DC: President's Council.

Garcia, C. (1994). Gender differences in young children's interactions when learning fundamental motor skills. *Research Quarterly for Exercise and Sport, 65(3),* 225.

Gibbons, S.L., Ebbeck, V., & Weiss, M.R. (1995). Fair play for kids: Effects on the moral development of children in physical education. *Research Quarterly for Exercise and Sport, 66(3),* 247–255.

Gill, D.L. (1992). Gender and sport behavior. In T.S. Horn (Ed.), *Advances in sport psychology* (pp. 143–160). Champaign, IL: Human Kinetics Publishers.

Gill, D.L. (1995). Gender issues: A social-educational perspective. In S.M. Murphy (Ed.), *Sport psychology interventions* (pp. 205–234). Champaign, IL: Human Kinetics Publishers.

Gould, D. (1993). Intensive sport participation and the prepubescent athlete: Competitive stress and burnout. In B.R. Cahill & A.J. Pearl (Eds.), *Intensive participation in children's sport* (pp. 19–38) Champaign, IL: Human Kinetics Publishers.

Greenberg, D. & Oglesby, C. (1997). Section IV: Mental heath dimensions. In the President's Council on Physical Fitness and Sport, *Physical Activity and Sport in the Lives of Girls* (pp. 1–16). Washington, DC: President's Council.

Greist, J.H. & Jefferson, J.W. (1992). *Depression and Its Treatment* (Rev. Ed.). Washington, DC: American Psychiatric Press.

Jaffee, L. & Manzer R. (1992). Girls' perspectives: Physical activity and self-esteem. *Melpomene: A Journal for Women's Health Research, 11(3),* 14–23.

Jaffee, L. & Wu, P. (1996). After school activities and self-esteem in adolescent girls. *Melpomene: A Journal for Women's Health Research, 15(2),* 18–25.

Koniak-Griffin, D. (1994). Aerobic exercise, psychological well-being, and physical discomforts during adolescent pregnancy. *Research in Nursing & Health, 17,* 253–263.

Kramer, M.M. & Wells, C.L. (1996). Does physical activity reduce risk of estrogen dependent cancer in women? *Medicine and Science in Sports and Exercise, 28,* 322–334.

Landers, D.M. & Petruzzello, S.J. (1994). Physical activity, fitness and anxiety. In C. Bouchard, R.J. Shepard, & T. Stephens (Eds.), *Physical activity, fitness and health* (pp. 868–882) Champaign, IL: Human Kinetics Publishers.

Martens, R. (1993). Psychological perspectives. In B.R. Cahill & A.J. Pead (Eds.), *Intensive participation in children's sports* (pp. 9–17). Champaign, IL: Human Kinetics Publishers.

Martinsen, E.W. & Stephens, T. (1994). Exercise and mental health in clinical and free-living populations. In R.K. Dishman (Ed.), *Advances in exercise adherence* (pp. 55–72). Champaign, IL: Human Kinetics Publishers.

Morgan, W.P. (1994) Physical activity, fitness and depression. In C. Bouchard, R.J. Shepard, & T. Stephens (Eds.), *Physical activity, fitness and health* (pp. 851–867). Champaign, IL: Human Kinetics Publishers.

National Cholesterol Education Program. (1991). *Report of the expert panel on blood cholesterol levels in children and adolescents* (NIH Publication No. 91-2732). Bethesda, MD: National Heart, Lung and Blood Institute.

National Federation of State High Schools Association (1995–96). *The National Federation of State High School Associations Handbook, 1995–96.* Kansas City, MO: NFSHSA.

Newsholme, E.A., & Parry-Billings, M. (1994). Effects of exercise on the immune system. In C. Bouchard, R.J. Shepherd, & T. Stephens (Eds.) *Physical activity, fitness and health: International proceedings and consensus statement* (pp. 451–455). Champaign, IL: Human Kinetics Publishers.

Nieman, D.C. (1994). Exercise, upper respiratory infection, and the immune system. *Medicine and Science in Sports and Exercise, 26,* 1057–1062.

North, T.C., McCullaugh, P., & Tran, Z.U. (1990). Effects of exercise on depression. *Exercise and Sport Science Reviews, 18,* 379–415.

Oler, M.J., Mainous III, A.G., Martin, C.A., Richardson, E., Haney, A., Wilson, D., & Adams, T. (1994). Depression, suicidal ideation, and substance use among adolescents: Are adolescents at less risk? *Archives of Family Medicine, 3,* 781–785.

Passer, M.W. (1988). Psychological issues in determining children's age readiness for competition. In F.L. Smoll, R.A. Magill, & M.J. Ash (Eds.). *Children in sports* (pp. 203–227).

Plaisted, V. (1995). Gender and sport. In T. Morris & J. Summers (Eds.), *Sport psychology: Theory, applications and issues* (pp. 538–574). New York: John Wiley & Sons.

President's Council on Physical Fitness and Sports (1997a). *Physical Activity and Sport in the Lives of Girls: Physical and Mental Health Dimensions from an Interdisciplinary Approach.* Washington, DC: Department of Health and Human Services.

President's Council on Physical Fitness and Sports (1997b). *Executive Summary of Physical Activity and Sport in the Lives of Girls: Physical and Mental Health Dimensions from an Interdisciplinary Approach.* Washington, DC: Department of Health and Human Services.

Reel, J.J. & Gill, D.L. (1996). Psychosocial factors related to eating disorders among high school and college female cheerleaders. *The Sport Psychologist, 10,* 195–206,

Sale, D.G. (1989). Strength training in children. In C.V. Gisolfi & D. R. Lam (Eds.). *Perspectives in exercise science and sports medicine, Vol. 2.: Youth, exercise and sport* (pp. 165–222). Indianapolis: Benchmark.

Sewall, L., & Michele, L.J. (1986). Strength training for children. *The Journal of Pediatric Orthopaedia Strabismus, 6,* 143–146.

Shephard, R.J. (1984). Physical activity and child health. *Sports Medicine, 1,* 205–233.

Singer, R.S. (1992). Physical activity and psychological benefits: A position statement of the International Society of Sport Psychology (ISSP). *The Sports Psychologist, 6,* 199–203.

Stager, J.M., Wigglesworth, J.K., & Hatler, L.H. (1990). Interpreting the relationship between age of menarche and prepubertal training. *Medicine and Science in Sports and Exercise, 22,* 54–58.

Stephens, D. & Bredemeier, B.J. (1996). Moral atmosphere and judgments about aggression in girls' soccer: Relationships among moral and motivational variables. *Journal of Sport and Exercise Physiology, 18(2),* 158–171.

Thome, B. (1993). *Gender play: Girls and boys in school.* New Brunswick, NJ: Rutgers University Press.

Weiss, M.R. & Ebbeck. V. (1996). Self-esteem and perceptions of competence in youth sports: Theory, research and enhancement strategies. In O. Bar-Or (Ed.), *The child and adolescent athlete* (pp. 364–382). Oxford, England: Blackwell Scientific Ltd.

Weiss, M.R., & Pettichkoff, L.M. (1989). Children's motivation for participation in and withdrawal from sport: Identifying the missing links. *Pediatric Exercise Science, 1,* 195–211.

Wells, C.L. (1991). *Women, sport and performance, 2ed.* Champaign, IL: Human Kinetics Publishers.

Wiese-Björnstal, D. (1997). Section II: Psychological dimensions. In the President's Council on Physical Fitness and Sport Report: *Physical Activity and Sport in the Lives of Girls* (pp. 49–69). Washington, DC: President's Council.

Williams, D.P., Going, S.B., Lohman, T.G., Harsha, D.W., Srinivasan, S.R., Webber, L.S., & Berenson, G.S. (1992). Body fatness and risk for elevated blood pressure, total cholesterol, and serum lipoprotein ratios in children and adolescents. *American Journal of Public Health, 82,* 358–363.

Women's Sports Foundation Report: *Minorities in sports* (1989). East Meadow, NY: Women's Sports Foundation.

Physical Activity and Ergogenic Aids

In the single paper included here, Melvin Williams gives an excellent review of activity and ergonomic aids.

Topic 22 Nutritional Ergogenics and Sports Performance

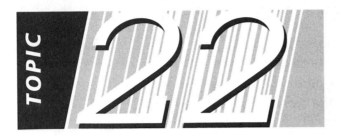

Nutritional Ergogenics and Sports Performance

Melvin H. Williams
Old Dominion University

A NOTE FROM THE EDITORS

The PCPFS *Research Digest* often focuses primarily on physical activity as it relates to good health and fitness. In this topic, we deviate a bit from that traditional theme. We asked Dr. Mel Williams to write about nutritional ergogenics and sport performance because the use of nutritional products in attempts to increase performance has become so widespread. We thought it was important to provide readers with a review of the latest evidence on these various products alleged to enhance performance.

This review shows that there is evidence to support the performance enhancement of a few supplements, but to use Dr. Williams's words " . . . supplementation with various essential nutrients or commercial dietary supplements will NOT, in general, enhance exercise performance in well-nourished and physically active individuals."

As editors, we solicited this paper for a second reason. Many non-athletes interested in increasing muscle mass or reducing body fat levels look to athletes for advice on dietary supplements. Even though they are not particularly interested in performance enhancement, they will mimic the behaviors of high profile athletes using the strategy ". . . if they use it, it must be good." This paper allows teachers, coaches, fitness leaders, and all other readers to find out the facts about dietary supplements. While some of the information in this paper is somewhat technical, Dr. Williams has made every effort to provide the information in a format that is easy to understand. Table 22.1 provides a good summary of the evidence available for the dietary supplements discussed in this paper.

INTRODUCTION

Most individuals participate in mild to moderate physical activity to improve their physical appearance or health. Many others, however, engage in high-intensity physical activity to prepare for sport performance. They are athletes.

Whatever the level of competition, be it for an Olympic gold medal or an age-group award in a local road race, the two major keys to successful athletic performance are genetic endowment and

Originally published as Series 3, Number 2, of the PCPFS Research Digest.

"First and foremost, a varied, healthful diet balanced in energy and nutrient content is the nutritional mainstay for most athletes. Although research suggests that a few forms of nutrient supplementation may enhance physical performance under specific circumstances, such supplements should complement a healthful diet, not substitute for it."

proper training. In order to optimize the genetic potential of the elite athlete, scientists at the United States Olympic Training Center design specific individualized physiological training programs to increase physical power, psychological training programs to enhance mental strength, and biomechanical training programs to provide a mechanical edge. Many of these training strategies are increasingly available to nonelite athletes to help increase their ability to perform their best athletically within their genetic potential.

Although there are multiple purposes for engaging in sport, one of the primary objectives of athletic competition is supremacy, to win the contest. The most appropriate means to achieve this objective is optimal physiological, psychological, and biomechanical training. However, some athletes believe that they have maximized their ability to improve their sport performance through training and may seek other methods to gain a competitive edge on their opponents.

Ergogenic aids, or ergogenics, are substances, strategies or treatments that are theoretically designed to improve physical performance above and beyond the effects of normal training. Some ergogenics are used during training to enhance the training effect over time, while others are used just before or during the sport event to provide an immediate competitive edge. In general, ergogenics are designed to enhance the athlete's physical power (physiological ergogenics), mental strength (psychological ergogenics), or mechanical edge (mechanical ergogenics).

Physiological ergogenics, particularly pharmacological and nutritional substances, are designed to increase physical power by enhancement of metabolic processes involved in energy production during exercise. For example, anabolic/androgenic steroids (drugs) and creatine monohydrate (nonessential nutrient) have both been used in attempts to increase strength and power.

Psychological ergogenics are devised to enhance mental strength by favorably affecting psychological processes before or during competition. For example, hypnosis and mental imagery have been used to induce psychological sensations of relaxation or stimulation, depending on the nature of the sport.

Mechanical ergogenics are used to provide a mechanical edge by improving energy efficiency. For example, a skintight racing suit will reduce wind resistance and help increase velocity at a given energy expenditure during sports such as downhill skiing and speed skating.

Within the regulations of the specific sport, use of most psychological and mechanical ergogenics is legal. However, use of many physiological ergogenics, particularly drugs and methods such as blood doping, is prohibited because they may provide an unfair competitive advantage or pose serious health risks to the athlete. A comprehensive list of prohibited substances and methods is available from the United States Olympic Committee (1996). Conversely, use of most nutritional substances is legal, and literally hundreds of dietary supplements have been promoted as ergogenic aids for sports performance. Table 22.1 provides a partial listing of individual nutrients or nutritional products that have been studied or marketed for their ergogenic potential. However, some commercial products include multiple ingredients. For example, Up Your Gas, advertised as a natural energy pill, includes the following among its many ingredients: Bee pollen, Cayenne Pepper, Ginkgo Biloba, Guarana, lnosine, Kola Nut, Korean ginseng, Niacin, Octacosanol, Spirulina blue-green algae, Vitamin E, and Yerba Mate.

First and foremost, a varied, healthful diet balanced in energy and nutrient content is the nutritional mainstay for most athletes. Sports nutritionists contend that athletes should obtain the energy and nutrients they need through wise selections within and among the various food groups,

TABLE 22.1 ▌▋▌ ▌▐▐▋▋▋ ▋▋ ▐▋▋▋▋▐ ▐▐ ▋▐▐▐ ▐▋▐ ▐▐ ▐▐▋▋▐▐ ▐▋▐▐▐▐▋▋▐▐ ▐▐ ▐▐▐▐ ▐▐▐▐ ▐▐ ▐▐ ▐▋▐▐▐▐ ▐▐ ▐▐▐▐▐ ▐▐

Efficacy of some purported nutritional ergogenics.

Nutritional ergogenics may be used in attempts to enhance physical power, mental strength, and mechanical edge for various sports. Research support for nutritional ergogenics may be classified as strong (meaning studies generally support effectiveness), uncertain (meaning some positive findings are available, but confirming research is needed), or weak (meaning little or no positive data are available). The following is a brief summary of the research-based efficacy of some purported nutritional ergogenics on physical power (PP), mental strength (MS), or mechanical edge (ME) in well-nourished subjects.

Strong evidence

Alkaline salts:	PP	aerobic endurance
Caffeine:	PP	aerobic endurance
Carbohydrates:	PP	aerobic endurance
Creatine:	PP	muscular strength
Water:	PP	aerobic endurance during heat stress conditions

Uncertain evidence

Alcohol:	MS	neuromuscular relaxation
Antioxidants:	ME	muscle tissue damage prevention
Aspartates:	PP	aerobic endurance
Choline:	PP	aerobic endurance
Dihydroxyacetone pyruvate:	PP	aerobic endurance
Glycerol:	PP	aerobic endurance
Phosphates:	PP	aerobic endurance
Vitamin E:	PP	aerobic endurance at altitude
Vitamins B1,B6, B12:	MS	neuromuscular relaxation

Weak evidence

Amino acids
  Arginine, ornithine, lysine
  Branched-chain (leucine, isoleucine, valine)
  Glutamine
  Glycine
  Tryptophan
Bee pollen
Carnitine (L-carnitine)
Ciwujia (Endurox)
Coenzyme Q_{10}, (Ubiquinone)
Conjugated linoleic acid (CLA)
Dehydroepiandrosterone (DHEA)
Ephedrine, ephedra (Ma Huang)
Fructose 1,6-diphosphate
Gamma oryzanol (Ferulic acid, FRAC)
Ginkgo biloba
Ginseng
Inosine
Medium chain triglycerides (MCTS)

Minerals
  Boron
  Chromium
  Iron
  Selenium
  Vanadium
Octacosanol
Omega-3 fatty acids
Polylactate
Protein
Smilax officianalis
Vitamins
  B-complex
    Thiamin (B_1)
    Riboflavin (B_2)
    Niacin
    Pyridoxine (B_6)
    Cyanocobalamin (B_{12})
    Folacin
    Pantothenic acid
  Antioxidants
    Beta carotene
    Vitamin C
Vitamin B_{15}
Wheat germ oil
Yohimbine (Yohimbe)

including whole grains, fruits, vegetables, and meat and milk products. Dietary supplements are designed to complement a balanced, healthful diet, not substitute for it.

The purpose of this review is to provide a broad overview of selected individual nutrients and dietary supplements purported to possess ergogenic properties. Space does not permit a detailed analysis of all specific studies, so most of the references cited are either principal studies or review papers that may provide the interested reader with more detail.

CARBOHYDRATE AND CARBOHYDRATE METABOLITES

Carbohydrate is the primary dietary energy source for high-intensity aerobic endurance exercise (>65–70% VO_2max), but endogenous supplies such as muscle and liver glycogen are limited and may become suboptimal within 90 minutes. Carbohydrate loading procedures may elevate endogenous glycogen stores, postponing fatigue and improving performance in which a set distance is covered as quickly as possible (such as a marathon) by 2–3 percent (Hawley et al., 1997). Additionally, numerous studies support the efficacy of carbohydrate supplementation prior to and/or during such prolonged aerobic exercise tasks to improve performance (Williams, 1998b).

Metabolic by-products of carbohydrate are theorized to provide a more efficient fuel than other carbohydrate sources. Several well-controlled studies by researchers at the University of Pittsburgh have shown that pyruvate, administered as dihydroxyacetone and pyruvate (DHAP), may increase muscle glycogen levels or blood glucose uptake by exercising muscles and enhance exercise performance in untrained subjects. However, these findings have not been duplicated by other scientists and the ergogenic effect of pyruvate for trained athletes is questionable (Anderson, 1997; Williams, 1998b). Other metabolites, such as fructose 1,6-diphosphate and lactate salts (polylactate) do not provide any ergogenic effect beyond that provided by more natural carbohydrate sources, such as glucose (Swensen et al., 1994; Williams, 1998b).

LIPIDS AND LIPID METABOLITES

Lipids represent an energy source for mild-to-moderate intensity aerobic endurance exercise (< 50-65% VO_2max), but unlike carbohydrate, endogenous stores of lipids as adipose and muscle tissue triglycerides are abundant. Triglycerides provide free fatty acids (FFA), the primary lipid energy source during exercise. Lipid dietary strategies or supplements attempt to increase FFA oxidation and reduce reliance on endogenous carbohydrate stores, sparing muscle glycogen use and delaying fatigue during prolonged exercise. Other supplements, such as L-carnitine and caffeine supplementation (discussed below) are theorized to exert similar effects.

Fat loading is a dietary strategy involving increased consumption of dietary fats, up to 70 percent of daily energy intake, in attempts to increase the contribution of endogenous fats as an energy source during exercise. Several preliminary studies have shown some beneficial effects of fat loading, but either the experimental design was not appropriate or the exercise tasks used do not appear to have any application to contemporary sports events (Williams, 1998b). In a major review, Sherman and Leenders (1995) noted that although the fat loading hypothesis is intriguing, the current scientific literature is not supportive.

Medium-chain triglycerides (MCT), oral water soluble supplements that may enter the circulation more readily than normal dietary fats, have been theorized to be a more efficient lipid energy source during exercise. However, recent research by scientists from the Netherlands has not shown any significant contribution of oral MCT to energy metabolism during exercise, and two recent studies have shown that MCT supplementation could actually impair 40-kilometer cycling performance (Williams, 1998b). Nevertheless, in a recent review, Berning (1996) noted that some preliminary research findings were promising, particularly when MCT were ingested with carbohydrate supplements during exercise. Confirming research is needed.

PROTEINS, AMINO ACIDS, AND RELATED METABOLITES

Protein supplements have been recommended to athletes to enhance nitrogen retention and increase lean body (muscle) mass, to prevent protein catabolism during prolonged exercise, and to support an increased synthesis of hemoglobin, myoglobin, oxidative enzymes, and mitochondria during aerobic training. Current research suggests that athletes may need slightly more protein than the Recommended Dietary Allowance (RDA). Values suggested for strength-type athletes approximate 1.6–1.8 grams per kilogram body weight, while recommended amounts for endurance athletes approximate 1.2–1.6 grams per kilogram body weight (Lemon, 1996; 1995). Such values may be obtained easily in a typical Western diet with adequate animal and plant protein. In general, research with protein supplements in excess of these dietary quantities has shown no beneficial effects on strength, power, hypertrophy of muscle, or physiological work capacity (Williams, 1998b).

Amino acid supplements have also been marketed to increase muscle mass and enhance aerobic endurance capacity via various mechanisms.

Arginine and ornithine have been used in attempts to increase human growth hormone (HGH) and/or insulin production, the theory being to increase muscle mass and strength via enhanced hormonal activity. Limited data are available, but a number of well-controlled studies, including several with experienced weightlifters, reported that amino acid supplementation elicited no significant increases in serum HGH, insulin levels, or various measures of muscular strength or power (Fogelholm, 1993; Kreider et al., 1993; Williams, 1998b).

Potassium and magnesium aspartates are salts of aspartic acid, an amino acid. They have been used as ergogenics, possibly by mitigating the accumulation of ammonia during exercise. The effect of aspartate supplementation on physical performance is equivocal, but about 50 percent of the available studies have indicated enhanced performance (Williams, 1998a). Additional research is needed to study their potential ergogenicity and underlying mechanisms.

Tryptophan (TRYP) and branched chain amino acids (BCAA) are thought to affect the formation of serotonin, a neurotransmitter believed to be involved in the etiology of central nervous system (CNS) fatigue during exercise. However, according to proponents of either TRYP or BCAA supplementation, the hypotheses underlying the serotonin effect on the development of fatigue are diametrically opposite.

In one hypothesis, TRYP serves as a precursor for serotonin, a brain neurotransmitter theorized to suppress pain. Free tryptophan (fTRYP) enters the brain cells to form serotonin. Thus, TRYP supplementation has been used to increase fTRYP and serotonin production in attempts to increase tolerance to pain during intense exercise, thus delaying fatigue. Limited data involving TRYP supplementation are available, but one study reported significant improvements in time to exhaustion at 80 percent VO_2max, accompanied by significant reductions in the psychological rating of perceived exertion (RPE). However, research with a more appropriate experimental design did not replicate these findings when subjects ran to exhaustion at 100 percent VO_2max. Moreover, other investigators reported no effect of TRYP supplementation on aerobic endurance performance at 70–75 percent VO_2max (Williams, 1998b). In a recent review, Wagenmakers (1997) concluded that TRYP supplementation had no effect on endurance performance.

Relative to the second hypothesis, some investigators believe that increased levels of serotonin may induce fatigue by depressing central nervous system functions (Newsholme et al., 1992). During prolonged aerobic endurance exercise, muscle glycogen may become depleted and the muscle may increase its reliance on branched chain amino acids (BCAA) for fuel, decreasing the plasma BCAA: fTRYP ratio. Because BCAA compete with fTRYP for entry into the brain, a low BCAA:fTRYP ratio would facilitate the entry of fTRYP to the brain, increasing serotonin formation and inducing fatigue. Hypothetically, BCAA supplementation may delay fatigue in prolonged aerobic endurance events by maintaining a high BCAA:fTRYP ratio to mitigate the formation of serotonin. Although several studies support this hypothesis both Wagenmakers (1997) and Davis (1996), in recent reviews, concluded not enough evidence indicates BCAA supplementation is ergogenic. Davis also noted that carbohydrate supplementation during exercise, by delaying the reliance on BCAA as a fuel, would serve the same purpose as BCAA supplementation.

VITAMINS

Research indicates that a vitamin deficiency may adversely affect physical performance, but the overall review of the literature supports the viewpoint that vitamin supplements are unnecessary for physically-active individuals who are on a well-balanced diet with adequate calories. Most studies report that athletes who consume high calorie diets containing the RDA of all nutrients have few vitamin or mineral deficiencies (Armstrong & Maresh, 1996). Several excellent studies have shown that multivitamin/mineral supplementation over prolonged periods, up to eight months, have no significant effects on both laboratory and sport-specific tests of physical performance (Singh et al., 1992; Telford et al., 1992). Nevertheless, vitamin/ mineral supplementation may be recommended for athletes consuming a low-calorie diet for weight control sports (Williams, 1998b).

Some studies have shown that specific vitamin supplements may benefit sports performance in events where excess anxiety may be disruptive. For example, thiamin (B_1), pyridoxine (B_6), and cobalamin (B_{12}) supplementation has been shown to enhance performance in pistol shooting, possibly because of beneficial effects on brain neurotransmitter functions (Bonke, 1986). Additional research is merited.

Supplementation with several antioxidant vitamins (beta-carotene, vitamin C, vitamin E) has been theorized to prevent muscle tissue damage associated with generation of oxygen free radicals during high-intensity exercise. However, recent reviews suggest that research regarding the value of antioxidant therapy for athletes is ambivalent. Some reviewers (Goldfarb, 1993; Kanter, 1995) note that further investigations are needed to determine the viability of antioxidant supplements in preventing exercise-induced lipid peroxidation and muscle damage. Conversely, other reviewers (Dekkers et al., 1996; Packer, 1997) indicate substantial research suggests that dietary supplementation with antioxidant vitamins has favorable effects on lipid peroxidation and exercise-induced muscle damage. All reviewers indicate more research is needed to address this issue and to provide guidelines for recommendations to athletes.

Antioxidant vitamins, particularly vitamins C and E, have also been theorized to enhance sport performance. Although vitamin C supplementation has been shown to improve physical performance in vitamin C-deficient subjects, research supports the general conclusion that vitamin C supplementation does not enhance physical performance in well-nourished individuals (Gerster, 1989). Vitamin E supplementation may increase tissue or serum vitamin E concentration, but a recent review indicates that there is no discernable effect on training or performance in either recreational or elite athletes (Tiidus & Houston, 1995). Nevertheless, Packer (1997) indicates that if antioxidant supplementation ameliorates exercise-induced muscle tissue damage, such supplementation may be beneficial in the long term. Additionally, some studies have shown that vitamin E supplementation may enhance exercise performance at altitude, but confirming research is needed (Williams, 1998b).

MINERALS

As with vitamins, research indicates that a mineral deficiency may adversely affect physical performance. Iron deficiency is the most common mineral deficiency among athletes, particularly female athletes in weight-control sports, and curing an athlete's iron-deficiency anemia with iron supplementation will return performance to normal. However, in general, research also indicates that mineral supplements, including multivitamin/mineral compounds, are unnecessary for physically-active individuals who are on a well-balanced diet with adequate calories.

Several minerals have been marketed as potent anabolic agents. Chromium is an insulin cofactor, and its theorized ergogenic effect is based on the role of insulin to facilitate BCAA transport into the muscle. Chromium has been advertised for strength-type athletes. The available research with chromium is limited, and the data available have not been subjected to a critical scientific review. Some early research data do suggest an increase in lean body mass and decreased body fat with chromium picolinate supplementation (Evans, 1989). However, this report was based on flawed studies. More contemporary research with better experimental protocols replicated these studies and have shown that chromium picolinate supplementation does not increase lean muscle mass or decrease body fat (Clancy et al., 1994; Hallmark et al., 1996; Trent & Thieding-Cancel, 1995). Other research also indicated different forms of chromium, such as chromium chloride, had no effect on body composition (Lukaski et al., 1996).

Boron and vanadium have also been advertised for their anabolic potential. However, the limited data available do not support an anabolic effect of either boron (Ferrando and Green, 1993) or vanadium (Fawcett et al., 1996).

Phosphorus is an essential nutrient present in the diet as a phosphate salt, or phosphate. Phosphate is a component of several high energy compounds, is essential for the functioning of several B vitamins, and is part of 2,3-DPG, essential for oxygen release from hemoglobin. An increased 2,3-DPG level is the prevalent theory underlying phosphate supplementation to endurance athletes. Current research is equivocal as to whether or not phosphate loading may improve physiological functions important to endurance performance. However, no study has reported decreases in performance, and several recent studies from independent laboratories have shown remarkable similarities relative to increased levels of VO_2max (about 10%) following phosphate supplementation. Increases in physical performance have also been documented in four of these studies (Cade et al., 1984; Kreider et al., 1990; Kreider et al., 1992; Stewart et al., 1990). However, a number of confounding variables in previous research have been identified and more controlled research has been recommended (Tremblay et al., 1994).

FOOD DRUGS

Although doping (the use of pharmacological ergogenics to improve sports performance) is prohibited, the International Olympic Committee does permit limited use of several nutritionally-related drugs, such as caffeine, alcohol, and alkaline salts.

Caffeine, found naturally in certain foods or beverages, such as cocoa, coffee, and cola drinks, consumed by athletes, has been studied extensively for its ergogenic potential. Caffeine is a stimulant that may improve various metabolic and psychological functions during exercise, and several recent reviews indicate that legal doses of caffeine may enhance performance in a variety of exercise tasks (Graham and Spriet, 1996; Spriet, 1995). Many studies that have evaluated the ergogenic effect of caffeine on prolonged aerobic endurance tasks greater than one hour have shown beneficial effects. For example, a series of studies from Guelph University in Canada has suggested caffeine may enhance prolonged aerobic endurance performance through increased levels of epinephrine and sparing of muscle glycogen (Graham & Spriet, 1991; Spriet et al., 1992). Other recent research suggests caffeine may exert an ergogenic effect in shorter endurance events through neurological mechanisms. For example, caffeine supplementation has been shown to improve performance in a 1,500-meter run, an event which is not dependent on muscle glycogen sparing (Wiles et al., 1992), and caffeine supplementation also has increased work output on a cycle ergometer at a set RPE (Cole et al., 1996). Because caffeine appears to be an effective ergogenic in legal doses, some investigators have suggested the IOC should reconsider the legal limits determinant for a positive drug test (Spriet, 1995).

Alkaline salts, such as sodium bicarbonate and sodium citrate, are described as antacids in the United States Pharmacopeia (USP) and have been studied as nutritional ergogenics. Taken orally prior to high-intensity anaerobic exercise, alkaline salts may increase the alkaline reserve and help buffer lactic acid in the muscle cell, an effect that theoretically could improve performance in exercise tasks dependent primarily on anaerobic glycolysis. Research indicates that alkaline salt supplementation will increase the serum pH and may enhance performance in exercise tasks, particularly repetitive exercise tasks, that maximize energy production for 1–6 minutes. Numerous laboratory and field studies support a positive ergogenic effect of sodium bicarbonate supplementation, and several comprehensive reviews (Linderman & Fahey, 1991; Williams, 1992), including a meta-analysis reporting an effect size greater than 0.40 favoring sodium bicarbonate when compared to placebo conditions (Matson & Tran, 1993), conclude that sodium bicarbonate is an effective ergogenic. Studies conducted subsequent to these reviews have provided mixed results but, in general, about half of these more recent studies have revealed ergogenic effects of sodium bicarbonate or sodium citrate on exercise performance. Some beneficial effects have even been noted on prolonged aerobic endurance tasks, a finding that merits additional research (Williams, 1998b).

DIETARY SUPPLEMENTS

Numerous dietary supplements are marketed to physically-active individuals. Advertisements insinuate that such supplements may improve energy production, increase muscle mass, decrease body fat, or induce some other possible ergogenic outcome. By and large, many commercial products have not been studied scientifically to validate such advertising claims. However, some data are available for several specific ingredients marketed individually or as part of a multiple-ingredient product.

Choline

Choline, an amine, is found naturally in a variety of foods. A sports drink powder containing carbohydrates, electrolytes, and choline has been marketed recently.

Choline is involved in the formation of acetylcholine, a neurotransmitter whose reduction in the nervous system may be theorized to be a contributing factor to the development of fatigue. Because plasma choline levels have been reported to be significantly reduced following events such as marathon running, choline supplementation has been theorized to prevent fatigue in aerobic endurance tasks. Research has shown that choline supplementation will increase blood choline levels at rest and during prolonged exercise, and some preliminary field and laboratory research has suggested increased plasma choline levels are associated with a significantly decreased time to run 20 miles. However, other well-controlled laboratory research has revealed that choline supplementation, although increasing plasma choline levels, exerted no effect on either brief, high-intensity anaerobic cycling tests or more prolonged aerobic exercise tasks (Williams, 1998b). These findings are equivocal and reviewers have recommended more research with choline supplementation, particularly research involving prolonged aerobic endurance exercise tasks (Kanter & Williams, 1995).

Coenzyme Q_{10} (Ubiquinone)

Coenzyme Q_{10} (CoQ_{10}), also known asubiqui-none, is a lipid with characteristics common to a vitamin. CoQ_{10} is found in the mitochondria in all tissues, particularly the heart and skeletal muscles. CoQ_{10} is also an antioxidant. CoQ_{10} supplementation has been used therapeutically for the treatment of cardiovascular disease because it may improve oxygen uptake in the mitochondria of the heart. Theoretically, improved oxygen usage in the heart and skeletal muscles could improve aerobic endurance performance.

Although research data suggests CoQ_{10} supplementation may benefit cardiac patients, several studies have shown that CoQ_{10} supplementation to healthy young or older physically-active subjects did not influence lipid peroxidation, heart rate, VO_2max, or cycling endurance performance (Braun, et al., 1991; Laaksonen et al., 1995; Snider et al., 1992; Weston et al., 1997). One study reported that CoQ_{10} supplementation was associated with muscle tissue damage and actually impaired cycling performance compared to the placebo treatment (Malm et al., 1996).

Creatine

Creatine is a nitrogen-containing substance, found naturally in small amounts in animal foods. Acute oral creatine supplementation, daily as creatine monohydrate for approximately 5–7 days, has been reported to increase muscle concentrations of total creatine, both as free creatine and creatine phosphate, a high-energy phosphagen. Several reviews indicate creatine supplementation may be an effective sport ergogenic (Balsom et al., 1994; Green-

haff, 1995). Subsequent to these reviews, numerous studies have reported a positive ergogenic effect of creatine supplementation, particularly in repetitive, short-duration, high-intensity, short-recovery isokinetic and isometric resistance tests or cycle ergometer protocols. However, in such tests, although some body parts are exercising, the total body mass is stationary. Thus, the ergogenic effect of acute creatine supplementation may be limited to laboratory tasks in which the body mass does not need to be moved.

Acute creatine supplementation also appears to increase body mass (Williams & Branch, 1998). In exercise tasks in which the body mass is moved, research generally has not supported an ergogenic effect of creatine supplementation on sprint swim performance (Burke et al., 1996) or sprint run performance (Redondo et al., 1996), and actually may be ergolytic (impair performance) in endurance running because of the acute increase in body mass (Balsom et al., 1993), which may simply be water associated with the oncotic effect of creatine in the muscle. Creatine supplementation has been shown to improve rowing performance (Rossiter et al., 1996), an exercise task in which the body mass is supported, and may theoretically enhance performance in cycling tasks for similar reasons.

Although acute creatine supplementation may enhance exercise performance under certain laboratory conditions, more research is needed to evaluate its efficacy to enhance actual sports performance. Additionally, well-controlled research is needed to evaluate the effect of chronic creatine supplementation on the training response and subsequent competitive sport performance.

Ginseng

Extracts derived from the plant family Araliaceae contain numerous chemicals that may influence human physiology, the most important being the glycosides, or ginsenosides. Collectively, these extracts are referred to as ginseng. Numerous commercial forms of ginseng products are available, including Chinese or Korean (Panax ginseng), American (Panax quinquefolium), and Russian/Siberian (Eleutherococcus senticosus), but the ginseng content may vary considerably (Cui et al., 1994).

Ginseng supplementation has been theorized to mitigate the stress of exercise and possess ergogenic qualities, but the underlying mechanisms have not been determined. Although some earlier studies reported ergogenic effects of ginseng supplementation on exercise performance, a recent comprehensive review by Bahrke and Morgan (1994) indicated that ginseng research with humans has been characterized by numerous methodological and statistical shortcomings. They concluded, in 1994, that there is an absence of compelling research evidence demonstrating the ability of ginseng to consistently enhance physical performance in humans, and that there remains a need for well-designed research.

Several well-controlled studies subsequent to the review by Bahrke and Morgan reported no significant effect of either Panax ginseng, Eleutherococcus senticosus Maxim L (regarded to be Siberian Ginseng), or a standardized ginseng extract on cardiovascular, metabolic, or psychologic responses to either submaximal or maximal exercise performance, or on maximal performance capacity (Dowling et al., 1996; Engels & Wirth, 1997; Morris et al., 1996).

Glycerol

Water ingestion is essential to help optimize body water balance and body temperature regulation during exercise under warm environmental conditions. Rehydration during exercise in the heat has been shown to decrease physiological stress as evidenced by a decreased heart rate response, lesser rise in the core temperature, and increase endurance performance. Hyperhydration before exercise may also be helpful, but has not been shown to be as effective as rehydration (Williams, 1998b). Glycerol (glycerin), an alcohol byproduct of fat hydrolysis, has been studied as a means to enhance the hyperhydration effect. Small amounts of glycerol are mixed with water in set proportions and the water is consumed following normal hyperhydration procedures. Glycerol capsules and a glycerol-containing sports drink are marketed to athletes.

Glycerol-induced hyperhydration, when compared to water hyperhydration alone, has been shown to increase total body water in some (Freund et al., 1995; Koenigsberg et al., 1995), but not all (Latzka et al., 1997) studies. Several studies have shown that glycerol-induced hyperhydration improves cardiovascular responses, temperature regulation, and cycling exercise performance under warm/hot environmental conditions (Lyons et al., 1990; Montner et al., 1996). However, other research has shown that both glycerol and carbohydrate supplementation improved cycling endurance compared to a placebo solution, suggesting carbohydrate supplementation was as effective as glycerol supplementation as a means to enhance performance (Lamb et al., 1997). Additional research is needed to resolve these equivocal findings, particularly so in sports such as distance running in which the extra body mass (water weight) must be moved as efficiently as possible.

Inosine

Inosine is a nucleoside with a variety of proposed ergogenic effects, including enhancement of aerobic endurance performance by facilitating the delivery of oxygen to the muscles during exercise. Although scientific research is limited, two well-controlled studies did use the recommended supplementation protocol for endurance athletes and reported no beneficial effects of inosine on cardio-vascular-respiratory or metabolic functions during submaximal or maximal exercise, nor was there any effect on time to complete a simulated three mile race on a treadmill. Both studies actually suggested inosine could be ergolytic for certain athletic endeavors involving anaerobic glycolysis (Starling et al., 1996; Williams et al., 1990).

L-carnitine

L-carnitine is a vitamin-like compound found naturally in animal foods, particularly meats, and may also be formed in the liver from various amino acids. L-carnitine facilitates the transport of fatty acids into the mitochondria for oxidation and also facilitates the oxidation of several amino acids and pyruvate, functions that theoretically could lead to a sparing of muscle glycogen during exercise and a decreased production of lactate. However, recent reviews of the available research do not support an ergogenic effect of L-carnitine supplementation on fuel utilization during exercise, maximal heart rate, anaerobic threshold, maximal oxygen uptake, time to exhaustion in various anaerobic or aerobic exercise tasks, or performance in either a marathon or 20-kilometer run (Heinonen, 1996; Wagenmakers, 1991; Williams, 1998b).

SUMMARY

Adequate dietary intake of carbohydrate, essential fatty acids, protein, vitamins, minerals and water is necessary to insure optimal physical performance, because a deficiency of any essential nutrient associated with energy production may impair physiological or psychological functions during exercise. As may be discerned from this review, supplementation with various essential nutrients or commercial dietary supplements will not, in general, enhance exercise performance in well-nourished, physically-active individuals. However, research tends to support an ergogenic effect for some nutritional ergogenics (including alkaline salts, caffeine, carbohydrate loading, and creatine) under certain conditions or for some athletes. Additional research is needed to evaluate the possible ergogenic effects of aspartate salts, choline, glycerol, MCT, phosphates, pyruvate, and certain vitamins (antioxidants; B_1, B_6, B_{12}; E) for specific conditions mentioned above.

Caution is advised when using any nutritional ergogenic in an attempt to enhance sport performance. As noted above, some products may impair performance. Also, improper amounts may cause various health problems. For example, supplements such as alkaline salts may cause gastrointestinal distress and diarrhea while others, such as ephedrine, have been associated with fatalities. Individuals who desire to use specific nutritional ergogenics should consult a sports nutrition expert or physician, and also experiment with their use in training before use in competition.

REFERENCES

Anderson, O. (1997). Pyruvate: Good for the alcoholic, the diabetic, the obese person—and the marathon runner? *Running Research News, 13* (10), 1, 9–11.

Armstrong, L., & Maresh, C. (1996). Vitamin and mineral supplements as nutritional aids to exercise performance and health. *Nutrition Reviews, 54,* S148–S158.

Bahrke, M., and Morgan, W. (1994). Evaluation of the ergogenic properties of ginseng. *Sports Medicine, 18,* 229–248.

Balsom, P., et al. (1994). Creatine in humans with special reference to creatine supplementation. *Sports Medicine, 18,* 268–280.

Balsom, P., et al. (1993). Creatine supplementation per se does not enhance endurance exercise performance. *Acta Physiologica Scandinavica, 149,* 521–523.

Berning, J. (1996). The role of medium-chain triglycerides in exercise. *International Journal of Sport Nutrition, 6,* 121–133.

Bonke, D. (1986). Influence of vitamin B1, B6, and B12 on the control of fine motoric movements. *Bibliotheca Nutritio et Dieta, 38,* 104–109.

Braun, B., et al. (1991). The effect of coenzyme Q_{10} supplementation on exercise performance, VO_2max, and lipid peroxidation in trained cyclists. *International Journal of Sport Nutrition, 1,* 353–365.

Burke, L., et al. (1996). Effect of oral creatine supplementation on single-effort sprint performance in elite swimmers. *International Journal of Sport Nutrition, 6,* 222–233.

Cade, R., et al. (1984). Effects of phosphate loading on 2,3 - diphosphoglycerate and maximal oxygen uptake. *Medicine and Science in Sports and Exercise, 16,* 263–268.

Clancy, S., et al. (1994). Effects of chromium picolinate supplementation on body composition, strength, and urinary chromium loss in football players. *International Journal of Sport Nutrition, 4,* 142–153.

Cole, K., et al. (1996). Effect of caffeine ingestion on perception of effort and subsequent work production. *International Journal of Sport Nutrition, 6,* 14–23.

Cui, J., et al. (1994). What do commercial ginseng preparations contain? *Lancet, 344,* 134.

Davis, J. M. (1996). Carbohydrates branched-chain amino acids and endurance: The central fatigue hypothesis. *Sports Science Exchange, 9* (2), 1–5.

Dekkers J., et al. (1996). The role of antioxidant vitamins and enzymes in the prevention of exercise-induced muscle damage. *Sports Medicine, 21,* 213–238.

Dowling E., et al. (1996). Effect of Eleutherococcus senticosus on submaximal and maximal exercise performance. *Medicine and Science in Sports and Exercise, 28,* 482–489.

Engels, H., & Wirth, J. (1997). No ergogenic effects of ginseng (Panax ginseng C. A. Meyer) during graded maximal aerobic exercise. *Journal of the American Dietetic Association, 97,* 1110–1115.

Evans, G. (1989). The effect of chromium picolinate on insulin controlled parameters in humans. *International Journal of Biosocial Medicine, 11,* 163–180.

Fawcett, J., et al. (1996). The effect of oral vanadyl sulfate on body composition and performance in weight-training athletes. *International Journal of Sport Nutrition, 6,* 382–390.

Ferrando, A., and Green, N. (1993). The effect of boron supplementation on lean body mass, plasma testosterone levels, and strength in male bodybuilders. *International Journal of Sport Nutrition, 3,* 140–149.

Fogelholm, G. M., et al. (1993). Low dose amino acid supplementation: No effects on serum human growth hormone and insulin in male weight lifters. *International Journal of Sport Nutrition, 3,* 290–297.

Freund, B., et al. (1995). Glycerol hyperhydration: Hormonal, renal, and vascular fluid responses. *Journal of Applied Physiology, 79,* 2069–2077.

Gerster, H. (1989). Review: The role of vitamin C in athletic performance. *Journal of the American College of Nutrition, 8,* 636–643

Goldfarb, A. (1993). Antoxidants: Role of supplementation to prevent exercise-induced oxidative stress. *Medicine and Science in Sports and Exercise, 25,* 232–236.

Graham, T., & Spriet, L. (1996). Caffeine and exercise performance. *Sports Science Exchange, 9,* (1), 1–5.

Graham, T., & Spriet, L. (1991). Performance and metabolic responses to a high caffeine dose during prolonged exercise. *Journal of Applied Physiology, 71,* 2292–2298.

Greenhaff, P. (1995). Creatine and its application as an ergogenic aid. *International Journal of Sport Nutrition, 5,* S100–S110

Hallmark, M., et al. (1996). Effects of chromium and resistive training on muscle strength and body composition. *Medicine and Science in Sports and Exercise, 28,* 139–144.

Hawley, J.A., et al. (1997). Carbohydrate-loading and exercise performance: An update. *Sports Medicine, 24,* 73–81.

Heinonen, O. Carnitine and physical exercise (1996). *Sports Medicine, 22,* 109–132.

Kanter, M. (1995). Free radicals and exercise: Effects of nutritional antioxidant supplementation. *Exercise and Sport Sciences Reviews, 23,* 375–398.

Kanter, M., & Williams, M. (1995). Antioxidants, carnitine, and choline as putative ergogenic aids. *International Journal of Sport Nutrition, 5,* S120–S131.

Koenigsberg, P., et al. (1995). Sustained hyperhydration with glycerol ingestion. *Life Science, 57,* 645–653.

Krelder, R., et al. (1993). Amino acid supplementation and exercise performance, *Sports Medicine, 15,* 190–209.

Kreider, R., et al. (1992). Effects of phosphate loading on metabolic and myocardial responses to maximal and endurance exercise. *International Journal of Sport Nutrition, 2,* 20–47.

Kreider, R., et al. (1990). Effects of phosphate loading on oxygen uptake, ventilatory anaerobic threshold, and run performance. *Medicine and Science in Sports and Exercise, 22,* 250–256.

Laaksonen, R., et al. (1995). Ubiquinone supplementation and exercise capacity in trained young and older men. *European Journal of Applied Physiology, 72,* 95–100.

Lamb, D., et al. (1997). Prehydration with glycerol does not improve cycling performance vs. 6% CHO-electrolyte drink. *Medicine and Science in Sports and Exercise, 29,* S249 (abstract).

Latzka, W., et al. (1997). Hyperhydration: Thermoregulatory effects during compensable exercise-heat stress. *Journal of Applied Physiology, 83,* 860–866.

Lemon, P. (1996). Is increased dietary protein necessary or beneficial for individuals with a physically active lifestyle? *Nutrition Reviews, 54,* S169–S175.

Lemon, P. (1995). Do athletes need more dietary protein and amino acids? *International Journal of Sport Nutrition, 5,* S39–S61.

Linderman, J., & Fahey, T. (1991). Sodium bicarbonate ingestion and exercise performance. *Sports Medicine, 11,* 71–77.

Lukaski, H., et al. (1996). Chromium supplementation and resistance training: Effects on body composition, strength, and trace element status of men. *American Journal of Clinical Nutrition, 63,* 954–965.

Lyon T., et al. (1990). Effects of glycerol-induced hyperhydration prior to exercise in the heat on sweating and core temperature. *Medicine and Science in Sports and Exercise, 22,* 477–483.

Malm, et al. (1996). Supplementation with ubiquinone-10 causes cellular damage during intense exercise. *Acta Physiologica Scandinavica, 157,* 511–512.

Matson, L., & Tran, Z. (1993). Effects of sodium bicarbonate ingestion on anaerobic performance: A meta-analytic review. *International Journal of Sport Nutrition, 3,* 2–28.

Montner, P., et al. (1996). Pre-exercise glycerol hydration improves cycling endurance time. *International Journal of Sports Medicine, 17,* 27–33.

Morris, A., et al. (1996). No ergogenic effect of ginseng ingestion. *International Journal of Sport Nutrition, 6,* 262–271.

Newsholme, E., et al. (1992). Physical and mental fatigue: Metabolic mechanisms and importance of plasma amino acids. *British Medical Bulletin, 48,* 477.

Packer L., (1997). Oxidants, antioxidant nutrients and the athlete. *Journal of Sports Sciences, 15,* 353–363.

Redondo, D., et al. (1996). The effect of oral creatine monohydrate on running velocity. *International Journal of Sport Nutrition, 6,* 213–221.

Rossiter, H., et al. (1996). The effect of oral creatine supplementation on the 1000-m performance of competitive rowers. *Journal of Sports Sciences, 14,* 175–179.

Sherman, W.M., and Leenders, N. (1995). Fat loading: The next magic bullet. *International Journal of Sport Nutrition, 5,* S1–S12.

Singh, A., et al. (1992). Chronic multivitamin-mineral supplementation does not enhance physical performance. *Medicine and Science in Sports and Exercise, 24,* 726–732.

Snider, I., et al. (1992). Effects of coenzyme athletic performance system as an ergogenic aid on endurance performance to exhaustion. *International Journal of Sport Nutrition, 2,* 272–286.

Spriet, L. (1995). Caffeine and performance. *International Journal of Sport Nutrition, 5,* S84–S99.

Spriet, L., et al. (1992). Caffeine ingestion and muscle metabolism during prolonged exercise in humans. *American Journal of Physiology, 262,* E891–E898.

Starling, R., et al. (1996). Effect of inosine supplementation on aerobic and anaerobic cycling performance. *Medicine and Science in Sports and Exercise, 28,* 1193–1198.

Stewart, I., et al. (1990). Phosphate loading and the effects on VO_2max in trained cyclists. *Research Quarterly for Exercise and Sport, 61,* 80–84.

Swensen, T., et al. (1994). Adding polylactate to a glucose polymer solution does not improve endurance. *International Journal of Sports Medicine, 15,* 430–434.

Telford, R., et al. (1992). The effect of 7 to 8 months of vitamin/mineral supplementation on athletic performance. *International Journal of Sport Nutrition, 2,* 135–153.

Tiidus, P., and Houston, M. (1995). Vitamin E status and response to exercise training. *Sports Medicine, 20,* 12–23.

Tremblay, M., et al. (1994). Ergogenic effects of phosphate loading: Physiological fact or methodological fiction? *Canadian Journal of Applied Physiology, 19,* 1–11.

Trent L., and Thieding-Cancel, D. (1995). Effects of chromium picolinate on body composition. *Journal of Sports Medicine and Physical Fitness, 35,* 273–280.

Wagenmakers, A. (1997). Branched-chain amino acids and endurance performance. In T. Reilly and M. Orme (Eds.), *The Clinical Pharmacology of Sport and Exercise.* Amsterdam: Excerpts Medica.

Wagenmakers, A. (1991). L-carnitine supplementation and performance in man. *Medicine and Sport Sciences, 32,* 110–127.

Weston, S., et al. (1997). Does exogenous coenzyme Q10 affect aerobic capacity in endurance athletes? *International Journal of Sport Nutrition, 7,* 197–206.

Wiles, J., et al. (1992). Effect of caffeinated coffee on running speed, respiratory factors, blood lactate and perceived exertion during 1500-meter treadmill running. *British Journal of Sport Medicine, 26,* 116–120.

Williams, M.H. (1998a). *The Ergogenics Edge: Pushing the Limits of Sports Performance.* Champaign, IL: Human Kinetics.

Williams, M.H. (1998b). *Nutrition for Health, Fitness, and Sport.* Dubuque, IA: WCB/McGraw-Hill.

Williams, M. (1992). Bicarbonate loading. *Sports Science Exchange 4,* (1),1–4.

Williams, M. H., and Branch, J. D. (1998). *Journal of the American College of Nutrition, 17* (3).

Williams, M., et al. (1990). Effect of oral inosine supplementation on 3-mile treadmill run performance and VO_2, peak. *Medicine and Science in Sports and Exercise, 22,* 517–522.

Index